THE EYE CARE SOURCEBOOK

JAY B. LAVINE, M.D.

Contemporary Books

Chicago   New York   San Francisco   Lisbon   London   Madrid   Mexico City
Milan   New Delhi   San Juan   Seoul   Singapore   Sydney   Toronto

Library of Congress Cataloging-in-Publication Data

Lavine, Jay B.
    The eye care sourcebook / by Jay B. Lavine.
        p.   cm.
    Includes bibliographical references and index.
    ISBN 0-7373-0395-6
    1. Eye—Care and hygiene—Popular works.   I. Title.

   RE51 .L28   2001
   617.7—dc21   2001028635

Contemporary Books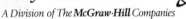

A Division of The *McGraw·Hill* Companies

1 2 3 4 5 6 7 8 9 0   DOC/DOC   0 9 8 7 6 5 4 3 2 1

ISBN 0-7373-0395-6

This book was set in Minion by Reider Publishing Services
Printed and bound by R. R. Donnelley—Crawfordsville

Cover design: Hebron Design
Art director: Laurie Young
Cover photo: PhotoDisc

McGraw-Hill books are available at special quantity discounts to use as premiums and sales promotions, or for use in corporate training programs. For more information, please write to the Director of Special Sales, Professional Publishing, McGraw-Hill, Two Penn Plaza, New York, NY 10121-2298. Or contact your local bookstore.

This book is printed on acid-free paper.

Contents

CONTENTS

CONTENTS

Foreword

THE EYES ARE MIRACULOUS MACHINES. THESE TINY PERFECT organs focus images from great distances, track movement, tell us about depth—and provide all this in vivid color. These miniature cameras are so complex, it's no wonder we entrust their care only to highly trained professionals. Unlike our skin, which we dab with salves and potions, or our hearts, which we strengthen with exercise and diets, our eyes are strictly the province of specialists with bewildering diagnostic instruments and treatments that are more astounding every day.

But even in this complex area of medicine, some of the most powerful interventions are those we make ourselves. Take macular degeneration, for example. This relentless damage to the retina is a leading cause of blindness in older people. Yet research shows that a few simple, but important, changes in diet can help us hold this disease at arm's length.

People who eat plenty of green leafy vegetables cut their risk of macular degeneration dramatically. The credit goes to powerful protectors, called *lutein* and *zeaxanthin,* hidden in plant foods. More protection comes from avoiding fatty foods. Whether because avoiding fats allows blood to flow more easily through the tiny vessels in the eyes or for some other reason, people who choose a lean vegetarian entrée instead of chicken salad do themselves a huge favor, not just for their hearts, but for their eyes, too.

Similarly, cataracts are strongly influenced by factors in our daily lives—things we can control. Too much sunlight wrinkles the skin, of course, but it also contributes to cataracts, as does smoking. And a measure of protection comes from diets rich in fruits and vegetables, because the vitamin C and other nutrients they contain pass into the lens and knock out the free radicals that would otherwise contribute to opacities. While ophthalmologists will gladly replace clouded lenses with new ones, they prefer to let patients keep their original equipment.

In this carefully written and detailed volume, Jay Lavine, M.D., tells you everything you need to know about caring for those most delicate instruments, your eyes. Dr. Lavine has made medical science so tangible and exciting, you'll want to read this book cover to cover. I strongly encourage you also to keep this book as a reference for the years to come. When the doctor uses strange terms, like *uveitis* or *pterygium,* the translation into plain English is at your fingertips, along with everything you need to know. Also included are crucial everyday topics—how to correct poor vision, remove a foreign body, or tackle vision-related headaches—and the latest, often surprising, tips, which can save you from going down many a blind alley.

Many professionals look to Dr. Lavine for advice on tough cases. Now readers from all walks of life can profit from his wisdom and experience.

Neal Barnard, M.D.
Author of *Food for Life,*
The Power of Your Plate,
and *Eat Right, Live Longer*

Introduction

THE EYE IS THE WINDOW TO THE BODY. WHERE ELSE IN THE body can we actually see a nerve that is an extension of the brain? Or internal blood vessels whose health often mirrors the health of blood vessels in other organs? Many bodily diseases cause changes in the blood vessels, nerves, and other tissues of the eyes. Even minor changes, which might well go unnoticed in other organs, often reveal themselves in the eye by their effects on vision. Other changes may not cause symptoms but may still be detected by a competent and conscientious physician.

The eye is the organ of sight, our most important sense. If we lose our sight, a part of us dies. We should therefore try to do everything possible to maintain this precious gift. With that in mind, the emphasis in this book is on prevention, the highest form of healing. All legitimate modalities of healing, including drugs and surgery, have their place, and we should feel fortunate that medical advances have facilitated the treatment of disease. But all drugs have side effects, and even successful surgery does not usually leave us the same as we were before we became ill. Furthermore, not all diseases are curable or even treatable. It seems intuitively obvious that it is preferable to prevent illness than to become sick and then have to be treated.

This sourcebook is intended to be a self-defense manual for today's health care environment. As patients travel down Medical Lane, the road sometimes seems more like a tunnel of love, with ghouls popping up in all directions. On one side are the fee-for-service doctors recommending surgery. Should patients believe them? On the other side the HMOs are saying that nothing more needs to be done. Should patients believe them? Out of nowhere, the specter of alternative medicine approaches, like the emperor with his new clothes, promising to get at the root of your problem. Is this promise real? How about the medical information on the Internet and in the mass media? Are the "experts" they're interviewing really expert? Clearly, a guide is needed to find the right path.

We live in the Disinformation Age. Doctors and hospitals hawk their wares like street vendors. Drug companies advertise their prescription drugs directly to the consumer, hoping that patients will dictate their own treatment rather than rely on the expertise of their physicians. All of these players in the medical arena know that if people hear something enough, they start to believe it. One of my goals in writing this sourcebook is to remind the educated reader that self-education and regard for reputation, ethics, and legitimate authority still constitute the best approach to obtaining quality eye care and taking care of one's own eyes.

It would be nice if we could learn all we needed to know about our eye condition from a visit to the doctor, but such is not the case, especially in this day and age of reduced doctor time per patient visit. To be sure, medical practice involves much more than just drugs and surgery. Any modality that can prevent, treat, or cure illness is in the domain of the physician. Nevertheless, the reality is that lifestyle change, especially in the area of nutrition, is too often ignored by medical practitioners.

You won't find any miracle cures on these pages, but you will learn about most major eye problems and how to treat them in the safest, gentlest, and most effective way possible. You will discover which foods can help prevent macular degeneration, the most common cause of poor vision among the elderly, and which nutritional approaches may have unwanted side effects. You will learn how to avoid unnecessary cataract surgery; how to obtain long-lasting relief from itchy, burning eyes; and how to reduce the need for laser treatment if you are diabetic.

Myths will be shattered. Did you know that many people with glaucoma have normal eye pressures and that exercise can lower eye pressures? Is refractive surgery as safe and free from complications as you may have been led to believe? Were you aware that dry eyes, a common cause of reading problems, don't usually feel dry?

The information on all of the various eye problems is grouped according to the part of the eye affected. In recognition of the increasingly important role of nutrition in the practice of medicine, I have included a primer on nutrition. You will often find that the foods that are best for your eyes are also the foods that benefit the rest of your organs as well.

CHAPTER ONE

Myths About Vision and the Eyes

THERE ARE MANY COMMON MYTHS ABOUT VISION AND THE EYES. This chapter discusses some of the most well known of them.

It Is Desirable to Detect Cataract As Soon As It Appears

There is no advantage to diagnosing cataract in its earliest stages. A cataract can be safely removed at any time and, in fact, should generally not be removed until it makes you unable to function in your everyday activities. Cataract is only a cloudiness of the lens; it is not a growth or tumor.

Cataracts Are Removed by Laser

Cataract is a condition in which the lens of the eye becomes cloudy. Cataract surgery entails removal of the lens. The only way to remove the lens is by performing conventional surgery. Laser is only used for secondary cataract, a clouding of a formerly clear membrane that remains in the eye after cataract surgery.

Eye Pressure Checks Diagnose Glaucoma

High pressure in the eye is the main risk factor for glaucoma, but 25 percent of people with glaucoma have normal eye pressures, and many people with elevated pressures do not have glaucoma. Other procedures must be performed to diagnose glaucoma.

Contact Lenses Help Keep Eyes from Changing

Contact lenses allow you to see clearly, just as glasses do. If your eyes are going to change, they do so whether you wear contact lenses or not.

Exercises Can Improve Your Vision

Special eye exercises have never been shown to change refractive errors, such as nearsightedness or astigmatism. Exercises may occasionally be of value in strengthening weak eye muscles, such as those that turn the eyes inward when you are reading.

Wearing Your Glasses Too Much Makes You Dependent on Them

Glasses only help you to see better while you are wearing them. They do not change the eyes. They may make you more psychologically dependent on them because you get used to seeing better while wearing them.

People Who Need Glasses Have Weak Eyes

People who need to wear glasses do so to allow the light to focus properly on their retinas. The need for glasses has little to do with the health of the eye, and it certainly does not mean that the eyes are "weak."

Reading in the Dark Harms Your Eyes

It may strain your eyes to read in the dark, but it won't cause any damage to your eyes or make you need to wear glasses sooner than you would otherwise.

Using Your Eyes Too Much Weakens Them

Eyes do not wear out from being used. They may feel strained from overuse, but such strain does not cause any permanent harm or permanent change in vision.

Children Often Outgrow Crossed Eyes

Eyes occasionally wander during the first six months of life. Constant crossing of an eye will not be outgrown and may reflect a serious problem. In such a case, examination by an ophthalmologist is mandatory.

Taking Vitamin Supplements Is the Best Way to Good Nutrition

Good nutrition results from eating a wide variety of vegetables, fruits, grains, and nuts. Besides the vitamins and minerals we need, plant foods contain phytochemicals, special substances that promote good health, including resistance to degenerative eye diseases. Supplements do not contain all of these important phytochemicals.

A Low-Carbohydrate, High-Protein Diet Helps with Weight Loss and Prevents Diabetes

This kind of fad diet is unsafe and unwise. Cutting back on calories helps you lose weight. As for diabetes, countries in which people typically eat a high-fiber, high–complex carbohydrate (starch) diet show the lowest incidence of the disease. In diabetics, a lower protein diet may help prevent kidney and eye complications.

Eating Whatever You Want in Moderation Is the Key to Good Nutrition and Healthy Eyes

Eating a variety of foods in moderation is the key to good health. But that does not mean that you should eat whatever you want. If foods A and B both supply required nutrients, but consumption of food B has some health risks associated with it, then why consume food B at all? Concentrate on health-promoting foods and enjoy them.

Most Eye Diseases Cannot Be Prevented

Recent research has revealed that a number of eye problems, including cataracts and age-related macular degeneration, may be prevented, primarily by nutritional means. A dark, leafy green vegetable a day may keep the ophthalmologist away.

CHAPTER TWO

What Should You Do If . . . ?

T HIS CHAPTER DISCUSSES A NUMBER OF "WHAT IF" EYE CARE
scenarios.

You Get Some Acid, Oven Cleaner,
or Other Chemical in Your Eyes?

Run, don't walk, to the nearest faucet and start splashing water in your eyes.
Theoretically, an eyewash might be slightly better, but plain old water does the
job just fine. The longer the chemical is in contact with your eyes, the more damage it does. Therefore, time is of the essence. Continue to flood your eyes with
water for at least fifteen minutes. It can take a good while to completely flush out
all the remaining chemicals. If your eyes then feel irritated or burn, or they seem
blurry, or if it was a strong acid or base that got in your eye, seek medical attention right away from either an ophthalmologist or an emergency room.

You Suddenly Lose Vision in One Eye?

If your vision has completely blacked out in one eye and remains that way, seek
emergency medical attention immediately. One major cause of sudden blindness in an eye is a central retinal artery occlusion. This is equivalent to a stroke
in the eye. The emergency measures employed to treat an occlusion such as this

are controversial, but if they are to have any effect, they must be begun as soon as possible. Without its blood supply, the retina can die very quickly.

Vision that is only partially lost or that takes hours to days to be lost can be due to a number of conditions but should still be checked out on an urgent basis. The optic nerve may have lost its blood supply from a shutdown of small blood vessels. Retinal detachment can cause loss of vision, but it generally begins in the periphery and gradually works its way across the field of vision.

If you lose your vision but it then returns within thirty to forty-five minutes, you may have suffered a *transient ischemic attack* (TIA), a warning sign that a stroke may occur in the near future. Usually the loss of vision occurs as a dimming of vision over a number of seconds, although occasionally it may appear as though a shade were slowly being drawn across the eye. A possible TIA requires urgent evaluation, because if you have a TIA you may need medication to reduce your tendency to form blood clots.

If your vision just becomes blurry but doesn't black out, try blinking a few times or rinsing the eye with some water. Sometimes excess mucus from the glands in the eyelids may spread over your cornea and cloud your vision for a short while. If the blurring is accompanied by funny patterns in your vision and a headache begins after the blurring subsides, you may have suffered your first migraine, assuming you are a child or young adult. If the blurring does not go away, have it checked out as soon as possible.

You Get a Foreign Body in Your Eye?

Do not rub the eye. Rubbing can cause the foreign body to become more deeply embedded or to scratch the cornea. Blink your eyes several times to try to wash the foreign body out. If that does not work, grasp your upper eyelashes between your thumb and forefinger and then pull the upper eyelid down over the lower eyelid, allowing it to contact the lower lid. This often dislodges a small foreign body adhering to the inside of the upper lid. If that doesn't work, try rinsing the eye with some water or eyewash. Repeat these steps as necessary. If you continue to feel as if a foreign body is in your eye, you should seek medical attention. Sometimes a foreign body sensation in the eye is not due to a foreign body at all but may instead be the first symptom of a developing eye infection (conjunctivitis).

You Can't Get Your Contact Lens Out?

First, don't panic. Although a contact lens can fall out of your eye, it can't travel behind your eye and get lost that way. The conjunctiva ends in a cul-de-sac as it reflects from the eyeball to the inside of the eyelid, so nothing can get past it. If you have a rigid contact lens and you know for sure that it is on your cornea, you can use a little contact lens remover (plunger) if you have one. But be careful. People sometimes think they still have a contact lens in their eye, but it has long since fallen out. They have a feeling of something in the eye simply because the eye has become irritated. Many a person has tried using a plunger in such a situation and ended up abrading the cornea because no lens was present.

Sometimes a contact lens travels up under the upper eyelid and gets caught there. Irrigating the eye with some saline or contact lens wetting solution may help free the lens. If you can't get it out, then your ophthalmologist or optometrist has to do it for you. But don't be surprised if you're told that there's nothing there! This problem is much more common, of course, in new contact lens wearers.

You See Floating Spots and Flashing Lights?

Black dots, lines, and cobwebs are called *floaters*. They may appear when the vitreous humor detaches itself from the retina. A white light flashing off to one side, more prominent in the dark, can be a symptom of traction on the retina by the vitreous. If you begin seeing floaters, white light flashes, or both, see an ophthalmologist as soon as possible, certainly within twenty-four hours. A retinal tear, which is an easily treatable lesion, might be present. Untreated retinal tears may lead to a retinal detachment, a much more serious problem requiring major surgery.

Your Eyelid Keeps Twitching?

The medical term for this common symptom is *lid myokymia*. It may occur when you're feeling tired, a condition that produces a little nervous stimulation that causes the eyelid muscle to twitch. A slightly dry eye or a little eyelid-associated irritation can also provoke lid myokymia. Consuming caffeine-containing beverages is another major risk factor, as illustrated by this anecdote.

During one hot summer, a man made an urgent appointment to see me because his eyelid began twitching. I remarked that he had probably been drinking a lot of soda. Sure enough, he entered my office carrying a can of cola!

Treatment of this harmless but annoying symptom includes elimination of caffeine or other stimulants from the diet and treatment of any underlying dry eye syndrome or eyelid inflammation (blepharitis) problem. Occasionally treatment can include a little antihistamine medication or, as a last resort, an old remedy called quinine.

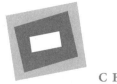

CHAPTER THREE

Anatomy of the Eye

THE EYE RESTS IN THE BONY SOCKET THAT WE CALL THE *ORBIT*. The rims of the orbit help protect the eye from injury. Fat in the orbit behind the eye serves as a cushion to keep the eye from being traumatized by the bones of the orbit when the eye or the head is jostled. The optic nerve, an extension of the brain, enters the back of the orbit through a bony canal and then enters the eye, where its nerve fibers become distributed over the surface of the retina. Also entering the orbit are the various blood vessels that supply all the parts of the eye, including its muscles, and the nerves that transmit messages back and forth between the eye and the brain.

It is sometimes helpful to think of the eye in terms of its coats or layers. The outer coat consists of the *cornea*, the clear window of the front of the eye, and the *sclera*, the tough, white tissue that begins where the cornea ends. The middle layer is the *uvea* (Greek for "grape," because of its coloration). The uvea includes the ciliary body; the iris, which surrounds the pupil; and the choroid, the blood vessel–rich layer in the back half of the eye. Finally, the retina forms the inner coat and is located beside the choroid. The retina is in contact with the *vitreous humor*, the gel-like substance that fills the interior of the back of the eye, while the cornea is in contact with the *aqueous humor*, the fluid inside the front part of the eye. We will now look at each part of the eye in more detail.

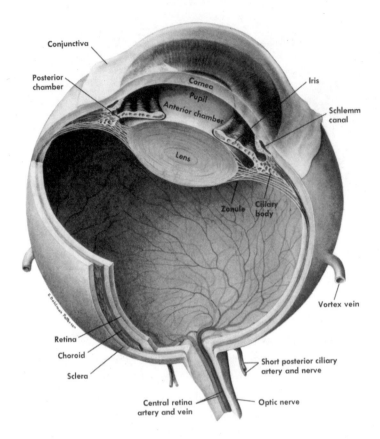

Conjunctiva

Posterior chamber

Cornea

Pupil

Anterior chamber

Lens

Iris

Schlemm canal

Zonule

Ciliary body

Vortex vein

Retina

Choroid

Sclera

Short posterior ciliary artery and nerve

Central retina artery and vein

Optic nerve

FIGURE 3.1 **The Human Eye**

Source: "The Human Eye," by C. Bohlman Patterson, in *Opthamology Principles and Concepts,* 8th edition, 1946, p. ii; reprinted with permission from The C. V. Mosby Company (Harcourt Health Sciences).

The Cornea

The cornea is transparent and fairly thin, only about half a millimeter in thickness near its center. It serves as a lens, changing the pathway of incoming rays of light, making them converge so that they ultimately focus on the retina. The cornea also has a protective function in terms of infection and foreign bodies that might enter the eye.

The outermost layer of the cornea is called the *epithelium* and is only about six cell layers thick. These cells may be thought of as the "skin" of the eye. They prevent most bacteria from entering the cornea or the interior of the eye. When some of the cells of the epithelium are lost, as occurs with a corneal abrasion, the cornea becomes susceptible to infection, and a corneal ulcer may form. The tear film, the layer of tears that coats the surface of the cornea, protects the epithelium, keeping it from drying out, and also contains antibodies and other substances that resist infection.

The corneal surface is extremely sensitive because of the numerous nerve endings there. If the eye is abraded and epithelial cells are lost, the exposed nerve endings produce sharp, fairly severe pain. Other insults to the surface of the cornea, such as overwearing a contact lens, can produce similar pain. Sensitivity of the cornea may be reduced in some circumstances, for example, with herpes infections of the cornea or in diabetics. Fluid buildup

The cornea's nerve endings make it one of the most sensitive tissues of the body.

(edema) in the epithelium can occur when the pressure in the eye becomes very high; when the endothelial (inner lining) cells of the cornea are not functioning properly; or as a result of injury, infection, or inflammation. This edema gives the corneal epithelium a cloudy appearance. The vision becomes blurred, and the person may see halos around lights.

The eye tends to replace lost epithelial cells very quickly, as they can divide rapidly and slide over to fill in any gaps. In diabetics, however, the epithelial cells may not "stick" down as well to the layer of the cornea behind them.

The middle layer of the cornea, called the *stroma,* makes up most of the thickness of the cornea. It is composed of collagen, the same protein that is in skin and nails. In the case of the cornea, however, the collagen is laid down in such a way that it remains transparent. The part of the stroma immediately next to the epithelium is fairly dense and is called *Bowman's membrane,* although it is not really a membrane. The corneal epithelial cells form over Bowman's membrane. If this "membrane" becomes damaged, the epithelial cells may have difficulty adhering to it.

If the stroma becomes damaged by injury (such as laceration), ulceration, or inflammation, it usually forms a scar in the affected area rather than returning to its pristine, transparent state. Such scarring interferes with vision if it occurs near the center of the cornea. It can also make the curvature of the cornea irregular, causing *irregular astigmatism,* a kind of blurring that ordinary eyeglasses do not correct very well. *Corneal edema,* or fluid buildup in the cornea, can thicken the stroma and sometimes even make it cloudy.

Along the back surface of the stroma is a thin membrane called *Descemet's membrane*. A single layer of cells, the endothelium, is present on Descemet's membrane. The endothelium represents the innermost layer of the cornea. The endothelial cells have a very important function. Because of the fluid pressure inside the eye, water is always trying to enter the cornea. If it did so, the cornea would lose its transparency. The endothelial cells constantly pump any water that gets into the cornea back into the anterior chamber of the eye. Although endothelial cells are lost with age and as a result of eye surgery or injury, they do not regenerate as the epithelium does. If too many are lost, the cornea develops edema.

The Sclera and Conjunctiva

The *sclera* is the tough white coat of the eye. It begins where the cornea ends and extends all the way around to the back of the eye. A small gap in the sclera allows the optic nerve to enter the eye at the very back. The sclera is also perforated by tiny blood vessels and nerves. Like the cornea, the sclera is composed of collagen, but since the collagen fibers are laid down differently, the sclera is opaque rather than transparent. Because of its density, the sclera imparts some rigidity to the eye. It can be lacerated by sharp objects or even ruptured by sharp blows to the eye, but it usually halts minor foreign bodies in their tracks.

Covering the sclera in the front part of the eye is a transparent, blood vessel–containing mucous membrane called the *conjunctiva*. The conjunctiva is reflected from the sclera onto the inside surface of both the upper and lower eyelids. In the area where the conjunctiva leaves the sclera and becomes the lining of the eyelids, a narrow pouch, or cul-de-sac, is formed. People who fear that their misplaced contact lenses may travel behind their eye will be reassured to know that this conjunctival

The conjunctiva is the only place on the outside of the body where you can see the blood vessels.

cul-de-sac is what prevents that possibility. The blood vessels in the conjunctiva are the thin, thready red lines you see over the sclera. When these blood vessels dilate, the eye develops its familiar bloodshot appearance. An interesting fact is that the conjunctiva is the one place in the body where the blood vessels are visible externally. The appearance of these vessels (for example, narrowing) can help indicate whether blood vessel damage is occurring in people with high blood pressure or diabetes. Inflammation of the conjunctiva is called *conjunctivitis*, and this is the term used to denote ordinary eye infections.

The Anterior Chamber

The *anterior chamber* is the fluid-filled space behind the cornea and in front of the iris. The watery fluid that fills the anterior chamber is called the *aqueous humor*. Aqueous humor is produced by the ciliary body and is continuously secreted into the *posterior chamber,* the small space behind the iris and in front of the lens. The aqueous humor flows from there through the pupil to enter the anterior chamber. The anterior chamber always maintains about the same depth, although it may become shallow or even "flat" as a result of abnormal events— for example, an injury that perforates the cornea, allowing the aqueous humor to leak out. Surgical complications, especially accompanying glaucoma surgery, can also cause a flattening of the anterior chamber. Whatever the cause, urgent action is often necessary to restore the anterior chamber to its normal depth.

When *iritis,* an inflammation of the iris, is present, white blood cells and protein can be detected in the aqueous humor. Bleeding *(hyphema)* may occur in the anterior chamber as well, most commonly as a result of injury.

The Trabecular Meshwork

In the angle of the eye, the region at the edge of the anterior chamber where the ends of the iris and cornea can be found, two important structures can be seen. One is a portion of the ciliary body, discussed next. The other is the *trabecular meshwork,* the series of drainage channels through which the aqueous humor percolates out of the anterior chamber. From the trabecular meshwork, the aqueous humor enters a channel called the *canal of Schlemm.*

When fluid cannot drain out, the pressure goes up.

From there, the fluid is transported through microscopic vessels and eventually reaches tiny veins near the surface of the eye. Clearly, if the angle closes down so that the aqueous humor cannot reach the trabecular meshwork and therefore has no way to exit the eye, the pressure in the eye becomes very high, in a form of glaucoma called *angle-closure glaucoma*. In the most common form of glaucoma, *chronic open angle glaucoma*, resistance in the drainage pathways is present at the microscopic level.

The Ciliary Body

The *ciliary body*, along with the iris and the choroid, are pigmented tissues that form the uveal tract of the eye. (*Uveitis* refers to inflammation of these structures.) As already noted, one of the functions of the ciliary body is to produce aqueous humor, the fluid that fills the anterior and posterior chambers. The ciliary body also contains the *ciliary muscle*, which is involved in a focusing mechanism called *accommodation*. When you change your gaze from distance to near, this muscle contracts, releasing tension on the zonules, the fibers that suspend the lens in place. As this occurs, the lens becomes more curved so that light coming from objects close to the eye is focused on the retina. Aging changes in the muscle result eventually in *presbyopia*, the difficulty in focusing on materials at the reading distance that most people experience when they reach their forties. Contraction of some of the ciliary body muscle fibers can also affect the drainage channels of the eye, allowing the aqueous humor to drain out of the eye more easily.

Aging changes in the ciliary muscle cause presbyopia, or "oldsightedness."

Some eyedrops used to treat glaucoma, for example, pilocarpine, lower the eye pressure by making these muscle fibers contract. Other glaucoma eyedrops lower eye pressure by suppressing the formation of aqueous humor by the ciliary body.

The Iris and Pupil

The *iris* is the pigmented ring of tissue that surrounds the pupil, the hole through which light travels toward the back of the eye. The color of the eye depends on the amount of pigment (melanin) in the iris. An iris with a large amount of pigment appears brown, whereas one with only a little pigment looks blue. Of course, there are varying degrees of pigment in the eyes of different people.

The iris contains muscles that dilate and constrict the pupil. It dilates in the dark and constricts in bright light. The pupil also becomes smaller when you look at something up close. Pupils vary in size from one person to another, although they tend to become smaller with age. Usually, a person's two pupils are about the same size, although small differences are common. If a pupil changes in size, the problem must be investigated. The change could be the result of a very benign problem or a more serious problem in the brain.

Iridology—diagnosing bodily diseases by the appearance of the iris— is a pseudoscience.

The iris itself can be involved with various diseases. Growth of abnormal blood vessels (*rubeosis iridis*) can occur in diabetics or after major vein occlusions of the retina, and these blood vessels can scar shut the trabecular meshwork area, resulting in glaucoma. When there is inflammation in the eye, the iris may stick down to the lens behind it or to the cornea in front of it, causing problems. Pigment can sometimes be lost from the iris, for example, in a form of glaucoma called *pigmentary glaucoma,* giving the iris a bit of a moth-eaten appearance. A pseudoscience called *iridology* is based on the belief that the appearance of the iris can be used to diagnose all sorts of bodily diseases. There is no scientific basis for iridology, however, and its ability to diagnose disease has been refuted in at least one study.

The Lens

The *lens* focuses incoming light rays onto the retina so that the image can be clearly seen. Its shape can change to allow the eye to focus both on objects in the distance and on those up close. In this respect, it is like a zoom lens on a camera. However, the ability of the muscle of the ciliary body to change the shape of the lens declines with age, finally resulting in the need for reading glasses, a condition called *presbyopia,* or "oldsightedness."

The lens is a transparent disk composed of protein and suspended in place by the *zonules,* fibers that are attached on their other end to the muscles of the ciliary body. The lens is similar in structure to an onion, with numerous layers formed by thin cells that continue to be laid down throughout life. The oldest portion of the lens is therefore the central portion. The inner core of the lens is called the *nucleus,* whereas the outer layers are called the *cortex*. The lens is entirely surrounded by a thin envelope called the *capsule*.

The most common abnormality involving the lens is *cataract,* a cloudiness in part or all of the lens caused by changes in the proteins of the lens. Thus, a cataract involving the nucleus is called a *nuclear cataract,* whereas clouding of the outer layers is called a *cortical cataract.* A foreign object entering the eye may damage the lens, and the end result may be a cataract.

Changes in the lens proteins make it become cloudy, a condition we call cataract.

Blunt injuries to the eye may not only cause cataract but also cause some of the zonules to break. The lens may then become dislocated, floating about in the eye.

The Vitreous Humor

The *vitreous humor,* or simply vitreous, as it is known for short, is the gel that fills the largest chamber of the eye, bounded by the lens in front and the retina in back. It is mostly water, but it contains hyaluronic acid and a special framework of thin collagen (protein) fibers. As the eyes age, a degenerative process occurs, and the gel liquefies. Eventually, about half of the vitreous may become liquid, and half remains as a gel. As the gel portion shrinks, traction is applied to those areas of the retina to which the vitreous gel is attached. Usually the vitreous separates itself from the retina without incident, but sometimes it causes a tear in the retina, the first step in the formation of a retinal detachment.

When *uveitis,* or inflammation inside the eye, is present, white blood cells form in the vitreous, and they can be clearly seen when the eye is examined. Cancer cells, for example, from lymphoma, may build up in the vitreous as well. Blood in the vitreous can be seen after eye injuries or as a result of bleeding on the surface of the retina, as is sometimes seen in diabetics.

The Choroid

The *choroid* is part of the uvea or uveal tract, the middle coat of the eye. It is located behind the ciliary body and is sandwiched between the sclera on the outside and the retina on the inside. The choroid is rich in blood vessels and supplies blood to the outer portion of the retina, which lies next to it. A layer called *Bruch's membrane* is shared by the choroid and the retina. The choroid can be damaged by blunt injuries to the eye, and its blood vessels may be affected by high blood pressure and other diseases. Inflammation of the choroid, *choroiditis,* is a form of uveitis. Scars that form in the choroid and adjacent retina *(chorioretinal scars)* as a result of inflammation can be quite easily seen on examination of the eye. Because of the choroid's rich network of blood vessels, cancers that originate in other parts of the body can occasionally spread to the choroid.

The Retina

The *retina* is a complex, multilayered structure that forms the inner coat of the eye. Incoming light rays are focused on the retina, which is similar to the film in a camera. The light energy is then converted into nerve impulses that transmit signals to the brain. The central part of the retina, called the *macula,* is responsible for our central (straight ahead) vision. The deepest layer of the retina, the *pigment epithelium,* lies next to Bruch's membrane, which separates the retina from the choroid. Breaks in Bruch's membrane from injury or from diseases can allow blood vessels from the choroid to grow in through the breaks, where they can leak and bleed and disrupt the retina.

Images are focused on the retina, which then transmits the signals to the brain.

The portion of the retina next to the pigment epithelium is called the *sensory retina.* Its deepest layer, lying next to the pigment epithelium, consists of the photoreceptor cells, called *rods* and *cones.* The cones, which are most densely concentrated in the macula, help make out sharp details and colors. The cones function mainly when a moderate to high amount of illumination is present. The rods, located away from the center of the macula, help perceive images at times when there is dim illumination

The rods and cones of the retina connect with other interconnecting cells, and ultimately the nerve impulses travel along the over one million nerve fibers in each eye that make up the optic nerve. A thinning of this nerve fiber layer can often be seen when the eye is examined, especially if a green (red-free) light is used.

The retina is interrupted in the area where the optic nerve enters the eye. Major blood vessels, the *central retinal artery* and the *central retinal vein,* enter the eye through the optic nerve and then undergo a branching pattern as they spread over the surface of the retina. The branches of the central retinal artery supply the blood for the inner layers of the retina. Abnormalities of the blood vessels caused by diabetes, high blood pressure, and other diseases can cause leakage of fluid and hemorrhage into the retina, which in some cases can blur vision. The retina is also subject to numerous other problems, including detachment, degeneration, infection, inflammation, injuries, and rarely tumors.

The Optic Nerve

The *optic nerve* is a cranial nerve, which means that it is part of the central nervous system, an extension of the brain. Each optic nerve contains about 1.2 million individual nerve cells, all of which travel with the optic nerve out the back wall of the eye, across the orbit, and into the brain. The nerve then courses through the brain, connecting with other cells, which ultimately reach the back

The optic cup aides in the diagnosis of glaucoma.

of the brain, the *occipital cortex*, where our consciousness becomes aware of what we are looking at. As the optic nerve fibers travel through the brain, they can be damaged by tumors, aneurysms, blood clots, high fluid pressure around the brain, and the effects of injuries. When damaged by problems such as these or by loss of circulation, certain vitamin deficiencies, or toxins, the optic nerve often loses its normal rosy color and becomes pale.

The portion of the optic nerve where it penetrates the back wall of the eye is called the *optic disk*. The center of the optic disk may contain a depressed area called the *optic cup*. Some people have no discernible optic cup, whereas others have fairly large ones. The optic cup is important because it usually increases in size when the optic nerve becomes damaged by glaucoma. Its appearance therefore helps in the diagnosis of glaucoma.

The External Eye Muscles

Six straplike muscles control eye movements. Four muscles are called *rectus muscles:* the *superior rectus,* which turns the eye upward; the *inferior rectus,* which turns the eye downward; the *medical rectus,* which turns the eye inward; and the *lateral rectus,* which turns the eye outward. The word *rectus* means "straight" in Latin, and these muscles travel in a straight path. They are attached to the bones at the back of the orbit and travel straight to the eye, where they attach to the sclera. These muscles work in combination so that the eye can move in any direction.

The muscles move the eyes, but the brain provides the coordination.

The other two muscles are the *oblique muscles,* which have somewhat complex actions. The *superior oblique* can turn the eye downward and rotate it inward, while the *inferior oblique* can turn the eye upward and rotate it outward. The reason for the rotating motion of the eyes is that when you tilt your head to the left or the right, the eyes have to rotate in the opposite direction to compensate somewhat for the head tilt.

Of course, the brain coordinates the movements of the eyes so that both eyes are always moving in tandem. If they did not work this way, you would see double. In fact, this is exactly what happens when a nerve controlling a particular muscle or a group of muscles becomes paralyzed. The eye muscles can be affected by many problems, including inflammation (orbital myositis, thyroid disease), muscle diseases like myasthenia gravis, injuries, and inherited muscular disorders.

CHAPTER FOUR

Eye History and Examination

W HEN YOU SEE YOUR EYE DOCTOR FOR A SPECIFIC PROBLEM, you describe the nature of the symptoms you are having. This is called the *history* of your present illness. Then your eyes are examined and appropriate tests performed. Although today's examinations employ sophisticated instruments and other gadgetry, the importance of the history should not be underestimated. In many cases, it may be more helpful in arriving at a diagnosis than the examination is. So when the doctor asks you what the problem is, don't say, "You tell me, you're the doctor!" Instead, describe your symptoms as well as possible. Be as succinct as you can: In today's health care environment, unfortunately the time you get with the doctor may be rationed. As Sergeant Joe Friday used to say, "Just the facts, ma'am."

Let us now go over the main components of the medical history.

The History

Chief Complaint

Just because you have a chief complaint doesn't mean you're a chronic complainer. The words *chief complaint* simply refer to the main reason for the appointment (for anything other than a routine examination). Examples may be "I have pain in my right eye" or "My vision became blurry after I had the headache." The doctor often records your chief complaint in your own words.

Present Illness

Present illness refers to the nature of your symptoms. After mentioning your chief complaint, you can go into more detail about your symptoms. Have you had a loss of vision or some change in your vision? Have you had pain, irritation, discharge from the eye, or light sensitivity? Have you been seeing floating spots or flashing lights in your field of vision? If you have pain, what is it like? Is it a sharp or dull pain? Exactly where is it located? Is it present all the time or just occasionally? How severe is it? Do you have any other symptoms while you are having the pain? How long has each of your symptoms been present? If you forget to mention anything relevant, your doctor should ask you about it.

Medical History

Many eye problems may be related to diseases of the body. It is especially important to know whether you have any history of diabetes or abnormal blood sugars, high blood pressure, arthritis, infectious diseases, immune system problems, cancer, or colitis. Needless to say, any previous eye problems should be fully disclosed.

Current Medications

When you are asked what medications you are taking, give a complete list, not just prescription drugs but also vitamins, herbs, and any other supplements. Vitamins in large doses can sometimes act like drugs, and herbal supplements can interact with many prescription medications. You should give the name of each medication, the dose, how many times a day you take it, what you take it for, and any other relevant information. If you take a large number of medications, bring a list containing all of this information to your appointment. That way, the doctor or the assistant can either photocopy it or transcribe it into your record, and completeness is ensured.

Many prescription drugs can affect your eyes. For example, the cortisone type of medication can cause cataracts or increase the pressure in your eyes, a large number of medications can cause dryness of the eyes, and others some-times have a direct toxic effect on certain structures of the eye.

Medication Allergies and Sensitivities

This is a very important category, because you don't want to be prescribed products that contain medications to which you are allergic. Allergies to sulfa drugs, antibiotics, and adhesive on surgical tape should be mentioned. Anything that has caused hives or wheezing is especially important. You should also mention side effects you've suffered other than allergy, for exam-ple, stomach upset from penicillin or erythromycin, nausea and vomiting from codeine, and so on.

Family History

Many eye conditions are more common in some families than in others. Have any of your close relatives been diagnosed with glaucoma? Do people in your family tend to get cataracts when they are in their forties or fifties? Have any relatives had a retinal detachment? It is also important to know whether dia-betes, high blood pressure, or allergies run in your family.

Social History

Many personal factors may have a bearing on your eye health. Do you smoke? Do you drink alcohol? If so, what kind and how much? What is your diet like? What are your current living arrangements like? Is anyone available who could help you instill eye medications, change your bandage, or help you get around after surgery?

The Eye Examination

Some procedures are used in virtually every eye examination, whereas some specialized procedures are used only on people who have certain problems. Of course, the completeness of the examination varies greatly from one ophthal-mologist to another. Once you know what should be included in your exam-ination, you can know how complete an examination you have had.

Visual Acuity

Visual acuity is a measure of how well you can see. It is an important part of every examination of the eye. Visual acuity measures the clarity of your vision, that is, your ability to see details when you look straight ahead at something. It does not measure your peripheral (side) vision. Visual acuity is tested at a distance, usually twenty feet (or the equivalent in a room equipped with mirrors), and can also be tested up close at the reading distance, especially in people over the age of forty.

Distance visual acuity can be measured in a number of ways. Most commonly, an eye chart with letters of the alphabet is used. A disadvantage of this method is that some letters are easier to discern than other letters of the same size. There are also number charts that feature the numerals from zero to nine. For children who are not yet able to read letters, the E game is used. The letter E on the chart is oriented in any of four positions, and the child must point to show which way the "arms" on the E are pointing. To test near vision, we generally use reading material with print of different sizes.

Distance visual acuity is typically tested with each eye individually: The right eye is tested first with the left eye covered up, and then the process is reversed. If you are wearing glasses, we generally test with the glasses on. You hold a device called an *occluder* to cover the eye not being tested. It is important to keep your face pointed straight ahead during this test, because it is very easy to use the covered eye without knowing it. As you read the letters on the chart, do not squint but do try to read them even if they are not clear. You will usually be right more often than you would expect.

After reading the eye chart, with or without your glasses, you will often be asked to look at the same letters through a little device called a *pinhole*. You may be surprised to find that the letters look much clearer through the pinhole. Improvement in vision as you look through the pinhole usually means that you need a change in glasses prescription (or glasses if you do not have them now). The pinhole lets in only the rays of light that are least affected by one's refractive error (nearsightedness, farsightedness, or astigmatism). Therefore, only the light rays providing the clearest image reach the eye. However, other eye problems, such as cataracts and scars on the cornea, can sometimes also allow improvement of vision with the pinhole.

The way you read the eye chart may provide other important clues. For example, if you consistently don't see letters on the right side, this may indicate a problem with the right side of your peripheral vision. There may be a serious underlying problem, such as a blind area caused by a stroke, a tumor, or an aneurysm.

Distance visual acuity is recorded as a fraction, with 20/20 being considered the standard for normal vision. The first number in the fraction refers to the distance at which the visual acuity was measured. If the first number is 20, then the person was standing twenty feet away from the eye chart. If a person's visual acuity is 20/40, that means that the smallest letters that person can see are twice the size of the letters that a person with 20/20 vision can see. Although 20/20 is considered the standard, most younger individuals with healthy eyes have better than 20/20 visual acuity either with or without glasses. For example, they may have a visual acuity of 20/15, 20/13, or even 20/10, which is about as good as it gets. If you have 20/10 visual acuity, you can see letters that are half the size of those on the 20/20 line.

Normal visual acuity for younger people is usually better than 20/20.

If you do not have at least 20/200 visual acuity with your better eye while you are wearing the best possible glasses, then you are legally blind. Some people mistakenly say they are legally blind without their glasses, but of course they are not legally blind. Occasionally, one hears of an ophthalmologist who tells a patient that he or she is legally blind in one eye. Obviously, such an individual does not know the definition of legal blindness.

Near visual acuity, which tests vision at the reading distance, is generally tested on both eyes at the same time. Thus, no occluder is used. If you wear reading glasses or bifocals, you should wear them for this test, which determines the smallest size of print you can read. Near visual acuity may not be routinely tested in younger people but should be in people over the age of forty, especially people complaining of difficulty reading. If you complain of difficulty reading and your near visual acuity is not tested as part of your eye examination, head for the nearest exit! I have reviewed the records of people who sought an eye examination because of difficulty reading but who never had their reading vision checked during the examination. Instead, they were simply told they needed cataract surgery! Believe it or not, this is not a rare occurrence.

The way you read the near vision chart may shed some light on the nature of your problems. For example, if you read easily at first, but the letters then start to become blurry, or if you have to blink your eyes repeatedly to read clearly, you may have a type of dry eye problem.

Differences between one's distance and near visual acuities may also provide information about underlying eye problems. Some types of cataract, for example, affect distance visual acuity more than near, whereas age-related macular degeneration may do the opposite. In some people who have both of these problems, it may be difficult to decide whether the reduction in vision is due primarily to the cataract or to the macular degeneration, and this is one way of determining which problem predominates.

Refraction

Refraction is the process by which your refractive error is determined. Your *refractive error* is essentially your glasses prescription for distance. If you have perfect vision at distance without glasses, then you have no refractive error. If a person with an eye problem has less than normal vision in each eye, the ophthalmologist often performs a refraction even if glasses are not going to be prescribed. The reason is that, in evaluating eye problems, it is often important to know just how well each eye is capable of seeing. The only way of accomplishing that is by performing a refraction.

Nearsightedness is the common term for the refractive error known as *myopia*. Nearsighted people can see things at close range, but beyond a certain point, everything appears blurry, and the farther into the distance they are looking, the blurrier things get. In a normal eye, the light rays entering the eye come to a focus on the retina in the back of the eye, just as a movie projector might focus an image on a screen. But in a myopic eye, the light rays come to a focus in front of the retina inside the eye.

Farsightedness is a misleading term commonly used for the refractive error called *hyperopia*. A hyperopic eye is out of focus at all distances, but the blurriness is worse at distance than at near. The problem is that the light rays coming from an object come to a focus behind the retina rather than right on the retina. Yet most hyperopic individuals see clearly when they are younger and only develop the blurriness as they become older. How can this be? Although the eye at rest is set to focus at distance, a focusing muscle (the ciliary muscle) in the eye acts like the zoom lens in a camera. When this muscle contracts, it changes the shape of the lens inside the eye and thereby changes the way the eye focuses. The eye uses this mechanism, called *accommodation,* to change its focus from far to near. As we become older, the ciliary muscle becomes weaker and weaker until it hardly works at all. This loss of ability to change focus with age is called *presbyopia* (described later). A young person, however, can use this focusing muscle to eliminate the blur caused by the hyperopia. By contracting this focusing muscle even when looking in the distance, that person can change the way the light rays focus in the eyes so that they focus on the retina and not behind it. But as the person becomes older and the focusing muscle weakens, the eyes lose the ability to compensate for the hyperopia, either partially or fully, and eyeglasses are then needed.

Sometimes older children or young adults, especially when under some tension, complain of blurry vision at distance and may appear to be myopic when a refraction is performed. However, they may be suffering from a *spasm of accommodation.* This occurs when the ciliary muscle has a certain degree of tightness or spasm. These individuals are accommodating, that is, using their near focusing mechanism even though they are looking into the distance. The diagnosis is suspected when they give variable answers as the refraction is performed. They seem to be focusing in and out, and they often remark as they look at the letters on the chart that they can sometimes see the letters for an instant but that the letters then blur up again. Spasm of accommodation can be confirmed by dilating the pupils with drops that temporarily paralyze the ciliary muscle (cycloplegic drops) and then performing another refraction. If spasm of accommodation is present, the apparent myopia should disappear. It is important not to overcorrect myopia or to prescribe glasses for people suffering from accommodative spasm, because that only strains the eyes. Reassurance and muscle relaxation exercises, as one might recommend for muscle tension headache, may be the best approach.

Astigmatism refers to another refractive error that may be present in either myopic or hyperopic individuals. Astigmatism is caused by the shape of the eye. Although the curvature of the front surface of the eye is almost perfectly rounded in a normal eye, the surface of the astigmatic eye curves more sharply in one direction than another. Thus, it is shaped more like a football than like a basketball. The result is that the light rays coming from all points on a given object you are viewing do not focus together on the retina, and this causes blurring. Fortunately, eyeglass lenses can correct the blurring.

Presbyopia, which you might call oldsightedness, refers to the gradual decline in ability to change the focus of the eye from distance to near. As mentioned previously, it is caused by a weakening in the ciliary muscle, which is responsible for this function. This weakening begins in early childhood, but it does not cause problems at the reading distance for most people until they are in their forties. Many people mistakenly refer to this problem as farsightedness. However, it is not farsightedness (hyperopia) at all. Presbyopia is simply part of the normal aging process, and it occurs in everyone—nearsighted people, farsighted people, and people with no refractive error at all. Nearsighted individuals who become presbyopic will have to wear bifocals (or perhaps just remove their glasses for reading). Farsighted individuals may initially need glasses just at the reading distance but will eventually need a glasses correction both for distance and for near. And individuals with no refractive error will continue to see normally for distance but will require reading glasses.

How is the refraction performed? First, an estimate of the refractive error can be made. If a person already has glasses or contact lenses, the prescription of the lenses can be determined with the aid of special instruments. This "old prescription" often functions well as a starting point. The ophthalmologist can also use an instrument called a *retinoscope* that focuses a light into the eye, a process called *retinoscopy*. By looking at a light reflex in the pupil of the eye while placing different lenses in front of the eye, the ophthalmologist can usually get a good estimate of the glasses prescription. Modern technology has produced a kind of computerized retinoscope called an *objective autorefractor*. This machine focuses light rays into the eye and then determines what combination of lenses makes the light focus properly on the retina.

Once the starting point is determined, the final refraction is performed. The ophthalmologist may place an apparatus called a *phoropter* in front of the eyes, and the lenses in the phoropter are then changed based on the patient's responses in reading the eye chart. The final glasses prescription is based on this refraction as well as on a person's previous prescription. The latter is kept in mind to avoid changing a prescription so much that it feels uncomfortable and causes problems. For people who cannot participate in the final refraction, such as infants, young children, or anyone else who cannot read an eye chart and give accurate responses, the results of the retinoscopy or the autorefractor reading can be prescribed directly.

It must be emphasized that refraction is an art as well as a science. If an ophthalmologist has a technician perform the refraction but does not check the final results, they may not always be satisfactory.

Visual Fields

The visual acuity measurement as described earlier only measures the ability to see details in the very center of one's vision. But peripheral (side) vision is very important as well. Many eye problems affect peripheral vision but leave visual acuity unchanged. The *visual field* refers to the entire area of vision, both peripheral and central. Formal visual field testing involves the use of an instrument called a *perimeter*. Both manual and computerized varieties exist. However, formal perimetry (visual field testing) of this nature is not generally part of a routine examination but is performed in certain instances. For example, it is performed in people with elevated eye pressures to rule out visual field loss caused by glaucoma. It is also performed in people who have other optic nerve problems; certain retinal problems; or loss of vision caused by brain problems, such as tumors, strokes, and aneurysms; and in anyone who has reduced visual acuity for which the cause is not evident.

Informal testing of visual fields, in contrast, is a part of a routine examination. There are a number of ways in which this test can be done. Each eye is covered in turn, as with visual acuity testing. In one method, patients look directly into the eye of the examiner sitting opposite them. As they do this, the examiner holds up a certain number of fingers off to either side, and the patients have to say how many fingers there are each time. In another method, an object is brought slowly in from the side, and the patients tell when they first see it.

Still another type of visual field testing is the *Amsler grid,* which contains vertical and horizontal lines in a checkerboard pattern. As the patients fix their gaze on a black spot in the center of the grid, they indicate whether the lines around the center are missing or distorted in any places. This test is especially valuable for detecting problems involving the macula, the center of the retina.

External Structures

The important structures around the eye all begin with the letter L—lids, lashes, lacrimal system, and lymph nodes. These are usually the first things checked after the visual acuity, visual fields, and refraction have been completed.

Are the eyelids swollen? Is the upper lid droopy? Is the eyelid skin reddened? Many ocular conditions affect the eyelids. *Blepharitis,* a very common inflammation of the eyelids, can cause all of these problems. A scratch on the eye may make the upper eyelid droop a little. Styes and their close cousins, chalazia, cause reddened bumps. Tumors of various kinds may form on the lids. An overactive thyroid gland may cause the eye to open more widely. Medications may affect the lids. Foreign bodies may lodge under the upper lid. Eyelids may turn in or out, causing uncomfortable symptoms. All of these as well as other problems are usually evident at the start of the examination.

What do the lashes look like? Some eyelid conditions, such as blepharitis, can make the lashes fall out or turn white. Some eyedrops can make the lashes darker and thicker looking. Misdirected eyelashes, the result of scarring from infections or injury, may scrape the surface of the eye.

The lacrimal system is concerned with the production and drainage of tears from the eye. Any swelling in the area of the lacrimal gland, which is located above the eye toward the temple, must be noted. An enlarged lacrimal gland may give the contour of the upper lid an S-shaped appearance. Swelling in the area of the lacrimal sac, which is located between the eye and the nose, must also be detected. Sometimes we press on the skin over the lacrimal sac to see whether pus can be expressed through the small openings *(puncta)* in the eyelid margins. Someone in whom the tear drainage system is blocked will have a teary eye, and the tears will often run down the cheek, a condition called *epiphora*. This is sometimes present in newborns whose tear (nasolacrimal) ducts haven't fully opened or in adults whose tear ducts have shut down.

The *lymph nodes* are bits of tissue that help the body fight infection. They enlarge greatly and even become tender with some types of infection. When an eye infection is present, we try to determine whether the lymph nodes have become enlarged. The *preauricular lymph node* is located right in front of the ear and receives drainage primarily from the upper eyelid on that side. The *submandibular lymph node* is located just beneath the angle of the lower jaw and receives drainage primarily from the lower eyelids. Lymph nodes may also become enlarged when they become infiltrated by cancer cells.

Motility (Eye Movement)

In this part of the examination, we make sure that both eyes move well in all directions, both individually and as a pair. We check the straightness of the eyes, both at distance and at near. When one of the nerves coming from the brain is malfunctioning, this testing can often determine which nerve is the problem. In some people, the eyes are straight when both are being used, but when one eye is covered, it wanders a bit. This can sometimes explain a person's unusual symptoms. Further testing, such as *fusion* (ability to use the eyes together) and *stereopsis* (depth perception), is done in special cases, especially in children with eye straightness problems.

Pupils

Testing the pupils is part of every routine eye examination. We examine the pupils for their size, shape, and the way they react to light. We keep the room illumination dim and have the patient look at a target across the room. Then we shine a small light from below toward the eyes to compare them. We then shine the light more directly into each eye to see whether the pupil becomes smaller (constricts), as it should. Patients should not look directly at the light as this is done, as the simple act of looking at something up close also makes the pupils constrict. Then we perform the "swinging flashlight test," in which the light goes back and forth between the two eyes. In a person with an optic nerve disorder, the pupil may enlarge a bit when the light is swung over to that side.

Pupils come in widely varying sizes, but there shouldn't be a large difference between sizes of a person's two pupils. Some people are born with such a difference, but usually one of a variety of problems, from previous eye surgery or injury in an eye to inflammation, causes a size difference. For example, an eye with inflammation inside of it *(iritis)* may have a pupil that is smaller than that in the other eye. Sometimes a small, distorted, or unreactive pupil is the result of scarring caused by previous cataract or other surgery inside the eye. A blunt injury to an eye may cause tears in the little muscle of the iris surrounding the pupil, resulting in a larger pupil that does not react well to light. Some medications can also affect the size of the pupils. Of course, there are many unusual problems that can affect the size of the pupils as well.

As just mentioned, the pupils usually become smaller when you focus on something up close. When someone's pupils do not constrict normally when light is shined into them, we usually check to see whether they constrict with near focusing. A number of problems, including diabetes and syphilis, can cause the pupils to react with focusing at near but not when a light is directed at them.

Slit Lamp Examination

The *slit lamp,* also known as a *biomicroscope,* is an instrument that provides light and magnification for examining the eye. The name comes from the fact that the light is often in the form of a long, narrow slit, which allows the structures of the eye through which it passes to be seen in cross section. Thus, the slit lamp provides excellent depth perception, permitting abnormalities in the eye to be localized precisely. A variety of sophisticated techniques— shining the light in from different angles or changing the size, shape, or brightness of the light—can be employed to allow subtle problems to come into view more easily.

For the slit lamp examination, you will be asked to sit forward and place your chin on the chin rest, which should be covered with some disposable paper for hygienic purposes. Your forehead must also come forward to touch the forehead rest. Although this procedure sounds easy, it can be difficult for elderly (inflexible), stout, or full-chested individuals, who have a hard time getting close enough to position their head properly. Here are some hints. Instead of just leaning forward while you are sitting back in the exam chair, slide your bottom forward so that you are sitting near the edge of the seat. If you are very short, try sitting on a thick phone book to get up to the required height if the seat cannot be adequately adjusted. Make sure that when you place your chin on the chin rest, your forehead doesn't tilt back away from the forehead rest; if it does, it will be difficult for the examiner to focus on your eyes properly. Most slit lamps also have bars to hold on to, much like the handlebars on a bicycle. Use them to stabilize yourself.

We examine the cornea, noting how clear it is, whether any scars or foreign bodies are present, and whether there are any scratches or other defects in the surface. We also look for evidence of fluid (edema) and for any other signs of dysfunction. Fluid in the cornea, for example, may be caused by a loss of the cells lining the inner surface of the cornea, by high pressure in the eye, or by inflammation. Sloughing off of epithelial cells on the outer surface of the cornea may be caused by the irritative effects of infections, by dry eye syndrome, or by medications used in the eye. Since contact lenses rest on the cornea, we can check the fit of the lenses and make sure they are not harming the cornea. We also look at the deeper layers of the cornea, especially in the area of the endothelium, the cells that line the back surface of the cornea. Tiny dots called *guttata* and wrinkles are signs of possible degeneration of the endothelium, which could ultimately result in edema of the cornea.

We check the *conjunctiva,* the clear membrane over the white of the eye, for redness, pigmentation, and growths. An infection or other inflammation will make the eye look red by causing the blood vessels in the conjunctiva to become dilated. Bleeding from the blood vessels will create a solid red spot on the eye.

We then look deeper into the eye, checking the *anterior chamber,* the fluid-filled space bounded by the cornea in front and the iris from behind. With the slit lamp, we can determine how deep the chamber is and whether any blood, inflammatory cells, or protein is present. We can see cells in the fluid using high magnification. Protein in the fluid causes *flare,* a cloudiness seen in the slit of light that travels through it, much like what you see in the light coming from a movie projector in a slightly dusty room. Flare and cells are caused by inflammation. Blood may occur after injury or may represent bleeding from abnormal blood vessels on the iris in people who have diabetes or other disorders affecting blood vessels.

Next, we check the *iris,* the brown or blue ring of the eye. The color depends on the amount of pigmentation present. We look for the presence of *rubeosis iridis,* the abnormal blood vessels mentioned earlier that can bleed and cause other problems. We also look for changes in the color of the iris, for growths, and for areas where the pigmentation has been lost. If there has been previous inflammation or surgery in the eye, the iris may be scarred down to the lens behind it in some places.

The lens of the eye lies right behind the iris. We look for cloudiness in the lens, the condition called *cataract.* The slit lamp helps us determine in exactly which layer of the lens any cloudiness is located. We also make sure that the lens has not been dislocated, that is, moved slightly out of position as the result of injury or some other factor.

We examine the *vitreous,* the gel that fills the large chamber of the eye behind the lens, to see whether any cells are present. Such cells may indicate inflammation or, rarely, a malignancy. Tiny pigment flecks may signal the presence of a recent tear in the retina. If bleeding from any cause occurs, that can easily be seen as well. The front part of the vitreous can easily be seen with the slit lamp, but to examine the back part, a special focusing lens must be placed in front of the eye. This lens may simply be held in place, or it may be placed on the front surface of the eye as a contact lens would be.

Pressure Check (Tonometry)

Checking the intraocular pressure is part of the routine examination, even in children, if possible. The *intraocular pressure* (IOP) is the fluid pressure inside the eye. There can be a number of causes for high or low pressures, but a high pressure is the main risk factor for glaucoma. The standard testing method is called *Goldmann tonometry.* An anesthetic (numbing) drop is instilled in the eye, along with a yellow dye called *fluorescein,* and the patient is then positioned at the slit lamp. A white plastic cone is advanced until it touches the surface of the cornea. The device measures exactly how much pressure it takes to flatten the cornea against it. The measurement is generally quite accurate, although it is limited by the fact that the rigidity of the wall of the eye is greater in some people than in others.

A recent study has shown that tonometers generally underestimate the true pressure reading in ethnic Chinese adults. Also, an accurate reading can usually not be obtained in someone whose cornea has an irregular surface. Although the plastic piece should be disinfected after each use, the test is usually not performed in people who have active infections on the surface of their eyes.

A common method for checking the pressure is the *noncontact tonometer,* an instrument that directs a puff of air at your eye. This method is good for screening purposes but is not as accurate as Goldmann tonometry. There are also some electronic tonometers that are fairly accurate.

Fundus Examination

The *fundus* includes the structures along the back wall of the eye, namely, the retina, the optic disk, and the retinal blood vessels. We dilate the pupil with dilating eyedrops to get the best possible view of the fundus. Eyedrops are available that can help the pupils return to normal more quickly. They do sting a bit, but ask for them if you are bothered by the effects of dilated pupils.

We use the *direct ophthalmoscope,* a handheld instrument, to examine the optic disk and the surrounding retina and blood vessels. The ophthalmoscope provides some magnification, but because we look through it with only one eye, there is some loss of depth perception. When better depth perception is needed, we examine the fundus with the slit lamp with a special lens held in front of the eye for proper focusing. When we need to look at the peripheral areas of the retina, we use a special head-mounted instrument called an *indirect ophthalmoscope*. This is a good way to find retinal tears, which can lead to retinal detachments if undetected and untreated. A special focusing lens with attached mirrors can also be used at the slit lamp to examine the far periphery of the retina.

Special Tests

When certain problems are suspected, special testing techniques are added to the examination. The most common of these are described next.

Gonioscopy If the examination reveals an elevated intraocular pressure, or if the patient's history reveals symptoms that suggest that the patient may be having intermittent spikes of pressure, a technique called *gonioscopy* is employed. Gonioscopy involves use of a special lens that allows us to see directly into the angle of the eye, the approach to the fluid drainage channels (trabecular meshwork). This lens is placed on the surface of the eye in the manner of a contact lens. The eye is already numb at this point from the drop that was instilled prior to the pressure check.

We perform gonioscopy for several reasons. First, we want to make sure that the angle is open and not closed. If it is open, we want to see how narrow it is. This tells us whether the angle is capable of closing under the right circumstances. We want to see whether there is an *angle recession,* a change in the appearance of the angle caused by a previous injury to the eye. An angle recession is a possible cause of high pressure. We also want to see whether there are any scarlike adhesions *(synechiae)* in the angle and whether any abnormal blood vessels have grown into the angle, as can occur with *rubeosis iridis,* a condition affecting the iris.

Ophthalmodynamometry *Ophthalmodynamometry* is simply a measure of the blood pressure in the blood vessels entering the back wall of the eye. It is sometimes performed in people who have had transient loss of vision in an eye. This transient blindness can sometimes indicate hardening of the arteries and high risk of a stroke. This technique can give us some idea whether any major arteries (including the *carotid arteries,* the large arteries traveling up the neck) carrying blood toward the eye are narrowed.

To do this test, the pupils are usually dilated so that the blood vessels at the back of the eye can be viewed through an ophthalmoscope. The ophthalmodynamometer is then pressed against the side of the eye, and, just like a blood pressure cuff on the arm, it measures how much pressure it takes to make the arteries in the eye start to pulsate. At this point, the pressure reading corresponds to the systolic pressure reading (the first or higher number) in a standard blood pressure determination. If the blood pressure in the eye is much lower than that in the arm, it tells us that there might be a problem, and the patient is then referred to the primary care physician or to a specialist for further evaluation and treatment.

Photo-Stress Test People who have a problem with their *macula,* the central part of the retina, sometimes say that when they enter a dark room after being out in the bright light, it takes a long time for them to regain their vision. The *photo-stress test,* sometimes called the *dazzle test,* uses this observation to determine whether mildly reduced eyesight is due to a macular problem or some other cause. A moderately bright light is shined directly into one eye (while the other eye is covered) for ten seconds. Then we determine how long it takes for the visual acuity to return to its prior level. A prolonged recovery time suggests a disorder of the macula such as age-related macular degeneration.

Color Vision Testing A disorder in color vision, such as inability to distinguish red from green hues, is most often an inherited condition seen primarily in males. To test color vision, we use a book containing color plates. Each plate contains numbers hidden in colored dots, which patients attempt to see. A scoring system is then used to determine whether a color deficiency is present.

Some eye diseases can affect color vision as well. Optic nerve problems commonly reduce the ability to discern colors, as can macular problems to some degree.

A more complex test is the *Farnsworth-Munsell 100 hue test,* in which the patient must place numerous colored tiles of varying hues in order. This test can provide valuable information but is not used by most ophthalmologists.

Convergence and Divergence Amplitudes Some people who complain of vision problems or headaches are found to have an *esophoria* or *exophoria,* eye muscle disorders in which the person's muscles must strain to keep the eyes straight. In such a situation, we can determine what we call *convergence* and *divergence amplitudes*. Prisms (special lenses) of varying strengths are held in front of the eyes to measure muscle strength. We measure the strength of the muscles that turn the eyes in toward each other and also that of the muscles that turn the eyes out away from each other. If weakness is found, certain eye muscle exercises may be prescribed to help strengthen the weak muscles.

Special Eyedrops Although some eyedrops, such as anesthetic (numbing) and dilating drops, are part of the routine examination, we sometimes use special drops to help make a diagnosis. For example, when unequal pupils are present, certain drops that either dilate or constrict the pupils may be used to help determine the cause of the problem and, in some cases, the location of the disorder in the nervous system. Often, this tells us that we are not dealing with any potentially serious problem, and we can therefore avoid any unnecessary testing, which might be unpleasant as well as expensive.

CHAPTER FIVE

Vision Correction

S LICED BREAD IS THE GREATEST THING SINCE EYEGLASSES. WE
don't normally think of eyeglasses as being among one of the
great medical advances, but they truly were. Think about it. Nearsighted people who had to stumble around, unable to see beyond arm's length, could suddenly see everything clearly. People who could no longer read could again read
the smallest print.

Think about it another way. What if the only way we had to correct refractive errors such as nearsightedness were the eye surgeries people now talk
about? And then, all of a sudden, someone came and said, "Look, you don't
have to have surgery now! With these new eyeglasses I've invented, you'll be
able to see everything, and you won't have to take a risk with surgery!"
Everyone would think that the eyeglasses were the most marvelous invention.
So with that perspective, the next time you complain about your glasses, just
be grateful you have them!

Refractive errors refers to myopia (nearsightedness), hyperopia (farsightedness), and astigmatism. Because of the curvature, length, and shape of the
eye, focusing does not always occur the way it should. Rays of light coming
from an object at which we are looking are supposed to come to a focus on the
retina. In myopia, they come to a focus in front of the retina, whereas in hyperopia, they come to a focus behind the retina. Astigmatism prevents the rays of
light from focusing sharply, and it may be present along with hyperopia and

myopia. Presbyopia, the difficulty focusing at near that comes with age, is a separate phenomenon and occurs in everyone; it is one of the most predictable things in life.

Eyeglasses represent the traditional way of correcting vision, whereas contact lenses are a newer approach. Surgery can be performed to change the shape of the cornea of the eye, although the surgical approaches employed are still in a state of evolution. We will examine each of these alternatives in turn.

Eyeglasses

Eyeglass or spectacle correction has been used for several centuries. Lenses are ground in such a way as to neutralize the refractive error found on examination. Myopia, hyperopia, and astigmatism can generally be corrected, although a type of astigmatism called *irregular astigmatism* cannot be fully corrected by eyeglass lenses. Irregular astigmatism may be caused by scarring or warpage of the cornea.

Prescription of glasses is an art. The lenses found on examination to correct each eye to the best possible vision are not necessarily the ones prescribed. The most important thing is to make sure that people will be happy with their new glasses. If you've ever had difficulty adjusting to a new pair of glasses, you know what I mean.

There is an art to prescribing eyeglasses.

The final prescription depends on a number of factors. How much difference is there between the two eyes? If there is too much difference between the lenses prescribed for each eye, the eyes may have difficulty working together. Lenses change the size of the image you see. A lens to correct myopia makes the image appear smaller, whereas one that corrects hyperopia makes the image appear larger. The stronger the lens, the greater this effect. Therefore, if the strength of the lenses for the two eyes differs, what one eye sees appears larger to the brain than what the other eye sees. If this difference is too large, the brain is unable to fuse the two images together, and that can play havoc with your ability to function with the glasses on. Sometimes the thickness and curvature of the lenses can be adjusted to lessen this difference, but manipulations such as these are almost a lost art.

Even if the eyes tolerate lenses of different strengths for distance vision, there can be a problem with the bifocal portion at the reading distance. When you look down toward the edge of a lens, as you do when you look through bifocals, the image of something you're seeing becomes displaced somewhat from where it really is. If this displacement is different between the two eyes, you may have difficulty using the two eyes together. Fortunately, there are ways of dealing with this bifocal problem. A common solution is called a *slab off,* which involves the removal of a thin slice of glass from the lower part of a lens, but it must be done by a competent optician.

If the lenses are of a high power (six diopters or more), the doctor prescribing them must specify on the prescription how far the lenses were from the eyes when the examination was performed. This is called the *vertex distance.* If it turns out that the lenses in the frames you select will be closer to or farther from the eyes than the vertex distance used in the examination, the optician has to adjust the power of the lenses to compensate for the difference. Many myopic individuals are aware of this phenomenon; if their lenses have become a little too weak for their eyes, they can push them closer to their eyes to obtain more power from them.

At this point, we should discuss the importance of the optician. An *optician,* although not a doctor, is a professional who fills an eyeglass prescription. Opticians have a knowledge of optics and should know all the ins and outs of eyeglasses. Opticians must carefully measure the distance between the eyes, both at distance and at near. They must make sure that each lens is perfectly centered in front of each eye. They must also place the bifocal at the correct height. They should check the old glasses to make sure that the transition to the new glasses will be a smooth one. In short, good opticians are highly skilled individuals who provide a very important service.

Did you know that exactly the same lens prescription can be filled with different lenses? A glasses prescription simply indicates the power of the lens. However, a lens of a given power can be made with different thicknesses and curvatures. If these change significantly from those of the old glasses, a person may have difficulty adjusting to new glasses.

An optician is a skilled professional, not just a salesman.

Unfortunately, it is very difficult to find highly competent opticians because the public has foolishly considered eyeglasses to be a mere commodity and placed the filling of a glasses prescription in the same category as buying a TV set. Rather than select a competent optician on the basis of reputation, most people simply shop for price and follow the misleading advertising of optical chains. Thus, good opticians have become an endangered species. Of course, the public's reliance on advertising rather than solid reputation has profoundly affected the practice of medicine as a whole, especially in the specialty of ophthalmology.

Be cautious about the selection of frames. Lenses of large size are sometimes popular from a fashion standpoint, but with lenses of higher powers, the large size can create problems. A certain amount of distortion is present as your eyes turn and you look through a lens away from its center. The distortion coming from the edges of large lenses can be distracting and uncomfortable. Also, large lenses are heavier and place more weight on your nose and ears.

Large lenses can cause distortion when you look to the side.

Glass or plastic lenses? Sounds like something you'd be asked at the grocery store. Both glass and plastic lenses can provide excellent vision, although some people feel that they see more clearly with glass. Glass is heavier. Plastic scratches more easily. Take your pick.

The newer polycarbonate lenses are lighter and thinner and are quite impact resistant. Polycarbonate scratches easily, so scratch-resistant coatings are applied to the lenses. Because polycarbonate lenses refract (bend) light rays differently from glass and plastic, some people, especially people with stronger lenses, have difficulty adjusting to the change.

Tint or no tint? Tinting is mainly a matter of comfort. Sunglasses are fine if you want them, although their reduced light transmission may affect vision a little bit. A neutral color like gray is generally preferred because it does not alter your color perception, but other colors are fine if you want them. The PhotoGray lenses made by Corning are glass lenses that have minimal tint indoors but darken when you go out in the sun. However, they take a little time to lighten after you go back indoors. PhotoSun lenses are sunglasses that become darker when there is a lot of sunlight. Currently available plastic lenses that darken in the presence of sunlight do not work as well as the glass lenses. If you don't wear prescription lenses but want sunglasses, be aware that the optical quality of sunglasses can vary greatly.

UV (ultraviolet) coating or not? After some studies showed that extensive exposure to sunlight might increase the risk of cataracts and possibly even macular degeneration, optical shops were quick to recommend that lenses be coated to prevent the transmission of ultraviolet light. There was more than altruism behind the recommendation. It was a good opportunity for additional profit, akin to the rustproofing and paint protectants pushed by new-car salespeople. For most people, UV coating is not worth the extra cost. People who should consider UV protection are those who spend a good deal of time in the sun; who are exposed to other sources of ultraviolet light; who have had cataract surgery without lens implants or with the older implants that did not absorb UV light; and who have *pterygia,* growths on the front surface of the eyes. (See "Pterygium," page 103, in chapter 7.)

Ultraviolet coating is not necessary for most people.

For people who need reading glasses only, the question often arises whether the inexpensive store-bought variety is satisfactory. Although such glasses vary in optical quality, most people find them to be quite satisfactory, especially if both of their eyes have about the same vision. Try them on and make sure there are no areas of distortion when you read with them. If possible, have your ophthalmologist recommend the power of lenses you should obtain. Generally, they range from +1.00 up to +3.00. Get lenses that allow you to read comfortably at your preferred reading distance. Overly strong lenses will not harm your eyes but give you less range of usable vision. In other words, you also want to be able to see at arm's length with the same glasses if possible. You also have to decide whether you are more comfortable with full-size reading glasses, which blur your distance vision while you are wearing them, or half readers, which allow you to look over them if you need to look up from your reading material and see in the distance.

Store-bought reading glasses may work just fine.

If you play a musical instrument, you want the glasses to focus on your music. The distance of your eyes from the music depends, of course, on the instrument you play. It is more important to see the music clearly than to see the conductor clearly. Single-vision lenses rather than bifocals or trifocals usually work best for musicians.

Musicians have special needs when it comes to glasses.

When you go for an eye exam, make sure you bring your measurement (distance between your eyes and the music) with you so that glasses of the proper strength can be prescribed. Single-vision lenses, as opposed to bifocals, may also be helpful if you spend a lot of time in front of a computer screen.

Bifocals represent a challenge for many people. No one absolutely must wear bifocals. If you have been wearing glasses for distance and now require added power at the reading distance, you can always obtain a separate pair of reading glasses. Or, if you're just moderately nearsighted, you can remove your glasses to read. But repeatedly putting glasses on and taking them off is certainly inconvenient.

Benjamin Franklin invented bifocals. He stuck two lenses together and—voilà—bifocals! Today's bifocals are easier to use than early ones. Although many types of bifocal segments are made, the flat top, which has a horizontal line on top and a half circle on the bottom, is the most satisfactory for most people. Of course, the optician must place the line in exactly the right place. The width of the bifocal segment should not be any wider than it needs to be. Otherwise, it will get in your way when you are walking and trying to look at the ground.

When you first start wearing bifocals, you should be able to see clearly at all ranges using either the distance vision portion of your glasses or the reading segment. However, as you age and the strength of the bifocal segment is increased, vision may become blurry at the intermediate range, that is, at arm's length. If that becomes too bothersome, *trifocals* can be prescribed. The trifocal segment, which is sandwiched in the middle, provides clarity two to three feet in front of the eyes. Trifocals are more difficult to use than bifocals, however, so you should obtain them only if you think you really need them.

Progressive addition lenses, which contain no line, are a useful alternative to bifocals. These lenses are much more than bifocals without a line. The lens gradually, progressively increases in strength as you move your gaze down the lens. Progressive addition lenses allow you to see clearly at all distances, and they are appreciated by people who don't like the line in traditional bifocals.

It takes time for most people to get used to progressive addition lenses.

All progressive addition lenses are not the same. There are different brands, and some brands may work better for you than others. Your best bet is to go to a good, reliable optician so that you don't get stuck with whatever is cheapest. These lenses must be fit very precisely. The distance between the center of the bridge of your nose and the center of the pupil of each eye must be measured by an electronic gauge. Even with the best fit, many people have difficulty adjusting to these lenses. There is a certain amount of distortion when you look toward the side through these lenses, and some people complain of a swimmy, woozy feeling. If you try the glasses for a few weeks, however, you will probably get used to them, and they will seem just fine (assuming they were made correctly).

Another problem some people experience has to do with their near vision. As you look down through the glasses to read, you have to be looking more or less straight ahead, not to the side. The "corridor" for reading vision on these lenses is not very wide, and you will experience distortion when you look outside of that corridor.

Contact Lenses

Contact lenses correct vision just as glasses do, and they have both advantages and disadvantages as compared with glasses. Although contact lenses that correct hyperopia magnify what you see somewhat, and those that correct myopia minify (make smaller) what you see, they do so to a much smaller extent than glasses do. This is especially helpful to people who have very strong prescriptions, such as very highly myopic individuals or people who have had cataract surgery without a lens implant. Also, if the two eyes have very different prescriptions, the size of the image that one eye sees won't be too much different from that of the other eye, and the eyes will probably be able to work together well. Contact lens wearers do not experience some of the distortions that eyeglass wearers experience as they look to one side or the other. Contacts also provide somewhat better peripheral vision, as there are no frames to get in the way.

On the negative side, contact lenses may not correct vision quite as sharply as glasses do. Rigid contact lenses typically provide *Wearing contacts carries with it a little risk.* slightly sharper vision than soft contact lenses, and soft contact lenses do not correct astigmatism well unless they are specially made for that purpose.

The main problem with contact lenses is that they have the potential to harm the eye. Contact lenses can produce minute corneal abrasions, and infection in the form of a corneal ulcer can set in. The risk is typically higher with soft contact lenses than with rigid lenses. It is also higher in people who wear their lenses on an extended wear basis, who smoke, and who do not observe good contact lens hygiene. Because contact lens wear causes some numbness of the cornea, the wearer may not recognize problems that develop until they have progressed beyond the early stages. Infectious corneal ulcers are a complication we take very seriously, because in many cases contact lens wearers have lost an eye as a result of corneal ulceration.

Rigid Contact Lenses

The first contact lenses were hard contacts, manufactured from a plastic called *polymethylmethacrylate* (PMMA). Standard hard contact lenses provide a high quality of vision, even correcting mild to moderate amounts of astigmatism. Their surface is fairly wettable: Tears form a nice, uniform layer over them, and they don't tend to smudge easily.

The main problem with hard contacts is that they are fairly impermeable to oxygen from the air. The cornea, which lacks blood vessels, needs to have oxygen delivered to it some other way. It receives some from the oxygen dissolved in the tears. But a hard contact lens can sometimes prevent the cornea from receiving adequate oxygen. The cornea then develops edema (fluid buildup), an unhealthy situation. A well-fitting contact lens reduces the likelihood of this complication, but it can still occur to some extent in anyone. Hard contact lens wear over many years can also induce some warping of the corneal surface. This can induce irregular astigmatism, a form of astigmatism that glasses do not correct very well. Ultimately, many people may become less tolerant of their hard contacts, and some may have to stop wearing them.

Because of the corneal problems associated with hard contact lenses, newer materials were developed that would allow more oxygen to be

Dry eyes may make contacts smudge.

transmitted to the cornea through the contact lens. Contact lenses made with these newer materials are called gas-permeable contacts. They are rigid like hard contact lenses, although a little more flexible.

Gas-permeable contact lenses have made rigid contact lens wear more comfortable and certainly more successful for many people. Corneal edema has become an uncommon complication. These contacts are not as durable as standard hard contact lenses, however. Furthermore, they do not "wet" as well as hard lenses. As a result, some people whose eyes are a little dry or who have a poor quality of tear film because of oil gland secretion problems may experience smudging of their lenses soon after they insert them. Sometimes rewetting drops can lessen this problem.

Soft Contact Lenses

Many people decide on soft contacts because of their comfort. Whereas a rigid contact lens at first feels as though there is something in your eye, it may be hard for you to tell that you even have a soft contact lens on. With time, rigid contacts usually become quite comfortable. However, they have to be worn routinely for that to happen. Soft contacts, in contrast, are ideal for people who don't wear their lenses every day. They do require more care than rigid contact lenses, and the disinfection routine is very important. The average life expectancy of a soft contact lens is about one year, assuming it hasn't been torn before then. With age, they develop deposits and yellowing and can start to affect vision and comfort adversely.

Soft contact lenses are *hydrophilic*. This means that they contain a certain percentage of water, ranging generally from about 35 to 70 percent. Because of the water content, they are soft, and they drape over the cornea like a second skin. Since water is continuously lost by evaporation, the water in the lenses must be constantly replaced by drawing off water from the tears. Therefore, people with dry eye syndrome, who have a lack of tears, may not do well with contact lenses and could even be harmed by them. As with rigid contact lenses, oxygen transmission through soft contacts can vary somewhat, but most modern soft contacts are quite permeable to oxygen, and corneal edema is rare.

Soft contact lenses correct myopia and hyperopia quite well. If a significant amount of astigmatism is present, then special lenses called *toric contacts* must be used. They are fairly successful if a good fitting has been obtained. The astigmatism is generally not corrected quite as well as with rigid contacts or glasses, however.

Contact Lenses in Presbyopia

Contact lens wearers often do quite well until they develop presbyopia, the difficulty with focusing at near that typically begins when they are in their early to midforties. What do they do then? Do they simply buy some reading glasses and put them on when they have to read? That's a perfectly acceptable solution, but many contact lens wearers want to stay away from glasses if they can. Special contact lenses have been designed for people with presbyopia. Many people like them and do quite well with them. However, they can sometimes be hard to fit, and there is often some compromise in vision. Therefore, before we try these special contact lenses, we generally first try a fitting technique called *monovision*.

With monovision, one eye is corrected for distance vision, and the other for near vision. It sounds crazy to people who have never tried it, but about 75 percent of people who are fit this way are successful and quite pleased with the results.

Monovision fitting can eliminate the need for bifocal contacts or reading glasses.

Most people (although not all) prefer to have their dominant eye corrected for distance. How do you determine which is your dominant eye? Take a sheet of paper and cut a hole in the middle about the size of a quarter. Then, with both eyes open, hold the sheet squarely in front of yourself with both hands and look at something across the room through the hole. Which eye were you using? That is your dominant eye. Just to be sure, repeat the procedure a few times and see whether you are consistent. Have you ever looked through a handheld telescope, into a kaleidoscope, or through a monocular microscope at school? Chances are you always use the same eye for these activities, and that's your dominant eye. For people who need the best possible depth perception, monovision may not work very well. But most individuals are hardly aware that each eye is focusing at a different distance.

Contact Lens Fittings and Follow-Up Care

First, be sure you really want to wear contact lenses. Don't be persuaded by some advertisement, a waiting room booklet, or an inducement from an optometrist or ophthalmologist. Remember, there is a little risk to your eyes from wearing contacts. Be sure you are motivated enough to comply fully with the lens care routine. For this reason, we often wait until children are at least twelve years old to prescribe contacts, because younger children may not have the maturity to take care of their lenses properly.

The eyes should be carefully examined before contact lens fitting is begun.

If you decide you do want contacts, you should first have a comprehensive eye examination. This should include a refraction (determination of your glasses prescription), a careful examination of all parts of the eye, and a pressure check. The curvature of the cornea should be checked with an instrument called an *ophthalmometer* or *keratometer*. A tear measurement test called a *Schirmer test* should also be done. In this test, a thin strip of special paper is hung over the edge of each of your lower eyelids for five minutes and the amount of wetting measured. If your eyes are too dry, you may not be a good candidate for contacts. If your eyes are extremely dry, the risk of eye infection and other problems is high, and you should not wear contact lenses.

Be aware of the costs involved. Most of what you will pay at first is for the service provided, the fitting. But how much will it cost you later on just to get replacement lenses? I feel that an ethical physician, like any professional, should charge only for services provided and should not make a profit on any items sold, such as contact lenses. Be aware, however, that most practitioners today view the sale of contact lenses and other supplies as a way of generating more profit. The amount you pay can vary widely from one office to another, as this story illustrates.

When my accountant came to me soon after I opened my practice, she requested a replacement for one of her hard contact lenses. The charge was thirteen dollars. Eight dollars was my cost for the lens, and five dollars covered ordering the lens and checking its several parameters once it came in. She was incredulous, wondering whether I was giving her an inferior lens, because she routinely paid a hundred dollars per lens at her previous ophthalmologist. I assured her I was using the highest-quality contact lens laboratory.

The next step is the actual fitting of the lenses. This is generally done at a separate visit because the drops instilled in your eyes during the examination interfere with the fitting and evaluation of the lenses. Fitting means trying lenses on your eyes. It is important to remember that contact lenses are not like glasses. To make sure they fit on the eye properly and will not harm the eye, and to provide the best possible vision, they must be placed on the eye and the fit analyzed. Ideally, the ophthalmologist does this, but many have technicians who do it instead. The lens must center properly and have the right amount of movement on the eye. The fit is checked by examining the eye through the slit lamp, and the vision is checked by having the patient read the letters on the eye chart. Naturally, how the lenses feel is also important. Ultimately, the lenses are prescribed, and you are instructed in their care if you have not previously worn contacts.

After wearing your new lenses for two weeks or so, you should return for a follow-up visit. At this time, you can report any problems you have been having. Your vision is checked and your eyes, especially the corneas, carefully examined. Even if your eyes feel fine, there may be evidence that the corneas are drying out under the lenses or that the lenses are not fitting properly and abrading the eyes. The curvature of the corneas should also be rechecked to make sure that has not changed. If it has changed, the lenses may not fit properly, and it may not be safe to continue wearing them. If the lenses are not right, then different lenses may have to be prescribed.

Follow-up visits assure that the contacts are not harming your eyes.

Even if you are doing well with the lenses, you should have at least one more follow-up visit, perhaps a month to six weeks later. After that point, have your eyes examined at least once a year, even if they feel fine. Recall that contact lenses numb the eye somewhat and you may not be aware of early damage that is going on.

Possible Problems with Contact Lenses

Numerous problems can occur over time with contact lens wear, although fortunately most of them are minor. Corneal ulcer, a deep infection in the cornea, is one of the serious ones we worry about the most. Allergy or sensitivity to chemicals in contact lens solutions is quite common. Allergy to *thimerosal,* an antiseptic containing mercury, occurs in about one out of every six soft contact lens wearers who use solutions containing that chemical preservative. Preservative-free solutions can help reduce the risk of these problems, but you must be careful not to allow the solutions to become contaminated.

Giant papillary conjunctivitis (GPC) is an allergic type of reaction in soft contact lens wearers. This may be a reaction to a person's own proteins that get deposited on the lenses. Individuals affected by GPC may notice irritation and discharge, and the contacts may sometimes be pulled upward by the upper eyelids. Contact lens wear may have to be discontinued for a while. Refitting with different lenses can then be done, but sometimes rigid gas-permeable contacts are the only ones that will not trigger this reaction.

Episcleritis, a sensitivity reaction in which the eye becomes red in one area, is more common in both rigid and soft contact lens wearers. (See "Episcleritis," page 101, in chapter 7.) Corneal edema (fluid buildup) from a lack of oxygen is more likely if the lenses, either rigid or soft, do not fit properly. In general, rigid contact lens wearers tend to have fewer complications than do soft lens wearers.

Refractive Surgery

The newest way to correct refractive errors is surgery. Why would people subject their eyes to the risks of surgery when their vision could be corrected by glasses or by contact lenses? A number of reasons could be given. First, the majority of people who have this surgery done are happy with the results. (For the time being, forget about the minority who are unhappy.)

Second, many young people feel there is something imperfect about themselves when they have to wear corrective lenses. Perhaps it is the influence of Hollywood celebrities, who exude the image of perfection. Perhaps it is because most young people have not yet experienced the onset of any of the bodily imperfections that come on with age.

Is refractive surgery for everyone? Whom will you listen to?

Third, there is the effect of advertising. Richard Warren Sears reportedly noted when he published his mail order catalog that most people will believe anything they see in print, even if it is an advertisement.

Fourth, when "everyone" seems to be doing something, the inference is that it must be okay.

Clearly, there are certain people for whom refractive surgery has some important advantages. For people who cannot wear contact lenses and whose work or leisure activities make wearing glasses impractical, refractive surgery can be the answer to their dilemma. For example, wearing glasses and going water-skiing do not exactly go together. But is refractive surgery right for everyone? That is the question.

We know who's having the surgery done, but who's doing the surgery? Were most of the early refractive surgeons the conscientious, ethical ophthalmologists who practiced medicine to help the sick? Or were they the aggressive surgeons who for years lured people to their offices in the hopes of persuading them to have cataract surgery, but who then began promoting refractive surgery as a way of compensating for the reduced reimbursement from cataracts? The advent of advertising in medicine was a boon to buccaneer surgeons, and, ultimately, because of economic pressures and the tendency to reach the lowest common denominator, this type of surgical practice became widespread.

The question is, whom do you want to take care of your eyes? The ethical physician who cares what your eyes will be like twenty years from now? Or the entrepreneur whose main concern is to keep his level of income up in the present health care environment?

Most refractive surgical procedures do a reasonably good job of bringing the vision to a normal or at least an acceptable level. Before we discuss the advantages and disadvantages of each procedure, a few considerations should be mentioned. First, refractive surgery does not keep your eye from changing. If you wear glasses or contact lenses and the refractive error of your eye changes, you can simply change your glasses or contacts and regain normal vision. But if your eye changes after refractive surgery, you must either obtain glasses or else undergo another refractive surgical procedure.

Second, even if you achieve satisfactory vision from the surgery, you will eventually develop presbyopia, difficulty focusing at near, when you reach your forties. What will

Know what refractive surgery will not do for you.

you do then? Put on reading glasses every time you have to see something up close and then take them off? Naturally, you can do that, but if your point in having the surgery was to get rid of your glasses forever, you will have fallen short of that objective.

Radial keratotomy was the first major refractive surgical procedure to be widely performed. A surgical knife is used to make deep incisions into the cornea in a spokelike manner. An ultrasonic device measures the thickness of the cornea so that the incisions will not be so deep that the cornea becomes perforated, with the knife entering the anterior chamber of the eye. The number and depth of the incisions performed in a given case depend on the degree of myopia to be corrected. The effect is to flatten the curvature of the cornea, thereby lessening or eliminating the myopia. Since different people heal differently, there is some variability in the results. For many people, there is also some fluctuation of vision for many months as the cornea heals. Because of the scars in the cornea, some people complain about glare problems or a star-burst effect when looking at lights at night. The surface of the cornea may also develop a somewhat irregular curvature, resulting in irregular astigmatism. This may limit how well the eye can see with glasses after the surgery if the individual ends up wearing glasses because of a less-than-satisfactory result. And there is some concern that the cornea will always be somewhat weakened and more liable to rupture if the eye gets hit hard. Because of the newer refractive surgical procedures, which are ostensibly safer and more reliable, radial keratotomy is rarely performed these days.

LASIK stands for *laser in situ keratomileusis*. In this procedure, the surgeon uses a very thin blade to create a flap in the cornea near its apex. A laser directed by a computer program vaporizes some of the cornea in the bed of the flap. The corneal flap is then laid back down, and the operation is over. Myopia, hyperopia, and astigmatism can be corrected with this procedure. Both under-corrections and overcorrections of the refractive error are possible. Obviously, people with higher refractive errors are more likely to be undercorrected. In studies of myopic patients, the incidence of significant undercorrection has ranged from about 10 to 60 percent, depending on how much myopia was present to begin with.[1] Often, a tiny amount of the myopia will return over the next six to twelve months. If the vision is sufficiently undercorrected, another LASIK procedure may be necessary to achieve the desired result.

Over 90 percent of people who are mildly myopic end up with 20/40 visual acuity or better as a result of the initial LASIK procedure, but the percentage can be much less for people with high degrees of myopia. About 60 percent of people with mild myopia will end up with 20/20 vision without glasses.[2] Bear in mind, however, that many younger people are able to see better than 20/20, either with or without glasses. For example, they may have 20/15 or even 20/10 vision. To them, or to someone like a jet pilot who needs the sharpest possible vision, 20/20 may seem blurry. And if you do end up with 20/40 vision, you will be able to obtain a driver's license without eyeglass restriction. But will you really be satisfied with 20/40 vision?

Growth of the surface epithelial cells of the cornea under the edge of the flap may occur, and sometimes the flap will "melt" (slough off) in those areas, but vision is not usually affected. *Flap microstriae,* tiny folds in the flap that can affect the quality of vision, may also occur. Flap-related complications have been reported to occur in over 5 percent of cases. Occasionally, another surgery is required to fix the flap. A somewhat unusual complication is inflammation of the cornea, even in the absence of infection, and this inflammation may produce tiny cloudy areas in the cornea.

Many people experience troublesome halos around lights or a starburst appearance of lights at night. These problems tend to get better with time, but in some studies, about one in three to one in four people complained of these symptoms six months to a year after the surgery. Because of irregularities that can occur in the curvature of the cornea, about 5 percent of people undergoing LASIK lose two or more lines of best spectacle-corrected visual acuity.[2,3] This means that if they decide they need to wear glasses, they may find that the glasses do not correct their vision to as good a level as before the surgery. Losing two lines means a drop in visual acuity from 20/20 to 20/30, or 20/15 to 20/25.

Some people's best correctable vision will be worse after LASIK.

A recent article by Joshua Ben-nun, M.D., of Israel[4] highlighted important concerns about potential long-term complications that may result from LASIK as well as *photorefractive keratectomy,* commonly referred to as *PRK* (discussed later). As we shall see, a flurry of recent reports in the medical journals has shown that many of these complications have already occurred. Dr. Ben-nun pointed out that the laser creates free radicals, activated forms of oxygen and other molecules that can attack proteins and DNA in our cells. They also destroy *keratocytes,* the cells that make up the thick middle layer of the cornea and ensure its structural integrity by producing substances that lead to collagen formation. Thus, even if no short-term damage is seen from LASIK or PRK, complications may eventually be seen years down the road. One case report described a severe thinning of the cornea ten months after surgery. A corneal transplant, a major surgical procedure, was required to restore this patient's vision. Will we see many more cases of thinning of the cornea, even years after the surgery was performed? Only time will tell. In another report, a blunt injury to the eye a year after surgery caused the flap to partially fold in on itself.

The effect of the laser on the cornea of the eye may also be the cause of a common side effect—dry eye syndrome. (See "Dry Eye Syndrome," page 66, in chapter 6.) Dry eye syndrome can not only cause comfort problems for the eye but also markedly affect vision. After laser treatment of the cornea, both the quantity of tears and the quality of the tear film are affected. In one study conducted six months after LASIK or PRK, tear secretion after LASIK as measured by the standard Schirmer test declined, on average, by 23.4 percent compared with test results obtained before surgery. The *tear breakup time*, a measure of tear quality, declined by 18.8 percent. PRK did not produce quite as much of a decrease in tear secretion as LASIK did. If this effect on tear production proves to be permanent, this side effect of LASIK will have profound implications, because the incidence of dry eye syndrome increases with age. People who have had LASIK may have a much higher than average risk of developing dry eye syndrome when they become older.

LASIK may also have an effect on the lens of the eye, both in terms of its structure and the biochemical substances it contains. The fear is that these changes could result in an increased risk of cataracts later in life.

The vitreous of the eye, located between the lens and the retina, is another area of concern. The framework of the vitreous may be damaged and become liquefied even before it would normally do so as a result of age. Potential problems that could result from this process include retinal tears and detachment and macular holes and pucker. Thus far, an increased risk of retinal detachment after LASIK seems to occur only in extremely myopic individuals, but it remains to be seen what will happen to mildly and moderately myopic people over time. When you consider that LASIK is being performed mostly on young adults, you realize that they have a long life ahead of them in which complications may develop.

What about any effects on the optic nerve? Already we are seeing problems, even in the short term. In one study, the thickness of the nerve fiber layer after LASIK was found to be less than before the procedure, indicating that nerve fibers may have been destroyed. At this point, the results are controversial because it is not clear whether the LASIK procedure itself alters the accuracy of the thickness measurements, but even the possibility of such an effect should give one pause. In another report, four people who had undergone LASIK suffered moderate to severe permanent loss of vision from optic neuropathy (damage to the optic nerve). Three of the patients were in the forty-eight to fifty-seven age range. The presumed cause of the damage was the high intraocular pressure to which eyes are subjected during the LASIK procedure.

Finally, LASIK results in a falsely low reading of the intraocular pressure of the eye as measured by the usual instruments. A high intraocular pressure is the main risk factor for glaucoma, and its measurement is, therefore, one of the ways to screen for glaucoma. Thus, people who have had LASIK who later develop glaucoma may suffer more optic nerve damage than the average person before their glaucoma is finally diagnosed.

PRK also employs a laser to reshape the cornea. However, it does not require a corneal flap, so there is no traditional "cutting" surgery involved. The end result is not much different from that of LASIK procedures, but there is more discomfort and a somewhat longer time period to obtain vision improvement. The reason is that it takes some time for the cornea to resurface itself with new epithelial cells, since the cells in the area of treatment are destroyed by the laser. People who have PRK can also experience problems with halos or starbursts around lights at night. In one study comparing PRK with LASIK, people who had PRK were more likely to suffer a decline of two or more lines in their best spectacle-corrected visual acuity.[5] For many of the potential complications from PRK, see the earlier discussion regarding LASIK.

Intrastromal corneal ring segments are a newer, investigational procedure at the time of this writing. These rings are made of a kind of plastic called *polymethylmethacrylate* (PMMA), the same material used for hard contact lenses and for many intraocular lens implants used during cataract surgery. This material is inert in the eye and does not cause inflammation, a fact discovered during World War II when British fighter pilots occasionally had PMMA fragments enter their eyes when their planes' canopies, which were made of PMMA, were hit by bullets and shells. These ring segments are surgically inserted into the periphery of the cornea to flatten the center of the cornea and thereby correct low degrees of myopia. Results seem to be comparable to those of the other refractive procedures. There can be complications as well. In one study, 5 percent of the patients lost two or more lines of best spectacle-corrected visual acuity. In addition, three months after the procedure, about one in five patients developed one or more diopters of astigmatism that had not been present prior to the surgery.[6] Further studies are being done.

Other techniques have been tried for the very highly myopic. One technique is to simply remove the lens of the eye, the same procedure that is performed for cataracts. This can be combined with a lens implant, in which an artificial lens is placed inside the eye, just as is done for people with cataracts. The main problem here is the risk to the eye. Myopic individuals have a high risk of retinal detachment to begin with, and this type of surgery increases the risk. All of the other risks associated with cataract surgery, including infection; damage to the corneal endothelium, the delicate cells lining the inside of the cornea; bleeding in the eye, and so on, are present. This procedure is not worth the risk. In a newer procedure, specially designed lens implants are inserted into the eye without removal of the eye's natural lens. These implants end up right next to the lens. Again, with invasive surgery of this nature, there are very definite risks, including the high risk of cataract formation. Because of the risks, this procedure is not recommended either.

In summary, all of the refractive surgical procedures can have complications, and we really do not know their long-term effects on the eye. The amount of vision correction is not completely predictable, and you should not expect to end up with perfect vision without glasses. Minor annoyances, such as glare and other effects from lights at night, may be present. Your vision may change with time, and you can inevitably end up with a near focusing problem (arms too short) like everyone else. Only you can decide whether refractive surgery (which I call recreational surgery) is in your best interests or not. Caveat emptor! P.S. I'm still wearing my glasses.

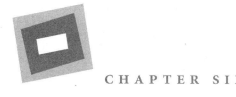

CHAPTER SIX

Eyelids and Lacrimal System

Blepharitis

Blepharitis is an inflammation of the eyelids. Several rows of oil glands run along the rims or margins of the eyelids in the area where the lashes begin. When these glands become irritated or inflamed, they produce extra oily, greasy material that becomes deposited on the eyelid margins and may get into the eye. The pores of the oil glands may also become plugged up. This plugging irritates the oil glands further, and a vicious cycle is created.

Blepharitis can be one of two types, or a combination: seborrheic, which may be associated with dandruff of the scalp or eyebrows; or staphylococcal, in which the glands harbor a low-grade infection that may flare up from time to time. Blepharitis is a chronic condition that may be very difficult to clear up. It is probably the single most common medical eye problem for which people see their ophthalmologists.

Blepharitis is probably the single most common medical eye problem.

Symptoms of Blepharitis

People who have blepharitis may experience any of the following symptoms: eye irritation, redness, tearing, feeling of something in the eye, itching, burning, occasional sharp pains, ache in or around the eye, sensitivity to light, blurring, "film" over the eye, crusting or mattering at the base of the eyelashes, and frequent stye or chalazion formation. (See "Chalazia and Styes," page 64.) The symptoms may be most noticeable upon awakening, because the eyes have been bathing in the irritating secretions of the oil glands all night.

The symptoms are often the worst upon waking in the morning.

During the day, these secretions are partially washed away by the blinking of the eyelids and the flow of tears. Some of the symptoms of blepharitis may also be caused by other eye problems, such as dry eye syndrome or allergic problems. Many people actually have both dry eye syndrome and blepharitis at the same time.

Causes of Blepharitis

The excess oil that gets into the eyes causes most of the symptoms of blepharitis. The oil and other components of the oil gland secretions have a direct irritating effect on the cornea. Cells on the surface of the lower part of the cornea, which is often bathing in these secretions, can slough off. The excess oil also creates a chemical imbalance in the tear film. This chemical imbalance results in an unstable tear film. This means that the tears cannot coat the surface of the eye very well. Normally, the tear film on the surface of the cornea should remain intact for at least ten seconds after a blink has spread fresh tears over the eye. But with

It's similar to water beading up on a piece of wax paper.

an unstable tear film, dry spots appear quickly, sometimes just one second after blinking. The process is similar to water beading up on a piece of wax paper. These dry spots are very irritating to the cornea and can cause sharp, needlelike pains. They can also cause blurring of vision, which is most noticeable during reading. When you read, you develop a little bit of a stare, and your eyes may blink only about half as often as they normally do. This gives those dry spots more time to form. Such blurring may be the only symptom of blepharitis.

Who Gets Blepharitis?

Blepharitis occurs most often in people who have oily skin. Diabetics may have a slightly higher risk of developing the problem. Some people have an underlying condition of the face called *acne rosacea,* or just *rosacea* for short. They tend to have tiny reddish bumps and corkscrewy blood vessels on the "blush" areas of the face. The skin changes are often most prominent on the nose. People with rosacea are very prone toward blepharitis, especially the staphylococcal type. Treatment of their underlying rosacea problem by a dermatologist can often help their blepharitis as well.

Problems Caused by Blepharitis

With the staphylococcal form of blepharitis, a wide variety of unusual problems may develop. The skin by the outer corner of the eye, where the eyelids meet, can become red and weepy in appearance, a condition called *angular blepharitis*. Sometimes the skin of the entire eyelids, especially the upper eyelids, develops this red, weepy appearance, called *eczematoid blepharitis* because it resembles the common allergic skin condition called *eczema*. Eczematoid blepharitis is felt to be a "hypersensitivity" or allergic type of reaction to the by-products of the bacteria that live in the oil glands.

Prompt treatment of blepharitis is important.

Another type of hypersensitivity reaction is the *marginal hypersensitivity ulcer*. This is a whitish area that appears just under the surface of the cornea but not far from its edge, right where the margin of one of the eyelids crosses the cornea. The corneal epithelium, the surface layer of cells, then breaks down, forming a shallow ulcer. If you ever see a white spot on your cornea, have it checked out right away. You may have the beginnings of an ulcer.

Episcleritis, a condition in which the deeper blood vessels in one part of the eye become inflamed and engorged with blood (see "Episcleritis," page 101, in chapter 7), is another type of hypersensitivity reaction occasionally seen in people with staphylococcal blepharitis. Even less common is *phlyctenular conjunctivitis,* in which a whitish nodule or bump appears at the edge of the cornea, with redness of the eye confined to that area.

Prompt treatment of blepharitis is important, particularly with the staphylococcal type, because otherwise a chronic infection may ensue as the bacteria become more deeply entrenched, making later eradication more difficult. With chronic infection, scarring may cause thickening of the eyelid margins, along with turning in or turning out of the eyelids and eyelashes.

Treating Blepharitis

The mainstay of treatment is known as *lid hygiene* or *lid scrubs.* First, apply warm compresses to the lids. To do this, hold a warm, moist washcloth against the closed eyelids, rewetting the washcloth with warm water every thirty seconds or so to keep it warm enough. Continue the warm compresses for about two minutes. Then take some mild baby shampoo that has been diluted about 50 percent with warm water, moisten a cotton-tipped applicator, and gently scrub the eyelid margins clean by wiping back and forth along their length, especially around the base of the eyelashes. This should include the upper and lower eyelids of both eyes if possible. The upper eyelids are more difficult, but by pulling up on the skin of the lid, you can often get the margin of the eyelid to pull away from the eye a bit. If the diluted baby shampoo seems too irritating, dilute it even more with water. The lid scrubs may be done anywhere from once a day (generally at bedtime) up to four times a day, depending on the severity of the condition. After completing a scrub, rinse the eyelids gently with warm water.

Makeup such as eyeliner can often aggravate the condition.

The margin of the eyelid gets all the attention. The goal is to remove oily material from the lid margin so that it will not get into the eye and so that the oil glands will become unplugged. Makeup such as eyeliner on the lid margins can often aggravate the condition, however. Makeup should be confined to the eyelashes and to the skin side of the eyelids.

Seborrhea of the scalp, more commonly known as *dandruff,* frequently accompanies seborrheic blepharitis. Clearing up scalp dandruff by using a good dandruff shampoo often helps relieve the symptoms of blepharitis.

There is some evidence that a high-cholesterol, high-fat diet may worsen the oil gland problems and increase the secretion of oils into the tear film.

Therefore, following a low-fat, low-cholesterol diet may have beneficial effects in people who suffer from blepharitis, just as it has beneficial effects with regard to so many other medical conditions.

In some cases, especially when staphylococcal blepharitis is present, a sulfa or antibiotic eye ointment is prescribed. The ointment should be applied very sparingly along the margin of the lower eyelids. A cotton-tipped applicator works well for this, or you can use your fingertip, assuming that your nails are short and you've just washed your hands. The ointment is applied *after* the lid scrub routine. If you use too much ointment, it blurs your vision. If the ointment is prescribed for once-a-day use, it is usually best to apply it at bedtime, when you won't notice the blurring. In some cases, the ointment may be prescribed for up to six weeks at a time. In more resistant cases, a combination antibiotic and corticosteroid (cortisone) ointment is prescribed for limited periods of time. You should not use this type of ointment on your own without a physician's advice because of the possibility of complications, especially with prolonged use.

You may wonder why antibiotic medication is sometimes used not only for the infectious staphylococcal form of blepharitis but also for the noninfectious seborrheic form. The reason is that although seborrheic blepharitis does not represent a true infection, there is often an overgrowth of bacteria in the affected oil glands, and these bacteria play a role in how these oil glands function. Suppressing these overgrown bacteria with medication can often make the glands function more normally and thereby quell the blepharitis. Dermatologists use the same principle to treat acne. In fact, antibiotics such as tetracycline and erythromycin are sometimes prescribed as a last resort, to be taken by mouth just as they are for acne.

If any of the hypersensitivity or allergic types of reactions, such as episcleritis, eczematoid blepharitis, phlyctenular conjunctivitis, or marginal hypersensitivity ulcer, is present, then special treatment, which usually includes the application of corticosteroid medication, may be needed. Again, such medication is available by prescription only.

Symptomatic treatment with over-the-counter artificial tear drops can be very helpful. These drops not only relieve irritation but also can help stabilize an unstable tear film that causes blurring and discomfort. The best drops for this purpose are the preservative-free ones, which come in tiny single-use plastic containers. The preservatives in regular artificial tear drops can irritate and even be toxic to the eye if used too frequently. If you have difficulty reading because of dry spot formation on the eye from an unstable tear film, you can use the drops every fifteen minutes if necessary. Try the different available brands and see which works best for you.

Although blepharitis is often a chronic, recurring condition, you can usually control the symptoms and prevent any complications just by keeping up with the lid hygiene routine. Additional treatment is generally reserved for flare-ups.

Chalazia and Styes

A *chalazion*, also known as an *internal hordeolum*, is a blockage of the pore of one of the oil glands that line the margins of the eyelids. The oil gland becomes "angry" when this happens, and it and the surrounding eyelid tissue become quite inflamed. At first, there may be pain in the area, along with mild redness and some diffuse swelling. After a few days, the swelling becomes more localized, forming a small "knot" in the area of the oil gland. In a small percentage of cases chalazia become infected, usually by a bacterium called staphylococcus. If that occurs, the swelling and redness become more intense, and the lymph node in the area of drainage from the lid becomes enlarged.

People with chronically inflamed oil glands are prone to develop chalazia.

For the upper lid, the lymph node is located just in front of the ear on that side, whereas for the lower lid, the lymph node is just under the angle of the jaw. Lymph nodes contain tissue that helps the body fight infection.

A *stye*, also known as an *external hordeolum*, is a cousin to a chalazion. It represents an abscess of a more superficial type of gland. Whereas a chalazion points toward either the skin or the underside of the eyelid, a stye points toward the margin of the eyelid, where its inflamed whitish head can be seen.

Who Gets Chalazia and Styes?

The people who are most prone to develop chalazia and styes are those who suffer from chronic blepharitis, an inflammation of the oil glands of the eyelids. (See "Blepharitis," page 59.) Blepharitis causes the oil glands to become overactive and to secrete a thick oil that can plug up the pores of the oil glands.

Therefore, for people who develop recurrent chalazia or styes, the best preventive measure is often to treat the underlying chronic blepharitis.

Treating Chalazia and Styes

The initial treatment for chalazia and styes is warm compresses. Wet a washcloth with water as warm as can be tolerated and then hold it against the area of the chalazion for ten minutes. Rewet it frequently during this period to keep it warm all the time. Perform this routine at least four times a day, more frequently if possible. It may be difficult to find time during the day to do this, but it really pays off. Use the warm compresses until the chalazion or stye is gone, usually for at least a *Warm compresses are the mainstay of treatment.* week but sometimes for several weeks. Application of antibiotic or similar ointments has never been shown to be of value in treating chalazia and styes.

If you have been using the warm compresses for a week or two but a well-localized chalazion is still present, an additional procedure can be performed. The ophthalmologist can inject a small amount of corticosteroid (cortisone) liquid into the chalazion with a very tiny needle. Injecting the liquid in this manner may build up enough pressure in the chalazion to force open the blocked-off pore, leading to a quick resolution of the problem. Even if this does not happen, the medication itself has an anti-inflammatory effect that can speed up the healing process. A single injection such as this usually has about a 50 percent success rate. Following the injection, continue the warm compresses until the chalazion appears completely gone.

If, after two to four weeks, the chalazion shows no sign of going away, we usually drain it, a minor surgical procedure. Some ophthalmologists perform the surgery much earlier than this, as soon as the chalazion becomes localized, but I think it is best to avoid even minor surgery, if possible.

The surgery should be performed under sterile conditions. The skin of the eyelids is wiped with an antiseptic solution such as povidone iodine, and a sterile plastic drape with a hole in the center is placed around the eye. The eyelid is then numbed by drops in the eye and a small injection of local anesthetic such as lidocaine under the skin of the eyelid. The eyelid is everted (turned over on itself), and a special clamp is applied to the lid to hold it in place. A small X-shaped incision is then made directly into the chalazion through the underside of the eyelid. The creamy contents of the chalazion are evacuated, and its interior is scraped to prevent recurrence. The opening into the eyelid is then enlarged so that the chalazion can continue to drain. The eye is generally left unpatched, and the warm compresses are resumed beginning the next day and continued until no sign of the chalazion remains. The surgery is usually curative.

In the unusual event that the chalazion becomes infected, antibiotic treatment by mouth generally becomes necessary. Otherwise, a *periorbital cellulitis,* a dangerous infection involving the entire eyelid, may develop, along with the possibility that it might spread to the orbit. Fortunately, infected chalazia usually respond quickly to appropriate antibiotic treatment accompanied by continued warm compresses.

Dry Eye Syndrome

The Importance of Tears

Drying out can be an ecological disaster for the environment, and the same is true for our eyes. The tears not only provide protection and comfort for the surface of our eyes but also are essential for good vision. To understand how dry eye syndrome can affect the eyes, we must first look at the nature of tears and the role they play in keeping the eyes healthy.

What Is the Tear Film?

To function normally, the cornea (front surface of the eyeball) must be covered at all times by a coat of tears called the *tear film.* This tear film consists of three distinct layers. Sandwiched in the middle is a watery layer produced by the main tear gland, located under the outer portion of the upper eyelid, and by many tiny tear glands, located all along the inside surface of the lid. The outermost layer of the tear film is an oily layer that helps keep the tears from evaporating. The oil is produced by glands near the margins of both the upper and lower eyelids. Finally, the innermost layer, the one that touches the eye itself, is composed of a substance called *mucin,*

With an unstable tear film, the tears bead up on the eye like water on a newly waxed car.

produced by mucus glands in the eyelids. The mucin acts as a detergent: It allows the tears to spread smoothly and evenly over the front surface of the eye. If this layer were not present, you would have an unstable tear film: The tears would bead up on the eye, and dry spots would be present between these watery islands. It would look very similar to what you see when water is sprayed on a car that has just been waxed.

What Is Dry Eye Syndrome?

There are two major types of dry eye syndrome, although many people actually have a combination of the two. The first is the aqueous deficiency form of dry eye syndrome. With this type, the tear glands are simply not making enough tears, so the middle, watery layer of the tear film thins out. Examination of the eye reveals a low level of tear fluid above the rim of the lower eyelid. A Schirmer test, in which a thin strip of special paper is hung over the edge of the lower eyelid and the amount of wetting achieved over five minutes is measured, can also be helpful in the diagnosis. Finally, special dyes can be instilled in the eye to show whether cells on the surface of the eye are sloughing off because of dryness.

Common symptoms include burning, irritation, itching, feeling of something in the eye, and light sensitivity. For many people, difficulty reading for more than a few minutes at a time may be the only symptom. In addition, many people with dry eyes complain of tearing—not what you might expect! Because of the dryness, the tear gland occasionally puts out a spurt of tears, and that's where the tearing comes from. Symptoms tend to be more marked in people

Difficulty reading for more than a few minutes may be the only symptom.

living in hot, dry climates. Aging is the most common risk factor for aqueous deficiency, but other risk factors include rheumatoid arthritis, lupus, Sjögren's syndrome, scleroderma, hypothyroidism (underactive thyroid gland), and estrogen deficiency, as with menopause or following total hysterectomy with removal of the ovaries. Most people, however, have no underlying disease.

The other form of dry eye syndrome is the unstable tear film type. This results in dry spot formation on the eye, as noted before. Every time you blink, a fresh coat of tears is swept over the surface of the eye. Therefore, we can diagnose an unstable tear film by measuring how long it takes after a blink for dry spots to appear (the *tear breakup time*). Normally, there should be no dry spots for at least ten to fifteen seconds. Symptoms with this type of dry eye syndrome can be similar to those seen with aqueous deficiency. Blurring can occur soon after you begin to read. That's because you have a bit of a stare when you read, and you blink only about half as often as you normally do. That gives the dry spots much more time to form. Some people also blink less often when they drive, so the blurring can occur with driving as well. A common cause of an unstable tear film is a malfunctioning of the oil glands of the eyelids. (See "Blepharitis," page 59.) The excess oil can create a chemical imbalance in the tear film, rendering it unstable. Some skin diseases that also affect the eye can destroy some of the mucous glands in the eyelids, and the lack of mucin can destabilize the tear film. Vitamin A deficiency can also do this. Although not common in the United States, vitamin A deficiency occurs in people who eat primarily grains and beans, as they lack the beta-carotene that the body converts to vitamin A.

Treating Dry Eye Syndrome

Treatment depends on the type and severity of dry eye syndrome. It is helpful to avoid exposing the eyes to wind or air coming in through the windows or the vents in a car. Eyeglasses can help protect the eyes from wind and lessen the amount of tear evaporation. Using glasses with side shields is even more effective. If you are able to choose where to live, try to avoid hot, dry climates.

Artificial tear drops are over-the-counter eyedrops that have been designed to replace the eye's natural tears. Even if you know the type of dry eye syndrome you have, it is impossible to know for sure which brand of artificial tear will work best for you. Therefore, it's best to try all of them and see which one feels best and provides the best vision and comfort. Unfortunately, their effect on the eye is fairly short lived. People who need to instill the drops more than two or three times a day should use preservative-free artificial tear drops. The chemical preservatives in regular artificial tear drops can irritate the eyes with frequent use. People who experience blurring with reading because of an unstable tear film may have to use the drops as often as every fifteen minutes while reading.

> *It is impossible to know for sure which brand of artificial tear will work best for you.*

Over-the-counter ointments represent another form of eye lubrication. The main drawback with ointments is that they blur your vision, so they are generally used only at bedtime. Mineral oil and petrolatum are the usual ingredients, but some lubricating eye ointments also contain lanolin. Lanolin comes from sheep's wool and can contain the pesticides that are sprayed on the sheep. These pesticide residues can irritate the eyes, so be aware of that potential problem.

Another lubrication option is Lacrisert. Lacrisert can be thought of as an artificial tear in solid form. It's a thin little pellet that you insert between your lower eyelid and your eye with the help of a flexible applicator. Insertion requires a little dexterity, but this can often be achieved with practice. The pellet can be inserted once or twice a day, and it gradually dissolves, slowly releasing the artificial tear substance. Sometimes people, especially those with very dry eyes, report a little irritation and a feeling of something in the eye after they insert the Lacrisert. One reason is that an extremely dry eye may not have enough moisture of its own to begin the process of dissolving the Lacrisert,

Extremely dry eyes sometimes require more extreme measures.

so it remains hard. One solution is to instill a few artificial tear drops after the Lacrisert is inserted. That is often enough to soften it and make it more comfortable.

Extremely dry eyes sometimes require more extreme measures. The openings *(puncta)* to the two tiny drainage canals *(canaliculi)* near the inner corner of the eye that allow tears to drain out of the eye can be sealed shut, either temporarily with tiny plugs or permanently by burning them shut with a thin wire cautery.

The results are often dramatic. People with red, painful eyes often find that their eyes have become white and comfortable within twenty-four hours. They feel so much better that they don't usually even notice any discomfort caused by the cautery. For eyes that are not so dry, however, there is the risk of developing a tear overflow problem.

Another temporary measure is using a moist chamber, a kind of inexpensive, close-fitting goggle that keeps the tears from evaporating.

Dry eye syndrome is a chronic condition, but new and improved treatments over the years have made it manageable for most people. Hopefully, we will soon find ways of treating the cause or even preventing the problem.

Lacrimal Problems

Lacrimal problems include disorders of the main tear gland *(lacrimal gland)* and the tear drainage system. The lacrimal gland lies behind the upper eyelid over the outside part of each eye. The tear drainage system includes the *puncta,* the two tiny openings in the margins of the upper and lower eyelids toward the inner corner of the eye; the *canaliculi,* the thin tubes that carry tears from the puncta to the tear sac *(lacrimal sac)* located in a little bony depression alongside the nose; the tear sac itself; and the tear duct *(nasolacrimal duct),* which carries tears from the tear sac into the interior of the nose.

Infant Tear Duct Problems

Infants are sometimes born with *congenital dacryostenosis,* a condition in which the opening of the tear duct into the nose is partially closed off. Most of the time, it has opened up before birth. However, if it remains shut, the tears cannot drain normally out of the eye, and the eye wells up with tears, which may even overflow and run down the cheek. This may occur in just one eye or in both. Because of the blockage, infection in the tear sac often occurs. Pus from the tear sac frequently moves backward through the canaliculi and out the puncta into the eye, which may become intermittently red from the mild infection.

Treating Congenital Dacryostenosis Treatment of congenital dacryostenosis should begin as soon as it is diagnosed. The mainstay of treatment is massage of the tear sac. With one finger, apply moderate pressure on the skin over the tear sac, located between the inner corner of the eye and the nose. As you press, pus may be expressed backward into the eye. As you continue pressing, slide the finger in a downward direction between the nose and the cheek. You are attempting to

Massage, massage, massage until it's better.

force the contents of the tear sac in a downward direction, which increases the pressure in the tear duct and hopefully encourages it to open up so that drainage into the nose occurs. You may repeat the process two or three times. If a mild antibiotic eyedrop has been prescribed for infection, instill it in the eye after completing the massage. Perform this whole procedure four times a day or as your doctor prescribes.

If Congenital Dacryostenosis Doesn't Get Better With time, most cases of congenital dacryostenosis resolve, although it could take months or even a year. If it does not get better on its own, a tear duct probing can be performed. In this procedure, the punctum of the upper lid (preferably) is dilated with thin, wirelike probes. A probe is then introduced into the punctum, advanced along the canaliculus until it enters the tear sac, and then threaded down the tear sac until it encounters the obstruction where it should be entering the interior of the nose. After a little pressure is applied with the probe, a little "popping" sensation is felt, and the probe enters the interior of the nose. This usually cures the problem. The timing of probing remains controversial. It can be done at two or three months of age without the use of anesthesia. However, some people claim that there might be an element of suffering for the infant. If one waits until the infant is over six months old, though, and has more difficulty keeping still, the procedure must be done under general anesthesia in the operating room, which entails a tiny degree of risk. It is even possible to wait until the infant is a year of age or more before resorting to the probing, but the chance of success declines in children over one year old.

With time, it usually gets better, but don't wait too long.

An unsuccessful probing can be repeated at a later date, but ultimately a more complicated procedure or even surgery may be necessary. So when to do the probing? I generally recommend doing it at one year of age if the problem has not resolved by then.

Adult Tear Duct Problems

The hallmark of a narrowing or obstruction of the tear duct in adults is *epiphora,* the medical term for tears running down the cheek. If people have an excess in tear production—for example, in an irritated eye—the tears generally do not run down the cheek if the tear duct is functioning normally. Adults may also get infections in the tear sac, just as infants do. The cause of the problem is different in adults, however. Although in rare cases a tumor may be causing the obstruction, most of the time we are simply dealing with a somewhat narrow tear duct whose lining has become swollen as the result of some irritation.

Evaluating Adult Tear Duct Problems When someone has a tearing problem, we often introduce a very thin probe into both the upper and lower canaliculi

71

to make sure no obstruction is there. If the canaliculi are open and the lids hug the eyes as they should, then we know that tears can get to the tear sac and that the problem is with the tear duct. What we can do at this point is prescribe an eyedrop that combines a sulfa drug or antibiotic (to fight infection) with a cortisone component (to combat inflammation). Such a drop might be used four times a day for two weeks. If the tearing problem goes away, then we taper off the drops and see whether the problem returns. If, however, the tearing problem is persistent, then further testing needs to be done.

In borderline cases in which we're not sure that there really is a tear duct problem, we might perform a five-minute dye disappearance test. In this test, a drop of a solution containing the yellow dye fluorescein is instilled in both eyes. After five minutes, we see how much of the fluorescein remains in each eye. An abnormal test result does not prove that there is a tear duct problem, however. For example, aging eyelids that do not hug the eye closely may not allow the tears to enter the puncta very well, thereby causing tears to well up in the eyes.

A more definitive test is called the *Jones test*. In the first part of this test, a fluorescein eyedrop is instilled in the eye as with the dye disappearance test. However, rather than just seeing how much dye remains in each eye after a few minutes, we advance a thin probe with some cotton wrapped around the tip into the nose in the area where the tear duct empties into the nose's interior. We then remove the probe and see whether the cotton has been stained with the fluorescein dye. If so, that is a normal result. If no dye is recovered in this way, we proceed with the second part of the Jones test. We irrigate the lower canaliculus with salt water, forcing the water into the tear sac and down the tear duct. If the yellow dye that had reached the tear sac is then recovered in the nose, we know that a partial obstruction or severe narrowing of the tear duct is present, and this is what we find in the majority of cases. However, if no dye is recovered in the nose, then either the tears are not reaching the tear sac (as with an eyelid problem or an obstruction of the canaliculi) or the tear duct may be completely obstructed. Once obstruction of the tear duct has been diagnosed, special X-ray tests may be done if there is any suspicion of a tumor or of any other abnormalities.

Treating a Tear Duct Obstruction The definitive treatment for tear duct obstruction is an operation called a *dacryocystorhinostomy*, or DCR. An incision is made alongside the nose in the area of the tear sac. A hole is drilled through the bone on the side of the nose, and a direct communication is made between the tear sac and the inside of the nose. The tear duct is thereby bypassed, and the procedure is successful over 90 percent of the time. If the canaliculi rather than the tear duct are blocked, however, then not only is a standard DCR performed, but a glass tube called a *Jones tube* is inserted through the eyelid tissue at its inner corner, with one end of the tube facing the eye and the other end traversing the hole in the bone and entering the interior of the nose. One must take care of the tube afterward to make sure it does not become plugged up.

Tearing as a Symptom

Tearing is a very common symptom. An eye infection, a scratch on the eye, or a foreign body in the eye will stimulate tearing. Even dry eye syndrome can paradoxically result in tearing, with the irritation caused by the dryness occasionally stimulating the tear gland to put out a spurt of tears. Tearing is especially common in elderly individuals. There may be many contributing factors. Dry eye syndrome along with a chronic blepharitis may be present. Aging changes in the eyelids may cause *ectropion,* a turning outward of the lid margin that denies the tears access to the lower punctum of the eyelid, where the tears enter the drainage system. *Entropion,* a turning inward of the lid margin, may be present, causing irritation of the eye. In some people, the tear duct may be somewhat narrower than in others. How, then, do we deal with a tearing problem in the older person?

Clearly, if there is some irritating factor, such as blepharitis, it should be treated. (See "Blepharitis," page 59.) Tearing is an extremely common problem, and by treating it with eyelid hygiene and occasional artificial tear drops, good improvement can often be obtained. But should surgery be performed?

Mild tearing is common in the elderly and does not necessarily require surgery.

Obviously, this depends on the individual case, but in the average person who has only mild symptoms that are an occasional annoyance, a conservative outlook toward surgery is warranted. Why subject yourself to the risks and uncertainties of surgery if you have a problem you can live with? If I had a very mild tearing problem, I would certainly think twice before undergoing surgery.

Inflammation and Enlargement of the Tear Gland

Enlargement of the tear gland is generally noticeable and may produce what is called an *S-shaped deformity of the upper eyelid*. This means that the margin of the eyelid toward the outside of the eye becomes pushed downward, while the eyelid toward the inner corner of the eye maintains its normal position, resulting in a gentle "S" curve to the eyelid margin. There are many reasons why the tear gland may become enlarged. It can be affected by both benign and malignant tumors. It may become enlarged by inflammation in Sjögren's syndrome as well as other autoimmune diseases (those in which the immune system attacks the body's own tissues). The term *dacryoadenitis* is used to refer either to inflammations of this nature or to infections of the tear gland. Swelling, pain, and redness are often present. If a bacterial infection is suspected, then antibiotics are given, generally with good results.

Common Eyelid Tumors

Growths on eyelids are very common. Some kinds of growths occur almost exclusively on the eyelids. Others often occur elsewhere on the body as well. We will review the ones that are seen most often.

Epithelial Inclusion Cyst

A very common finding on the eyelids is the *epithelial inclusion cyst*. It looks like a tiny white bead in the skin. The "white bead" represents the contents of one of the glands of the skin. These are simple to remove if you choose to do so. A very tiny incision is made in the skin over the white bead, which is then easily "shelled out." They generally do not recur.

Oil Gland Tumors

A *chalazion* is a pea-sized lump in the eyelid, often accompanied by inflammation, that results from a blocked oil gland. (See

Some cancers can masquerade as a chalazion.

"Chalazia and Styes," page 64.) They are benign. However, there is a rare kind of cancer that can begin in an oil gland and can sometimes masquerade as a chalazion. Therefore, if what appears to be a chalazion persists and continues to grow, despite both medical and surgical treatment, it may be wise to biopsy it just to make sure it is not malignant.

Xanthelasma

Middle-aged and elderly people may sometimes develop a yellowish, raised growth on the lids, most commonly in the half of the eyelid toward the nose. This is a *xanthelasma,* a cholesterol deposit in the skin. Some people who develop a xanthelasma do not have high blood cholesterol levels, but others do. Therefore, if you have a xanthelasma, it is a good idea to have your cholesterol level checked if it has not been done in the past few years. Xanthelasmas are only a cosmetic problem and do not cause harm. If removal is desired, they can be cut away with surgery or removed by application of a weak acid to the area. This, of course, should be done only by a physician experienced in the technique.

Papilloma

Papillomas are warty, benign growths that often appear between the eyelashes. The bigger they become, the more difficult they are to remove and the more likely they are to recur. Therefore, papillomas that are growing should be surgically removed by an ophthalmologist. So-called *skin tags,* which look like microscopic fingers of skin that grow out from the lid away from the eyelashes, are also papillomas but are much easier to treat.

Molluscum Contagiosum

Molluscum contagiosum is a virus infection that produces small, round, white nodules that are often hidden among the eyelashes. It can cause a chronic inflammation on the surface of the eye that goes away once the nodule is removed. Often, even partial removal of the nodules does the trick as the immune system takes over. People with immune system problems such as acquired immunodeficiency syndrome (AIDS) may develop many of these nodules, which can be very resistant to treatment.

Basal Cell Carcinoma

The most common cancers on the eyelids are *basal cell carcinomas*. These cancers are related to excessive sunlight exposure, so they are common on all areas of the face. There is some evidence that a low-fat diet can reduce the risk. Fortunately, most people today have heard about the dangers of excessive sun exposure and are using sunscreens, wearing hats, or just limiting their time in the sun.

A low-fat diet may lower the risk of these cancers.

Of course, ultraviolet-absorbing glasses, either sunglasses or regular, also provide protection. Basal cell carcinomas may be round or irregularly shaped lesions, often with a somewhat shiny surface traversed by tiny, thready blood vessels. The center part of the tumor may eventually become ulcerated.

Any lesion with a suspicious appearance should be biopsied. The biopsy is really a very simple procedure. The area is numbed, and a small blade is used to shave off the part of the tumor extending above the level of the surrounding skin. No attempt is made to remove the tumor completely at this point. The tissue removed is then examined by a pathologist. If it is a benign lesion, nothing more need be done. But if it turns out to be a basal cell carcinoma, complete removal is required. Although we don't normally think of basal cell carcinomas as a cause of death, in rare cases, they can spread to the area behind the eye and even to the brain.

Surgical removal of a basal cell carcinoma near the margin of the eyelid usually involves a pentagonal block resection. This means that an entire segment of the eyelid, roughly in the shape of "home plate," is removed in the area of the tumor. It is then sent to the pathologist, who confirms the diagnosis on the spot. The pathologist also indicates whether any of the tumor extends right up to the edge of the segment of removed tissue. If so, additional eyelid tissue may have to be removed. It is well known that, unlike most

Eyelid growths that look suspicious can be easily biopsied.

cancers, many basal cell carcinomas do not regrow even if they have not been completely removed. However, when we're dealing with the eyelid, there is less margin for error than elsewhere, and it is generally advisable to try to remove 100 percent of the tumor. Once the tumor removal is complete, the remaining portions of the eyelid can be sewn back together. If a large portion of the lid has been removed, this may necessitate advanced plastic surgical techniques.

An alternate way of removing a basal cell carcinoma is to use a technique called *Mohs's micrographic surgery*. Some dermatologists have been specially trained in this technique. Very thin slices of tissue around a tumor are removed and immediately examined under the microscope for the presence of residual tumor cells. The area is carefully mapped out to ensure complete removal. This technique, which is often used in more difficult cases, aims for 100 percent removal of the cancer with the least possible loss of normal tissue. Plastic surgical techniques may then be used to repair the defect in the eyelid, either at the time of the Mohs's surgery or later. Mohs's micrographic surgery has an unparalleled success rate in terms of tumor recurrence.

Squamous Cell Carcinoma

Squamous cell carcinoma is the other common skin cancer and is also related to sunlight exposure. It is less common than basal cell carcinoma but is more aggressive and invasive. The surgical techniques used to treat basal cell carcinoma are used here as well, but it is even more important to assure that a squamous cell carcinoma has been completely removed.

As with basal cell carcinoma, a low-fat diet may help reduce the occurrence of the squamous cell variety. In a recent study, consumption of citrus peel (rind, zest) was found to reduce the risk of squamous cell carcinoma of the skin by 34 percent. Researchers suspect that a substance called *limonene* in the oil of the peel may be responsible for the anticancer effect. If you eat citrus peel, you should probably get some that was grown without pesticides.

Ectropion and Entropion

Ectropion is a condition in which the margin of the eyelid turns outward. *Entropion,* in contrast, involves a turning inward of the eyelid margin. Most cases of ectropion and entropion involve the lower lids.

Causes of Ectropion

Ectropion generally occurs in older individuals as aging causes the lower lid to elongate and become lax. When the margin of the lower eyelid is not in contact with the eye, the tears are not able to find their way into the tear drainage openings (puncta). A stagnant pool of tears forms between the eyeball and the lower lid and can cause symptoms such as tearing and irritation. An ectropion does not have to be treated if it is not causing any symptoms, but if it remains for a long time, the skin of the eyelid can shrink. Repair at that point can be more difficult, sometimes requiring a skin graft.

Correcting Ectropion

Many surgical techniques have been developed to treat ectropion. One common method is to remove an entire segment of the lid to shorten it. This is usually done on the side of the eyelid away from the nose. If the ectropion is very mild and is causing a little tearing because the opening (punctum) to the tear drainage system in the rim of the lower lid has fallen away from the eye, a few simple techniques may help. In one technique, tiny burns are placed on the inside surface of the lid on the side toward the nose. This results in a scar that draws the lid margin inward. The other method is to surgically remove a small ellipse of tissue from the inside of the lid. This procedure, along with the scar that results, can draw the lid margin inward and allow the tears to drain out of the eye more normally.

Causes and Symptoms of Entropion

With entropion, irritation of the eye occurs because of the scraping of the eyelashes against the eyeball. Entropion often results from aging. First, there is the increased horizontal laxity of the lower lid, as discussed with ectropion. Second, there may be a defect in the retractor muscle of the lower eyelid. I would compare it to an old piece of cloth that, as a result of wear and tear, has become stretched and thinned out. These two factors together create a muscle imbalance in the eyelid that allows it to turn in against the eye. An entropion can also occur in any condition in which there is inflammation or irritation of the eye.

An irritation in the eye or eyelid can cause a muscle spasm that results in entropion.

The irritation causes the muscle in the eyelid to go into spasm, and the result is an entropion. However, even in this situation, aging changes in the eyelid often contribute to the problem. Finally, scarring caused by injuries, chemical or thermal burns, or certain types of infection can also cause entropion.

Treating Entropion

As with ectropion, there are a variety of ways of dealing with entropion. One should first check the eye closely for any irritative problems, such as dry eye syndrome or blepharitis. Treating any such underlying problems may cause the entropion to resolve and no surgery to be necessary. A stopgap measure that is sometimes used, especially with severe entropions caused by scarring, is placing an extended wear soft contact lens on the eye. It acts as a bandage to shield the eye from the eyelashes. Bandage contact lenses such as this increase the risk of corneal infection, however.

One common surgical technique to reverse the entropion is called a *base-down triangle procedure*. A wedge of tissue in the shape of a triangle is removed from the inside of the lower lid. It is a simple procedure and often effective in mild cases. Another technique is the removal of an entire segment of the eyelid to shorten it, as is done for ectropion. This corrects the age-related horizontal elongation of the lid that contributes to the problem. Finally, an approach favored by many is to locate the lid's retractor muscle and repair any defect in it, for example, where it attaches to the eyelid. This method attempts to restore the anatomy of the eyelid to its original state.

Ptosis

Ptosis generally refers to a drooping of the upper eyelid. Some infants are born with ptosis of an eyelid, but for most people, it is something acquired during life. Mild ptosis may be nothing more than a cosmetic problem. More severe ptosis may interfere with vision, however, especially the upper half of one's field of vision. Occasionally, the drooping eyelid may even change the curvature of the upper part of the cornea and cause blurring of vision in that way.

Causes of Ptosis

Ptosis has many possible causes. The ptosis in newborns is usually caused by a defect in the *levator muscle,* which is responsible for elevating the upper eyelid when you look up and for just keeping it open. In people of all ages, the development of ptosis may indicate a nerve problem. Nerve problems may be due to serious conditions in the brain, such as tumors, strokes, and aneurysms, but can also be caused by injuries, diabetes, and migraine, to name just a few possibilities. Nerve problems causing ptosis in adults often cause other problems at the same time. For example, ptosis can be caused by a palsy of the oculomotor nerve, also known as the *third cranial nerve.* A palsy of this nerve usually causes at least some eye movement problems and may also cause the pupil to be enlarged. Another kind of nerve problem, *Horner's syndrome,* causes mild ptosis along with a slightly smaller pupil on the affected side. It can be caused by either serious or not-so-serious problems.

In older people, ptosis is often caused by a weakening of the *levator aponeurosis,* a tendonlike sheet that connects the levator muscle to the structures of the eyelid. An uncommon cause of ptosis is *myasthenia gravis,* a muscle disease that causes weakness and sometimes involves only the muscles around the eyes.

Timing of Surgery

In children, surgery must be performed early if the ptosis is severe enough to cover most of the pupil and thereby cause the vision in the eye to deteriorate, a condition called *amblyopia* (lazy eye). In moderate cases, the levator muscle can undergo a strengthening procedure called a *levator resection.* In more severe cases in which the levator muscle is hardly functioning, a sling procedure may need to be done. It often involves taking some fibrous tissue from the thigh (called *fascia lata*) and using it to suspend the upper eyelid from the muscle of the forehead.

In adults, surgery can be planned once the cause of the problem has been established. For example, if there is any suspicion that myasthenia gravis may be the cause, it

Careful measurements must be taken when surgery is contemplated.

must be ruled out by appropriate testing or by consulting with a neurologist. People with myasthenia gravis often find that their problem becomes worse when they are fatigued or toward the end of the day, although even ordinary age-related changes in the eyelid may sometimes be worse later in the day. A

Tensilon test can be performed, in which the drug Tensilon is injected into a vein. If the person has myasthenia gravis, the ptosis gets better right after the injection. Since the ptosis in myasthenia gravis responds to medical treatment of the disease, it is important to diagnose this problem before doing any surgery.

In the patient with ptosis, we measure not only the height of the *palpebral fissure* (the distance between the edge of the upper lid and the edge of the lower lid) but also the distance traveled by the edge of the upper lid as the person's gaze changes from looking down to looking up. This latter measurement determines how well the levator muscle is functioning and what type of surgery is appropriate. In some cases, when it appears that the ptosis may be affecting vision, we perform a visual field test to see how much of the upper field of vision is being blocked by the droopy eyelid.

For mild ptosis in an adult, the *Fasanella-Servat procedure* is a time-honored operation that produces very predictable results. It involves removing a few layers from the inside surface of the eyelid. One possible objection to this surgery is that the tissue removed includes some tiny tear glands from the inside of the upper lid, possibly predisposing people to a dry eye syndrome later in life.

A problem with aponeurosis of the levator muscle can be corrected with special techniques. One clue that there may be such a problem is that the horizontal crease in the upper eyelid becomes less prominent, moves higher on the lid, or disappears. The crease is the area where part of the aponeurosis normally attaches to the skin of the lid.

When older people develop ptosis because of a defect in the aponeurosis but still have a levator muscle that functions well, the defect in the aponeurosis can be repaired or the aponeurosis strengthened, often with good results. When the muscle is not functioning well, a resection of the levator muscle, a strengthening procedure, can be done. In the more severe cases, a sling procedure as described earlier can be performed. In all of these procedures, there is a certain amount of unpredictability. This means that the ptosis problem may sometimes be undercorrected or overcorrected, in which case additional surgery may be necessary. Too much correction, especially with a muscle that does not function well, may result in too much exposure of the eye and a drying out of the surface of the eye.

Cornea and Conjunctiva

Corneal Abrasions and Lacerations

A common eye injury involves the loss of some of the epithelium, the outermost layer of cells of the cornea. A scratch of this kind is called an *abrasion*. Abrasions can be caused by fingernails, the edge of a sheet of paper, rubbing the eye when a foreign body is in it, or simply anything that contacts the surface of the cornea. These injuries tend to be very painful. Common symptoms include sharp pain, light sensitivity, watering, feeling of something in the eye, or a "sticking" feeling in the eye. The blood vessels in the conjunctiva become engorged, resulting in a reddened appearance, and the upper eyelid may become somewhat droopy.

In the treatment of abrasions, considerations include relieving pain, promoting healing, and preventing infection. Fortunately, abrasions tend to heal quickly, more so in the young than in the elderly. The epithelial cells on the surface of the cornea surrounding the abrasion multiply rapidly and slide in to fill up the space where the abraded cells were lost.

Treating Abrasions

The traditional method of treating corneal abrasions involves keeping the eye patched shut until it is all healed. Generally, antibiotic ointment or drops are instilled in the eye before patching to reduce the risk of infection. That's because the epithelium, like the skin, is the main barrier against infection from bacteria. A dilating eyedrop is sometimes instilled to put the eye at rest and to relieve the spasm that occurs in the injured eye when light enters either eye. However, patching has several disadvantages. First, patching one eye results in a loss of depth perception, making it difficult to drive or engage in other functions. Second, the tightness of the patch can be uncomfortable. Finally, keeping the eye shut deprives it

It may often be better not to patch the eye shut.

of oxygen, which is necessary for healing. Special types of patches have been devised that allow the eye to remain slightly open or that exert less pressure on the eye, but these are harder to apply.

Recent studies have shown that patching may be of no benefit in many cases, at least with regard to smaller corneal abrasions. The eye can be left unpatched, and antibiotic ointment can be instilled several times a day. The ointment helps prevent infection and also keeps the surface of the eye moist, thereby promoting healing.

Although some ointment ingredients could possibly retard healing a bit, overall the eyes do well in this manner, and they certainly receive more oxygen than they do when they are patched. Nevertheless, in each case, the doctor must use judgment in deciding which technique will work best.

Although anesthetic eyedrops, which numb the surface of the eye, could eliminate the pain caused by a corneal abrasion, they should never be used to treat these. They are to be used only by the doctor to eliminate the severe light sensi-

You should never use anesthetic eyedrops in your eyes.

tivity that interferes with the eye examination. The numbing effect of these drops lasts only a very short time, and their continuing use has a toxic effect on the cornea that can result in a corneal ulcer, an eye-threatening condition.

Why Abrasions Recur

An occasional complication of a corneal abrasion is a *recurrent abrasion,* sometimes called a *recurrent erosion.* This occurs more often when a thin sharp object, such as a fingernail or a sheet of paper, abrades the eye. A person with a recurrent abrasion usually experiences sudden pain, watering, and light sensitivity on awakening from sleep. Apparently, the epithelial cells in the area where the abrasion occurred sometimes do not heal properly. During sleep, the eye may become slightly dry, and the epithelial cells of the cornea may stick to the closed eyelid. When the lid opens, off come the epithelial cells, and the result is another abrasion. These recurrent abrasions are treated the same way as the original abrasions were treated, but additional techniques must often be used to keep them from recurring. For

Recurrent abrasions often require special techniques.

example, lubricating eye ointment can be instilled in the eye at bedtime for a period of time. Sometimes a thin contact lens called a *bandage lens* is placed on the eye and left in place for at least several weeks. It keeps the inside of the eyelid from coming into contact with the cornea and may allow better healing to take place. Finally, more invasive methods, such as laser treatments or pricking the surface of the cornea in multiple places with a needle, may be necessary.

Treating Corneal Lacerations

When a cut on the cornea goes through the epithelium and into the thick middle layer, the stroma, we call it a *laceration*. Such a laceration may go only partway through the cornea or through the entire thickness of the cornea. The latter possibility is much more serious, because the fluid *(aqueous humor)* inside the eye can leak out, and bacteria can get into the eye, resulting in an infection that could cause loss of the eye. When a full-thickness laceration occurs, an X ray of the eye is taken to make sure that no foreign body got into the eye. A tetanus booster shot may be given. The laceration must then be repaired (with microscopic stitches) in the operating room with the patient under general anesthesia. Antibiotics are given to lower the risk of infection. Although such a laceration could result in loss of the eye, the results are often very good, especially if the laceration does not cross the center of the pupil. In contrast, a laceration that goes only partway through the stroma layer of the cornea may not need stitches at all if the laceration is not very deep.

Superficial Foreign Bodies

Although tiny foreign bodies can lodge themselves in either the cornea or the conjunctiva, we most often see them in the cornea. They may become embedded more easily in the cornea, and those in the conjunctiva may cause fewer symptoms. Undoubtedly, many foreign bodies become more deeply embedded as the result of eye rubbing after the foreign body contacts the surface of the eye. There is usually a feeling of something in the eye, although sometimes minutes or even hours may elapse before that feeling is present. Although the eye is very sensitive, it is poor at localizing symptoms. Therefore, the person with a foreign body in the cornea will often complain of feeling something under the upper eyelid, often in its outer portion. After a while, watering of the eye, redness, and light sensitivity may occur, and a sharp pain may be present as well.

By far the most common type of corneal foreign body is a tiny piece of steel. It can enter the eye while a person is welding or working under a car, or it may just blow into the eye. When it lodges in the cornea, it immediately starts to rust. Interestingly, even galvanized steel, which is not supposed to rust, generally rusts somewhat. As it rusts, the rust seeps into the cornea, deeper and deeper. When that occurs, removal of the metal alone leaves a so-called rust ring in the cornea. If the rust ring is not removed also, the cornea may not heal properly and may become increasingly inflamed. Therefore, early removal is helpful. Since other types of corneal foreign body do not rust, their removal is generally much easier.

Corneal foreign bodies are removed while we look at the eye through a slit lamp. After the eye is numbed with drops, the foreign body and associated rust can often be removed with the bevel or edge of a needle normally used for injections, such as those used for TB skin tests. Occasionally, a kind of motorized drill with a small burr may be used to remove as much of the rust as possible. Since the cornea numbs easily, the entire process is painless. At the completion of the procedure, antibiotic drops or ointment is instilled in the eye, and the eye may sometimes be patched. Follow-up examinations are usually necessary to make sure that the eye is healing properly and that no infection is setting in.

Although it can be uncomfortable to have a foreign body in the cornea, never use anesthetic (numbing) eyedrops to relieve the discomfort. These drops are toxic to the cornea and increase the risk of developing a corneal ulcer.

Sometimes a tiny foreign body will become embedded on the inside surface of the upper lid. The symptoms may be very similar to those caused by a corneal foreign body. When the ophthalmologist examines the cornea, multiple, fine vertical scratch marks are often seen on the upper cornea. The cornea is being lightly scratched every time the eye blinks. To locate the foreign body, we have to evert the upper lid (turn it over on itself so that the inner surface is visible). The foreign body is usually easy to see through the slit lamp and can be removed without difficulty.

Corneal Clouding

The cornea is a marvel of nature. When it is working properly, its crystal-clear structure allows it to be transparent. This transparency is maintained by the cornea's endothelial cells. These cells form a single layer that lines the inner surface of the cornea, facing the fluid inside the eye. Their function is to pump any water that gets into the cornea back into the interior of the eye. This is a never-ending job, because the fluid pressure inside the eye is always trying to force fluid into the cornea. As we get older, we very gradually lose these endothelial cells, which are not replaced. Fortunately, we are born with many more of these cells than we need. However, some people lose so many cells that fluid buildup, called edema, develops in the cornea. A waterlogged cornea becomes thickened and cloudy. Vision can become blurred, and lights appear as though they have halos around them. Edema of the cornea can also cause tiny blisters to form on the outside of the cornea, creating inflammation and discomfort.

Causes of Endothelial Cell Loss and Edema

In some people, the loss of these endothelial cells is a genetically transmitted disorder called *Fuchs's dystrophy*. Other problems can also accelerate the loss of endothelial cells. Eye injuries, both mechanical and chemical (acid and base); surgery (including cataract); inflammations and infections in the eye; and high intraocular pressures (see chapter 10) can also cause the endothelial cells to malfunction or die off. People who have Fuchs's dystrophy have a mild tendency toward higher eye pressures, and this can exacerbate their problem. The effects of eye surgery, especially cataract surgery, represent a large number of the cases of corneal edema that we see today.

Diagnosing Endothelial Cell Problems

The condition of the endothelial cells and the presence of corneal edema are determined during examination of the eye with the slit lamp, also known as the biomicroscope. Careful examination of the back surface of the cornea where the endothelium is located may reveal the presence of guttata, tiny dots, in that area. People with Fuchs's dystrophy have such dense guttata formations that the back surface of the cornea has a beaten metal appearance. Thin, vertical wrinkles may also be visible in the endothelial layer. By shining the light of the slit lamp in at the correct angle and by using high magnification, the ophthalmologist can actually see the endothelial layer directly. It looks something like the tile floor in an old bathroom. If many endothelial cells have been lost, the remaining cells become enlarged and sometimes irregular in shape as they fill in the remaining space. A special instrument can also be used to actually estimate the number of endothelial cells in a given area. An indirect measure of how well the endothelial cells are doing their job is to measure the thickness of the cornea. It becomes thickened even before any edema becomes obvious, and this means that the endothelial cell function is compromised. Edema itself may be very subtle or quite obvious to the doctor, depending on its severity.

Treating Corneal Edema

If the edema is very mild, its effect on vision may be minimal. Any blurring or halos around lights may be most noticeable soon after you awaken in the morning. This occurs because less oxygen gets to the eyes while they are closed during sleep. One treatment you can try is to hold a hair dryer at arm's length and direct air of moderate warmth toward the eyes. The heat causes a little of the water in the cornea to evaporate, thereby bringing about improvement in vision.

Another helpful technique is using over-the-counter eyedrops and ointment that contain hypertonic saline. Saline is nothing more than salt water that, in this case, comes in a 5 percent strength. Hypertonic saline may sting a little because of the high salt content, but it works by drawing water out of the cornea. The ointment, which can blur vision, is generally used only at bedtime. The drops can be instilled every few hours. Very frequent use, say, more often than every two hours, should be avoided because the chemical preservatives in the drops can be mildly toxic to the cornea. If the drops sting too much, a 2 percent strength is also available.

If the surface of the cornea has developed tiny blisters from the edema and is painful, a special soft contact lens called a bandage lens can be placed on the eye, where it remains continuously. Sometimes such a lens can even draw a little fluid out of the cornea. Unfortunately, in some cases it can make the edema worse, and there is always the risk of developing an infection in the cornea with such a lens in place.

Ultimately, if the blurring from the corneal edema is becoming disabling, a corneal transplant, a major operation, can be performed. The central part of the cornea, measuring less than a third of an inch across, is taken from the eye of someone who has donated his corneas and is sewn in place after the central cornea from the person receiving the transplant is removed. The operation has a high success rate, on the order of 90 percent, but rejection or edema of the transplanted cornea, infections, and other complications can occur. A cataract operation with lens implant can be performed at the same time in someone who also needs cataract surgery. For people who have previously had cataract surgery, the lens implant can remain in place, or it can be replaced with a different lens implant if the physician feels that the original implant was contributing to the decompensation (clouding) of the cornea. After a corneal transplant, the stitches must be left in for a long time, a year or even more. It usually takes at least a year for the eye to heal and for the vision to stabilize with this type of surgery. Sometimes, mild distortion of the cornea, depending on how it heals, may affect the final vision by causing astigmatism, but the blur caused by astigmatism can often be corrected by eyeglasses.

If the blurring becomes disabling, a corneal transplant can be performed.

Other Corneal Problems That Cause Clouding

Many inherited conditions called *dystrophies* can affect the cornea. Fortunately, most of these are quite rare. A common but usually very mild condition is called *map-dot-fingerprint dystrophy*. It usually occurs in people of northern European descent. Its name is derived from its appearance when the cornea is examined through the slit lamp. Near the center of the cornea, just deep to the surface layer of cells, one may see several fine, wavy lines reminiscent of a fingerprint. In other people, there may be an irregular area that looks like the outline of a country on a map. Sometimes, tiny, whitish dots may be seen as well. Map-dot-fingerprint dystrophy may affect vision in the most severe cases, but for most people, it is just a comfort problem. The irregularity

One common condition occurs in people of northern European descent.

near the surface of the cornea sometimes causes a slight breakdown in the cornea's epithelium, and this may feel like a small scratch on the eye.

Other irritative eye problems, such as blepharitis and dry eye syndrome, may, if present, be contributing to the surface irregularity. Treating these other conditions may take care of the symptoms. A mild hypertonic saline eyedrop, as described earlier, may also help flare-ups to resolve more quickly. If you are told you have this type of dystrophy, it should not be a major cause for concern. Most people who have it are not even aware of it, and it is simply brought to their attention by a conscientious ophthalmologist who has taken the time to do a very careful examination.

Several dystrophies that affect the thick, middle layer of the cornea, the stroma, include *granular, lattice,* and *macular dystrophies.* These produce cloudy patches in the cornea that can affect vision. The macular form is the most severe of these, followed by lattice. In people in whom vision is severely affected, a corneal transplant operation may be necessary.

Keratoconus is a bulging, stretching, and thinning of the cornea. It occurs in teenagers and young adults and has a genetic basis. Affected individuals may have a history of seasonal allergies or may have close relatives with such a history.

The irregularity in the cornea produced by keratoconus causes a focusing error called *irregular astigmatism.* Irregular astigmatism, unlike regular astigmatism, cannot be fully corrected by eyeglasses. Therefore, people with keratoconus need to be fitted with rigid contact lenses if they desire to see more clearly. The fitting process can be difficult in more advanced cases, and special types of contact lenses are sometimes required. When contact lenses are no longer effective, corneal transplantation, with a success rate of well over 90 percent, can be done.

Keratoconus occurs in the young, often those with a history of allergy.

Corneal Infections and Ulcers

Infections of the cornea are quite serious because they threaten the entire eye. They may be caused by bacteria, viruses, fungi, and other organisms. The herpes viruses usually produce superficial infections, although they can still cause scarring and loss of vision. (See chapter 13.) Fungus infections are among the most dreaded but fortunately are fairly rare. Infections caused by bacteria have become more common in the past thirty years because of contact lens wear.

The cornea's epithelium is the first barrier against infection, just like the skin. Usually a break must occur in this layer for infection to occur. Another defense against eye infection is the antibodies in the tears. That's why people who have dry eye syndrome are at higher risk for infection.

A corneal abrasion can allow bacteria to enter and begin multiplying. A foreign body that lodges in the cornea also breaks the surface and can allow bacteria to enter.

People who wear contact lenses often suffer tiny abrasions that they may not even notice. The abrasions occur as the lenses are being inserted and removed. Soft contact lenses, which contain water, may be contaminated by bacteria. Their use entails a higher risk of infection than does rigid contact lens wear. That is why proper disinfection techniques and handling of contact lens solutions are so important. Wearing soft contact lenses on an extended wear basis, that is, not removing them at night, increases the risk. Being a smoker also increases the risk—possibly related to tars on the fingers (or on the lenses themselves) that encourage bacteria to stick to them.

Extended wear contacts increase the risk of infection.

How Ulcers Form

Once the bacteria start to grow in the cornea, a small, superficial cloudy spot called an *infiltrate* appears at the site of entry. This spot is caused by edema and the migration of white blood cells, part of the immune system, into the area. Soon the surface layer of cells sloughs off in the area over the infiltrate.

The infection then continues to eat away at the cornea, causing an ulcer. Corneal ulcers can become quite deep and, if left untreated, cause a perforation of the cornea.

Prompt diagnosis and treatment are essential.

If this happens, fluid from inside the eye leaks out, the bacteria gain entrance to the interior of the eye, and the eye may be lost. Thus, prompt recognition of the infection, identification of the cause of the infection, and treatment are essential.

Determining the Cause of Infection

If an ulcer is already present, it must be cultured. An anesthetic eyedrop is instilled in the eye to numb it, and a thin platinum spatula that has been sterilized with a flame is used to scrape the surface of the ulcer. The scrapings are then smeared directly onto culture plates if available and sent to the laboratory. Otherwise, the scrapings can be sent to the laboratory in a special tube and then smeared onto the culture plates. The laboratory incubates the plates, storing them at a set temperature and watching closely for the growth of bacterial colonies. If any appear, the type of bacterium (or fungus) is identified, and special tests are performed to determine the antibiotics to which it is most sensitive. However, it can take twenty-four to forty-eight hours or more to obtain culture results, and we don't want to wait that long to begin antibiotic treatment. Therefore, a little of the scrapings is smeared directly on a glass slide, treated with special stains, and viewed right away under the microscope. This can often give a clue as to which bacterium is causing the infection, and an appropriate antibiotic can then be selected.

Treating Corneal Ulcers

Systemic antibiotics—those taken by mouth or injected—are generally not helpful in treating corneal ulcers. Treatment consists of very frequent instillation of antibiotic eyedrops. In some cases, we may fortify standard eyedrops by adding very concentrated solutions of the antibiotic to them. This extra strength is sometimes needed to combat the infection. In addition, antibiotic solutions are sometimes given by injection, once or twice a day, under the conjunctiva, the clear membrane over the white of the eye. This sounds painful, and sometimes it can be. But these shots are only given until it is clear that the infection is being brought under control. The eye is examined once or twice a day, and if it appears that the ulcer crater is healing in, then we know that things are moving in the right direction and that the choice of antibiotic was correct. If things are not going well, then another antibiotic can be tried. The choice of antibiotic is then guided by the results of the culture.

Preventing Corneal Ulcers

The best approach to the problem of corneal ulcers is prevention. If you feel that you've scratched your eye, have it checked right away so that prophylactic sulfa or antibiotic treatment can be given. If you see a white spot on your cornea, have it checked out right away. If you wear contact lenses, disinfect them exactly as you are supposed to. Keep the case clean. Discard old or possibly contaminated solutions. Wash your hands thoroughly before inserting or removing the contacts. Enjoy your contacts, but remember that there is a risk to using them.

Conjunctivitis

Conjunctivitis is an inflammation of the conjunctiva, the nearly clear membrane that covers the white of the eye as well as the inside surface of the eyelids. The inflammation causes the blood vessels in the conjunctiva to dilate, giving the familiar appearance of bloodshot eyes.

Causes of Conjunctivitis

When we think of conjunctivitis, we usually think of infection, but allergies (see "Allergies and the Eye," page 98) and various irritants can also cause inflammation. For example, injuries, foreign bodies, chemicals such as acids, and contact lens problems are other possible causes. But if your eyes become red and irritated and there's no obvious reason, it's a good bet that you've contracted an infection.

If we feel that an infection is present, we must first determine the type of infection. The term *pinkeye* that you may sometimes hear does not have a precise meaning, because any infection will cause a pink eye. Viruses, bacteria, and fungi can all infect the eye. The treatment depends on the type of infection, so we must first look for the clues that point us in the right direction.

Determining Whether an Infection Is Viral or Bacterial

Viral infections *(viral conjunctivitis)* are by far the most common type. They are often caused by the viruses that cause colds. The cold symptoms may occur before, during, or after the eye infection. Therefore, if someone with infected eyes has a sore throat or has had a sore throat in the preceding week or so, it's likely that viral conjunctivitis is present. It's also common to hear that one or more people in the person's family or other immediate environment has had conjunctivitis or a cold recently.

Viral conjunctivitis usually involves both eyes, but it may take several days before the second eye is involved. The second eye usually has milder symptoms than the first. The most common symptoms are burning, irritation, scratchiness, tearing, mild itching, light sensitivity, and a feeling of something in the eye. The eyelids may be crusted somewhat or even stuck shut when you awake in the morning, but the discharge during the day is watery, not puslike. With bacterial infections, in contrast, we often see a thick discharge during the day, although in some cases the discharge may be scanty.

When we examine the eyes, we look for a number of features that are characteristic of viral conjunctivitis. The eyes tend to have a glassy look because of the excess of tears. We feel for a little knot of tissue called a lymph node (gland) just in front of the ear and below the arch of the upper jawbone. These lymph nodes, which *An eye with a viral infection often has a glassy look.* are part of the immune system and help fight infection, usually enlarge with viral infections but not with bacterial infections.

Sometimes we can actually feel the enlarged node; other times we may not actually feel it but may find that the area where the node should be is somewhat tender when we press on it. Next, we pull down the lower eyelid (something you can do also) and compare the degree of redness of the conjunctiva on the inside surface of the lid with that on the white of the eye. In viral conjunctivitis, the conjunctiva on the inside of the lid is often much redder. Not only that, but the conjunctiva lining the inside of the lid will have a granular appearance, as compared with the smooth, glassy appearance it normally has. When we examine it through the slit lamp, which magnifies its appearance, we see that the granular appearance is caused by the cropping up of numerous tiny, translucent bumps called *follicles*. These follicles contain lymphoid tissue, just as the lymph nodes do. Bacterial conjunctivitis usually does not cause significant lymph node enlargement or formation of follicles.

We also use the slit lamp to look more closely at the conjunctiva over the white of the eye. With some forms of viral conjunctivitis, we may see not only the dilated blood vessels but also small hemorrhages where a little blood has actually leaked out. Examination of the cornea of the eye is also important. Usually, no abnormalities are seen until we instill a little dye called *fluorescein* in the eye. It's called fluorescein because it fluoresces and shows up as a bright green when a special blue light is shone on the eye. This dye is taken up by the cornea wherever the surface cells of the cornea have sloughed off. With viral infections, we sometimes see numerous pinpoint dots of fluorescein all across the cornea.

By combining the history (symptoms related by the patient) with what we find when we examine the eye, we can usually tell that a viral infection, as opposed to a bacterial infection, is present. That's important, because the treatment for the two types of infection is different. Of course, there will always be some infections that appear to be in a gray area and for which the cause is not obvious.

> *We can usually tell whether it is a viral or a bacterial infection.*

Treating Viral Conjunctivitis

For most viral infections, there is no specific treatment to eradicate the virus. The infection just has to run its course, and that is generally anywhere from four days to two weeks. Viral infections are usually highly contagious. They are generally spread by hand-to-hand contact. People with the infection rub their eye (or nose or mouth) and either touch someone else or touch something that someone else touches. So when we examine someone with such an infection, we make sure to clean off everything that person has touched, including the doorknob on the way in! We also advise the patient not to touch anyone else and not to share the same washcloth with anyone else. Treatment is symptomatic: Over-the-counter eyedrops such as artificial tear drops or decongestant eyedrops (the ones that reduce the redness) can be helpful. Holding a cool, moist washcloth over the closed eyelids can also be helpful.

The eyelids and eyelashes should also be kept as clean as possible. Antibiotics are ineffective against viral infections

Why not treat with antibiotic or sulfa eyedrops? Very simple—these drops only fight off infections caused by bacteria, not those caused by viruses. Using such drops when they are not needed is not only a waste of time and money but can also be harmful in a number of ways. First, people can develop allergies to antibiotics when they use them in their eyes. That prevents them from being able to use the same antibiotic in the future. There may also be toxic reactions to some antibiotics. Second, if an infected eye stays red, it may be hard to determine whether it is still red because the infection is not going away or because an allergic reaction to the drops is occurring. Third, we should remember that just as we don't like to use antibiotics by mouth unnecessarily for fear of destroying the "good" bacteria that live in our intestines, we also don't want to get rid of the "good" bacteria that live in the conjunctiva of our eyes. Getting rid of such good bacteria can allow bad bacteria to multiply, and we may then have a much more serious infection to deal with. Fourth, use of antibiotics when they are not needed helps bacteria develop resistance to antibiotics, which then become useless when we really need them. That's why you should never ask your doctor to prescribe an antibiotic for you if you don't really need it. Finally, use of antibiotic drops can lead to a false sense of security that the infection is being treated. The infected person may then touch other people and continue to spread the infection.

A common dilemma occurs when children in school who develop viral conjunctivitis are sent home and told they can only return once they have begun treatment with antibiotic eyedrops. Unfortunately, such drops usually end up being prescribed. This should not be done for all of the reasons just mentioned. Teachers, school nurses, and others (including some doctors) need to be educated about the appropriate treatment of viral infections.

Steroid (cortisone) medication should not be used.

Eyedrops that contain corticosteroids (cortisone) should not be used to treat viral conjunctivitis. They impair the immune system and allow the virus to remain alive and active for a longer period of time.

Furthermore, a herpes simplex type of viral conjunctivitis may be indistinguishable from the usual types of viral infections, and using a corticosteroid-containing eyedrop in the presence of herpes simplex definitely worsens the prognosis. In the specific situations in which corticosteroid eyedrops are indicated, they should be prescribed only by an ophthalmologist, although they are abused by many ophthalmologists as well.

What If the Conjunctivitis Does Not Get Better?

If the conjunctivitis does not get better in the expected two weeks, we may suspect another type of infection. For example, there are eye infections caused by a primitive type of bacterium called *chlamydia*. It may look very similar to a viral conjunctivitis, but rather than resolve on its own, it continues on as a chronic infection. The conjunctiva lining the inside of the eyelid can be swabbed and a special test performed to confirm the diagnosis. Chlamydia is usually transmitted as a venereal disease, and it may also be seen in newborns to whom it is transmitted as they pass through the birth canal. Chlamydial infection is usually treated with antibiotics by mouth. This clears up not only the eye infection but also any chlamydial infections elsewhere in the body.

If someone with conjunctivitis has been using an eyedrop for symptomatic relief, it is also possible that an allergy to some component of the drop has developed. If we suspect that this is occurring, we discontinue use of the eyedrop and see whether the eye then improves.

Treating Bacterial Conjunctivitis

Many cases of bacterial conjunctivitis resolve on their own without treatment. The body's immune system takes over and eradicates the infection. Nevertheless, we usually treat these infections to make them go away more quickly. However, infections caused by the staphylococcus (or staph) bacterium may not resolve on their own. This type of infection is often associated with chronic blepharitis, a low-grade chronic inflammation of the oil glands in the eyelids.

The oil glands tend to harbor the staph bacteria. If a staph infection of the eye is not treated, it may become chronic, and then it is much more difficult to eradicate in the future. Another exception would be certain very virulent bacteria, such as the one that causes gonorrhea. Bacterial infections such as these require intensive treatment.

Antibiotics help clear the infection more quickly.

If the bacterial conjunctivitis is related to chronic blepharitis, we often see very little discharge. Treatment of the underlying blepharitis is the key here. (See "Blepharitis," page 59, in chapter 6.) The conjunctivitis component is generally treated as well with either sulfa or antibiotic eyedrops.

Sulfa eyedrops are often effective because they are available in high strengths for use in the eyes. However, they have some disadvantages. First, sulfa drugs are inactivated by a chemical (para-aminobenzoic acid) found in puslike discharge, so they may not be a good choice if much discharge is present. Second, some people are allergic to sulfa drugs. Finally, these drops tend to sting a bit.

Many antibiotic eyedrops are available, and they are all fairly effective. Cost factors as well as the chance of toxic or allergic side effects help dictate the choice. If the discharge is smeared on a glass slide for analysis under the microscope and is also sent for culture, we can determine which bacterium is causing the infection. That may help guide our choice of antibiotic. Many ophthalmologists do not routinely perform such a culture before beginning treatment, but I think it is a good idea, at least in those cases in which there is a great deal of discharge. Performing a culture later on, after antibiotic treatment has been begun, is less likely to allow identification of the infecting bacterium.

Getting Eyedrops into a Child's Eyes

For many children, it may not be difficult. Calm reassurance may be all that is necessary. I usually explain that we're going to put a little, cold drop of water in the eye. Drops do feel a little cold, and cold has a numbing connotation. When you are expecting a cool or cold sensation, you anticipate it and are less likely to mind any stinging that may accompany it.

But if you can't gently pry the child's eyelids open, it's best to avoid a fight, which will only make it worse the next time around. Instead, try the following technique. Have the child lie down on his or her back and with eyes closed. Place two or three eyedrops in the little well between the inner corner of the eyelids and the bridge of the nose. Sooner or later, the child's eye will have to open. When that happens, at least some of the drops will go in the eye! You may lose a little of the medication, but better than not getting it in at all.

Allergies and the Eye

The hallmark of eye allergy is itching. Itching may be one of the symptoms of other problems, such as blepharitis and dry eye syndrome, but with allergies it is by far the most prominent. Allergies occur in response to *antigens*—substances that cause the immune system to react. The cells of the immune system release substances that cause itching, dilation of blood vessels, swelling, hives, and other effects, such as wheezing. The antigens may come from the air or be introduced into the eye by the fingers or instillation of eye medications.

Hay Fever

Hay fever is one of the most common eye allergies. It is seasonal, occurring only when pollen or other offending substances, such as molds, are present in the air. Dust, animal dander, and chemicals may also be problematic. Itching and scanty mucous discharge are common. The conjunctiva may swell, as may the eyelids. The eye may or may not become red. Sneezing and itching of the throat are often present as well.

Treatment is aimed at reducing or preventing the symptoms in the safest way. Obviously, avoidance of the source of allergy, if possible, is the ideal approach. Air filters and avoidance of cigarette smoke can also be helpful. Rubbing the eyes should be avoided, as this can increase the itching, swelling, and redness. Simply splashing a little cool water in the eye from time to time washes out some of the antigen adhering to the tissues of the eye and soothes the eye as well.

Artificial tear drops, preferably preserva-tive free, sold over the counter as a lubricant for the eye, can accomplish the same thing. As the next step, over-the-counter drops contain-

Over-the-counter drops may be all that is necessary to relieve symptoms.

ing both an antihistamine (pheniramine or antazoline) and a decongestant drug can be used. The antihistamine counters the effects of *histamine,* one of the chemicals released from the cells. The decongestant constricts the blood vessels in the eye, which can also help control symptoms. Decongestant-containing eyedrops should not be used on a long-term basis, however. The eyes become "hooked" on them, and rebound redness occurs when their blood vessel–constricting effects begin to wear off.

Various prescription remedies are also available. Levocarbastine (Livostin) and emedastine (Emadine) are antihistamines that are used alone without a decon-gestant. Some drugs of the nonsteroidal anti-inflammatory class, such as ketorolac (Acular), are available as eyedrops and can effectively combat the symptoms as well. This class of drug was originally used for the treatment of arthritis.

The antihistamine drugs mentioned before work by blocking the action of histamine after it has already been released by the cells. Other drugs work by preventing the release of histamine and other substances from the cells involved in allergic reactions. These preventive drugs include cromolyn sodium (Opticrom and Crolom), lodoxamide (Alomide), nedocromil (Alocril), and permirolast (Alamast). For optimal effectiveness, they are gen-erally used continuously during the allergy season, as they do not affect the symptoms caused by histamine once the histamine has been released. A recent study showed that lodoxamide was superior to cromolyn sodium in the treat-ment of vernal conjunctivitis (described on page 101). Olopatadine (Patanol) and ketotifen (Zaditor) have a dual effect: They not only prevent the release of histamine; they also block its action.

Corticosteroid (cortisone) medication is well known for its anti-inflammatory and antiallergic properties. It is also well known for its many side effects. Corticosteroid eyedrops are very effective at relieving allergic symptoms, but with long-term use they can cause cataracts of the posterior subcapsular type, and they can raise the pressure in the eye, causing a transient secondary glaucoma. They can also reduce the resistance of the eye to infection and can allow the growth of bacteria and fungi that are dangerous to the eye. Thus, these drops are used only when necessary and then only on a short-term basis.

When allergy or any other source of irritation affects the eyes, congestion and overactivity of the tiny oil glands in the eyelids may occur. This produces an inflammation of these oil glands. Some people are predisposed to this type of problem because of the way their oil glands operate. This oil gland inflammation, or blepharitis, can produce symptoms of its own, exacerbating the allergic problem. These symptoms include burning, feeling of some-

The oil glands may remain inflamed even after the allergy is gone.

thing in the eye, tearing, crusting on the eyelid margins, and eyelashes stuck shut on awakening in the morning. Even worse, the blepharitis may become self-perpetuating and persist even after the allergy has resolved. Treatment of blepharitis entails carefully cleaning the eyelashes and margins of the eyelids with water and diluted baby shampoo anywhere from one to four times a day. (See "Blepharitis," page 59, in chapter 6.)

Acute Allergic Reactions

Whereas hay fever normally begins almost imperceptibly, we occasionally see someone who suddenly develops extreme itching and swelling in one eye. The swelling may be so severe that the conjunctiva balloon outward and almost hang over the edge of the lid. This kind of reaction may occur after you touch a plant or blossom and then later rub your eye. The appearance of the eye when this happens can be frightening. If this happens to you, try to rinse the eye out with cool water right away. If you have any antihistamine pills for allergy or antihistamine/decongestant eyedrops, use them. Hold a cool, moist washcloth over the closed eye. In some cases, we may instill a corticosteroid drop as well. The good news is that this condition resolves very quickly because the foreign substance (antigen) that got in the eye gets washed out and there is no continuing exposure to the antigen. Generally, the eye looks much better in twenty-four hours and is almost back to normal in forty-eight hours.

A different kind of reaction can sometimes occur when people are outside, perhaps in their yard, and a tiny bit of organic matter, dirt or plant, gets in an eye. Rather than itching or swelling, one sector of the white of the eye becomes red, and there may or may not be any other symptoms. This redness may persist for days or weeks but usually goes away on its own. (See "Episcleritis," below.)

Vernal

Vernal keratoconjunctivitis, as it's officially known, is a type of allergic problem that occurs in children, especially boys, and may persist into adulthood but often improves with time. It produces a great deal of itching, mucous discharge, and tearing, and it is most prevalent when the temperatures are warm. It may affect the inside lining of the eyelids or the conjunctiva right at the edge of the cornea. The disease causes the formation of small, blood vessel–containing bumps in these areas that can easily be seen on examination. A form of scarring may occur on the upper part of the cornea, and, in the most severe cases, an ulcer may even form in this area.

Filtering the air or moving to a different environment can help.

Treatment of vernal is similar to hay fever treatment. Avoiding exposure to the pollen or dust by filtering the air or moving away from a hot, dry climate can help. Preventing the release of histamine is the goal of medical treatment, and this involves the continuing use of drops like cromolyn sodium and lodoxamide, as described earlier. As a last resort, corticosteroid drops can be used on a short-term basis to get the disease back under control.

Episcleritis

Episcleritis is an inflammation on the surface of the eye that, like conjunctivitis, causes the blood vessels to be dilated, thereby giving the appearance of redness. But the appearance differs from conjunctivitis in two important ways.

First, usually only one portion of the eye is involved, for example, the side toward the nose or the side toward the temple, whereas in conjunctivitis, the white of the eye becomes red all over. Second, episcleritis involves primarily the deeper blood vessels, those next to the sclera, the white coat of the eye. Conjunctivitis, in contrast, involves mainly the more superficial vessels. Episcleritis may cause discomfort or a feeling of irritation, or there may be no symptoms at all. It generally occurs in young adults, and either one or both eyes may be involved.

Two types of episcleritis exist: simple and nodular. *Simple episcleritis,* the more common form, presents pretty much as just described. *Nodular episcleritis* looks similar, but on close inspection, one can see one or more small bumps (nodules) that have formed in the conjunctiva in the area of redness.

In some cases, it may not be obvious on first examination whether one is dealing with episcleritis or conjunctivitis. Two techniques can help differentiate between the two. First, the doctor can numb the eye with an anesthetic eyedrop and then lightly manipulate the conjunctiva with a cotton-tipped applicator. In episcleritis, the dilated blood vessels, which are deep down and attached to the sclera, do not move as the conjunctiva moves over them. In conjunctivitis, the blood vessels move. A second technique is to instill a vasoconstrictor (decongestant) eyedrop in the eye. These are the familiar over-the-counter eyedrops for "getting the redness out." Some of the redness may go away with conjunctivitis, but there will be no change with episcleritis.

Causes of Episcleritis

The cause of episcleritis is often obscure, but it represents a derangement of the immune system. You might think of it as a strange kind of allergic reaction. Some people with episcleritis have an underlying medical problem, such as rheumatoid arthritis or lupus. But most people with episcleritis have no such problems. Occasionally, a small piece of dirt or decaying material from the backyard may get in someone's eye and trigger the reaction. Other people may have an underlying chronic blepharitis. (See "Blepharitis," page 59, in chapter 6.) Substances produced by the bacteria that become overgrown in this condition can cause a number of allergic types of reaction in the eye, one of which is episcleritis. Wearing contact lenses seems to increase the risk of episcleritis as well.

Treating Episcleritis

Treatment depends on the form of episcleritis and whether symptoms are present. Simple episcleritis often goes away on its own after a few weeks. Therefore, if there are no symptoms, no treatment is needed. Episcleritis rarely causes any damage of a permanent nature to the eye, so such a "hands off" approach is often best. However, if it fails to improve on its own or if significant symptoms are present, then treatment with mild anti-inflammatory drops such as prednisolone (a cortisone medication) usually does the trick. The drops must be tapered gradually; stopping them suddenly may cause a rebound in the inflammation. Nodular episcleritis responds to this treatment as well. Unfortunately, episcleritis has a tendency to recur, especially if an underlying eye or general medical problem is present.

Episcleritis often goes away without treatment.

Pterygium

A *pterygium* is similar in appearance to a pinguecula (see "Pinguecula," page 105), but instead of remaining in the conjunctiva, it begins to grow over the cornea. As with pingueculae, they are generally seen on the side toward the nose. The most aggressive, rapidly growing ones contain many blood vessels. Older, more slowly growing pterygia may be lacking in blood vessels and often reach a point where they are no longer growing. Extensive exposure to the ultraviolet radiation from the sun as well as the irritative and drying effects of wind and dust are probably the causes. Pterygia are much more common in sunny and tropical areas than they are in places where the sun exposure is less.

Ophthalmologists who practice in the midwestern and northeastern portions of the United States generally regard pterygia as harmless growths that rarely require surgical removal. People in the Sun Belt areas, in contrast, sometimes see aggressively growing pterygia that may distort the curvature of the cornea or even grow over the pupil of the eye, obstructing vision. Clearly, active pterygia such as these should be removed.

When to Remove Pterygia

In general, if a pterygium is not growing rapidly or causing any problems, it is best to leave it alone. Up to 40 percent of pterygia grow back after being removed, and these recurrent pterygia sometimes grow more rapidly than they did before removal.

Newer surgical techniques are improving the results and lowering the recurrence rate, but a conservative philosophy about removing these growths is best. In general, a pterygium that has grown a distance of less than 1 millimeter onto the surface of the cornea should simply be observed. If it is 1 millimeter or more onto the cornea and is showing signs of active growth, with a "juicy," blood vessel–rich appearance, it should be removed. Waiting longer only results in a still more aggressive pterygium that is all the more likely to grow back.

Small pterygia that are not growing rapidly do not require surgery.

Removing Pterygia

A pterygium can be surgically removed in a variety of ways. One of the more promising approaches involves transplanting a piece of conjunctiva into the area where the pterygium is removed. This piece of conjunctiva comes from elsewhere on the eye where it is not needed. In addition to surgery, other treatments are sometimes performed to reduce the chance of a recurrence. For example, chemicals like thiotepa or mitomycin C, which interfere with rapidly growing cells, can be applied to the eye. Alternatively, a type of radiation called *beta radiation* can be applied to the eye immediately after the surgery. The problem is that all of these approaches can have side effects. For example, severe thinning of the sclera, the white coat of the eye, may occur many years after beta radiation, at least according to some studies.

Preventing Pterygia

As with everything in medicine, the best approach to pterygia is prevention. People who spend a great deal of time in the sun should wear glasses that absorb the ultraviolet rays of sunlight. Many of the better sunglasses have this type of protection, and regular prescription glasses can be made to block out the ultraviolet as well. Glasses or goggles to protect the eyes from the drying effect of wind and the irritating effect of dust can also be helpful to people who work or play in windy environments.

Pinguecula

A *pinguecula* is a white or yellowish irregular bump that appears over the white of the eye on either side of the cornea, although most commonly on the side toward the nose. It actually forms in the conjunctiva. The conjunctiva in these areas undergoes a kind of degeneration after years of exposure to sunlight and to wind. Thus, pingueculae frequently occur in people who work outdoors, especially in hot, sunny climates. As opposed to a pterygium (see "Pterygium," page 103), a pinguecula does not grow onto the surface of the cornea.

A pinguecula may go unnoticed for a very long time. Sometimes people with a slightly reddened, irritated eye notice a whitish bump, which prompts them to see their doctor right away. They complain that a growth has suddenly appeared on their eye. Of course, the pinguecula didn't suddenly appear. It was there all along but couldn't be seen because its color was similar to the color of the white of the eye. When the eye became reddened, however, the pinguecula stood right out because the thickened, opaque tissue did not become red as the rest of the eye did! A little reassurance is all that is needed in this situation.

Pingueculae may grow very slowly over the years. They occasionally become irritated, and over-the-counter artificial tear drops or decongestant drops can be used, although sometimes a very weak steroid (cortisonelike) eyedrop is prescribed. Surgical removal is rarely needed, but if they become so large that they interfere with contact lens wear or if their cosmetic appearance becomes unacceptable, they can be easily removed as an office procedure.

Subconjunctival Hemorrhage

A *subconjunctival hemorrhage* is simply a small spot of blood that collects between the conjunctiva and the sclera. It may cover only a small area or the entire white of the eye. Typically, people don't even know it's there until they look in the mirror and get the shock of their lives! These hemorrhages don't cause pain, but sometimes people begin to imagine a pain or ache after seeing what the eye looks like. The only real feeling that may be present is an occasional feeling of something in the eye.

Most of the time there is no obvious cause for a subconjunctival hemorrhage. Sometimes a hard sneeze or a bout of coughing causes a tiny blood vessel to break. Any trauma to the eye, including small foreign bodies, can cause the bleeding. Less commonly, an underlying eye problem is present. Some severe forms of viral conjunctivitis (viral infection of the eye) can cause hemorrhages. In this situation, the ophthalmologist can see dilated blood vessels on the eye, as in any case of conjunctivitis. However, conjunctivitis generally causes pain, watering, and occasional light sensitivity, so it is usually obvious that an infection is present. Sometimes we can see dilated, deep blood vessels in only one segment of the eye. This is called episcleritis (see "Episcleritis," page 101), a kind of allergic reaction on the eye. Episcleritis may cause no symptoms at all, but usually a person with the condition sees the localized dilated blood vessels on the eye before the hemorrhage occurs.

A subconjunctival hemorrhage is one of those things that look much worse than they are. No harm comes to the eye from it. The treatment is simple reassurance. It takes up to three weeks for the red spot to go away. Some people make up a good story about someone hitting them in the eye. But if it becomes too much of a "conversation piece," you may require sunglasses to get you through the three weeks!

CHAPTER EIGHT

Eye Muscles

THE ADVANTAGE OF HAVING TWO EYES THAT WORK TOGETHER is something that most of us don't normally think about—until one eye is patched shut after an injury. Have you ever tried to drive a car with just one eye open? It's not easy, unless you're used to it. Having two eyes that work together allows a kind of depth perception that most of us have learned to rely on. Without it, we have great difficulty judging distances. Even if our eyes do work together most of the time, we may experience headache and other symptoms if we have weak eye muscles that become strained as we try to keep our eyes straight and aligned with each other. If, as adults, one of our eyes suddenly turns in or out, we have double vision, which makes it impossible to function until one of the eyes is covered. Since eye straightness problems are more common in children than adults, we will begin by focusing on the common pediatric eye muscle problems. In most cases, these are problems that are recognized right after birth or in early childhood. It should be emphasized that in any person, child or adult, in whom an eye suddenly deviates and stays that way, immediate medical attention is imperative. The problem could be the result of a nerve palsy and reflect a serious problem in or around the brain.

Esotropia

Esotropia, or crossed eyes, may appear any time from soon after birth to when a child is several years old. *Infantile esotropia* (or *congenital esotropia*), which is noticed right after birth, is caused by a developmental problem in the brain, which in some cases may be inherited. It is normal for the eyes to wander a bit in a new-born infant, but persistent turning in of an eye is not normal. Children do not outgrow it. An eye examination to determine the cause is essential. In some cases, the problem may be not with the brain but rather in the eye itself. If an infant's eye sees poorly for any reason at all, it usually turns in, because this is the position of "rest" for an infant's eyes. Normally, the eye muscles have to work somewhat to keep the eyes straight, because if both eyes see well but one turns in or out, double vision occurs. If one eye sees poorly, however, double vision is not recognized, so there is no stimulus for keeping the eyes straight. Poor vision in an eye can have many causes. It may even be due to a malignant tumor in the eye, which is, fortunately, a rare occurrence. An early eye examination will rule out such problems or diagnose them while they are easier to treat.

> *Children do not outgrow persistent crossing of an eye.*

How do you know whether your child's eyes are straight? Some infants have what we call *pseudoesotropia.* The wide bridge of their nose and the folds of baby eyelid skin that cover the white of the inner part of their eyes make it look as though they have esotropia. It may be obvious that true esotropia is present if the degree of crossing is large, but it may be difficult for the layperson to tell in other cases.

> *The* Hirschberg test *is an easy way to test for straightness of a child's eyes.*

Here is the way ophthalmologists determine whether both eyes are seeing well and are straight. Hold your hand in front of one of the child's eyes while holding something the child wants to look at with the other hand. If one eye has poor vision, the child will object when the good eye is covered. Obviously, in older children, vision tests can be performed. To test for straightness, do the *Hirschberg test.* Shine a penlight or very small flashlight at the child's eyes in a dimly lit room so that the child looks at the light. The light causes a small light reflex to appear in each of the dark pupils. Normally, that light reflex should appear just a little off center in the pupil—displaced slightly inward toward the nose. In any case, it should appear in the same position in the two eyes. If the light reflex appears in the outer part of the pupil of one eye while the child is looking at the light, then that eye is probably crossed.

The examination for infantile esotropia includes an assessment of the health of each eye to rule out any structural problems or tumors. Dilating drops are instilled in the eyes so that the doctor can better examine the retina and optic nerve and estimate the refractive error. Most infants are mildly hyperopic (farsighted). We also determine whether the same eye is crossed all the time or whether the eyes alternate in that respect. If only one eye crosses, then that eye will develop *amblyopia,* commonly termed *lazy eye.*

Treating Infantile Esotropia

Surgery is the only treatment for infantile esotropia. Surgery can involve a weakening of the medial rectus muscle in each eye. The *medial rectus muscle* is the muscle that turns the eye inward. This type of surgery is called a *recession.* The muscle is severed from its attachment to the eyeball and then sewn back on several millimeters farther back, thereby "recessing" the muscle.

Why should both eyes be operated on if only one of the eyes is turning in? The answer is that we are really dealing with a relationship between the two eyes that is controlled by the brain and not with a problem of the muscles themselves. Many authorities favor this type of symmetrical surgery.

Alternatively, the medial rectus muscle in one eye may be recessed while the lateral rectus muscle, the one that turns the eye out, is resected. Resection is a procedure in which a segment of muscle where it attaches to the eyeball is removed and the remaining muscle is then sewn back on in the same place. This puts the muscle "on stretch," which has the effect of strengthening it.

Timing the surgery is controversial, but it is generally done around six months of age. The infant will probably never develop an advanced type of depth perception, but the

The goal of surgery is to get the eyes to fuse.

goal is simply to get the eyes to fuse—to work together so that they remain straight. If the eyes can lock into this kind of position, then the surgery has been successful.

In some cases, the surgery may undercorrect or overcorrect the crossing. If that happens, then further surgery is necessary. In other cases, the eyes may not fuse but still look good from a cosmetic standpoint. If this occurs, the situation is simply carefully monitored to see whether the position of the eyes changes over time.

In some children, the eyes may seem straight for the first few years of life, but then intermittent crossing occurs. At first, it may occur only occasionally, especially when the child is feeling tired or sick. Then it may start to become more frequent. If crossing of an eye occurs even occasionally, it is time to get it checked out. This type of esotropia often turns out to be what we call *accommodative esotropia*. *Accommodation* refers to the adjustments the eyes undergo when they shift their focus from distance to near. Three things occur: (1) The ciliary muscle inside the eye changes the shape of the eye's lens to allow it to focus close up. (2) The eyes converge: They both turn in so that they can focus together on the object they're looking at. (3) The pupils become smaller to increase the depth of focus.

Hyperopia (farsightedness) is a common cause of esotropia in young children.

In the child with accommodative esotropia, one of two problems (or a combination of the two) exists. First, the child may be highly hyperopic (farsighted). This means that when the eyes are at rest, vision is blurry because incoming light rays are focusing behind the retina instead of right on the retina. The eye then accommodates as just described (even though it may be looking at something in the distance) to focus the light onto the retina. However, this accommodation causes not only a change in focusing of the lens but also a convergence of the eyes, because these muscular activities are linked to each other. The eyes try to use their other muscles to oppose this convergence action, but if they are not able to do so, the convergence takes over, and one of the eyes turns in.

The other possibility is that the child is not highly hyperopic, only moderately so, but there is an abnormality in the accommodative mechanism such that a given amount of change in focus of the eye's lens stimulates a much greater degree of convergence than it should. This effect can also overcome the effort assumed by the opposing eye muscles to keep the eyes straight, and the eyes then cross.

If the child with intermittent accommodative esotropia shows crossing only rarely, say, once a week, then nothing may need to be done about it. But if the crossing occurs at least once a day, the brain starts to employ some unhealthy adaptations in its attempt to avoid double vision. It begins to suppress the image coming to it from the crossing eye, and it starts to get used to the crossing of the eye. Ultimately, amblyopia can develop. We don't like these brain adaptations to take hold because they may ultimately make it more difficult to keep the eyes straight and working together properly.

Eyeglasses are used to treat accommodative esotropia. Dilating drops temporarily paralyze the muscle of accommodation in the eye so that we can determine the full amount of hyperopia. An instrument called a *retinoscope* helps us make that determination. Glasses that correct the farsightedness are then prescribed. In some cases, it may even be necessary to prescribe bifocals to keep the eyes straight when they are looking at things up close as well as in the distance. The goal of the glasses is to keep the eyes straight at all times. This may help vision as well for the following reason. Some children with accommodative esotropia may purposely keep their vision a little blurry, because when they accommodate to see more clearly, their eyes cross. Less accommodation keeps their eyes straight, but they can't focus as well. Eventually, some children, especially those who overconverge their eyes with a given amount of near focusing, may be able to have glasses of reduced strength or even be able to go without glasses. Children who have very high hyperopia (farsightedness) will probably continue to need glasses even if the hyperopia decreases somewhat with age, as it often does.

Eyeglasses usually straighten the eyes in children with accommodative esotropia.

Amblyopia

Amblyopia (reduced vision) results from changes in the brain that occur as the brain suppresses (blocks out) what the crossed eye is seeing. It does this as a way of avoiding double vision. Unfortunately, an infant who remains amblyopic in one eye throughout childhood will have poor vision in that eye throughout life, as amblyopia can only be corrected in young children. The way we usually treat amblyopia is to patch the good eye. This forces the amblyopic eye to be used, and the vision should improve. We must be careful, however, not to patch the good eye too long, because the good eye can then become amblyopic! In a young infant whose visual acuity cannot be tested directly, the endpoint is to have the two eyes alternate—either one may cross at a given time, and there is no apparent preference for either eye. The eyes can be alternately patched until surgery so that the amblyopia does not recur before then. Below, we will discuss amblyopia that results from other causes.

Other Causes of Amblyopia

We have already mentioned that an eye that is esotropic much of the time may develop amblyopia. Amblyopia can actually occur in any situation in which one eye is not aligned with the other one. It can even occasionally occur in cases in which there is minimal or virtually no deviation of one of the eyes. We call this a *monofixation syndrome*—because of some unknown abnormality in the brain, the two eyes do not work with each other properly. Even though the eyes may appear to be straight, the brain still suppresses what one of them is seeing, and the result is amblyopia. This type of amblyopia responds to patching of the good eye just as the eye with a large esotropia does. Thus, even if a young child's eyes are straight, it is important to measure the child's visual acuity just as soon as that child is able to cooperate with eye chart testing. If amblyopia is not detected until the child is older, it may be too late to fully restore the vision in the amblyopic eye.

Amblyopia is treated by patching the good eye.

Amblyopia can occur for other reasons as well. If there is a large difference in the refractive error between the two eyes, the more out-of-focus eye may develop amblyopia. For example, if one eye is much more hyperopic than the other, or has much more astigmatism than the other, this eye may develop what we call *refractive amblyopia*. Prescription of appropriate eyeglasses is necessary, and a little patching of the good eye at first may be needed as well.

An eye that is not permitted to see well because of some obstruction may also become amblyopic. One example would be a droopy upper eyelid that covers most of the pupil of one eye. An eye injury that causes a cataract or a scar in the cornea can also cause amblyopia. Treatment in these cases is directed at removing the obstruction and performing some patching to improve the vision in the weaker eye as much as possible.

Amblyopia may even be present in a child whose eyes appear straight.

Exotropia

Exotropia, or turning out of an eye, is often intermittent at first but may sometimes become constant over time. It may be noticed only occasionally at first, for example, when a child is tired or sick, staring at something in the distance, daydreaming, or in bright sunlight. It may first be noticed when the child is only a few months old. As the child gets older, it may or may not cause symptoms. A common symptom would be a feeling of tiredness in the eyes. Some blurring of vision may occur as the child uses accommodation to try to control the eyes. The convergence that is part of accommodation keeps the eyes straight, but the change in focusing that occurs along with it causes the blurring.

Treatment of this disorder depends on how frequently it occurs, whether it is causing any symptoms, and how far the eye turns out. Orthoptic therapy, which involves the use of special eye exercises, may be tried if the degree of turning out of the eye is not very large. If the eye does turn out fairly far to the side, then surgery is necessary. Such surgery is not needed if the turning out is only occasional and not causing any symptoms.

Exotropia may also occur in children who originally had esotropia. The exotropia may occur immediately after surgery to correct the esotropia. This is called an *overcorrection,* and additional surgery is probably required to straighten the eyes. Sometimes, a person who had a small esotropia as a child ultimately becomes exotropic as an adult. Because such a person has never developed *fusion* (alignment of the eyes), the deviation of the eyes can change with age as the eye muscles change. Similarly, an adult who has lost vision in one eye often develops an exotropia in that eye, since that is the normal position for an adult eye at rest when there is no stimulus (such as double vision) to keep the eyes straight. In people whose eyes do not fuse or work together, surgery to correct exotropia can be done for cosmetic reasons, but there is no guarantee that the eyes will always remain straight thereafter.

Eye exercises may sometimes be helpful.

Convergence Insufficiency During Reading

People who have a tendency to lose the alignment of their eyes when they are reading are said to have a *convergence insufficiency.* Their eyes are usually perfectly straight when they are looking at something in the distance, with no tendency for the eyes to deviate in either direction. However, when they are looking at something close up, the process of accommodation, in which the eyes not only change their focus but also converge, does not work properly. The eyes do not converge as strongly as they should, and it requires considerable effort to keep both eyes focused on the reading material. Occasionally, one of the eyes just "gives up" and turns out, losing its alignment with the other eye.

Convergence insufficiency is a very common cause of reading problems in adults. When they try to read, their eyes tire quickly. The words may start to run together or go double. Headaches and feelings of eye irritation may also occur. For people whose schooling or work requires them to read extensively, these symptoms can be disabling.

Convergence insufficiency is easy to diagnose. Even if the eyes are perfectly straight at the reading distance, there may be a tendency for them to turn out. We call this *exophoria* (described later in this chapter). Exophoria that may be part of convergence insufficiency is detected by having people focus at an object at the reading distance. As they do so, we alternately cover and uncover each eye. If an eye starts to turn out while it is covered but then returns to proper alignment when it is being used with the other one, then exophoria is present. Another test is to have someone focus on an object at the reading distance while we move that object closer to the eyes. We see how *Pencil push-ups can strengthen the weak eye muscles.* close we can move it without having one of the eyes start to turn out. Normally, we should be able to get fairly close to the nose. These tests, which are often part of a routine eye examination, make it easy to diagnose convergence insufficiency.

Convergence insufficiency is treated with eye exercises, not surgery. *Orthoptists,* technicians who specialize in eye muscle exercises, can prescribe appropriate exercises. A very simple but effective exercise is what we call *pencil push-ups.* With pencil push-ups, we try to strengthen the medial rectus muscles, the muscles that turn the eyes in and are therefore involved in convergence. To begin the pencil push-up routine, hold a pencil a few feet in front of your eyes while you focus on something on the wall across the room. Suddenly shift your focus to the tip of the pencil. As you do this, your eyes converge. Then focus back on the wall. Go back and forth like this a dozen times. Then bring the pencil an inch or two closer and repeat the process. Do about twenty-five of these sets every day. As the days and weeks go by, gradually move the pencil closer and closer to your face. With time, you will strengthen those medial rectus muscles, and your reading symptoms should diminish. Pencil push-ups are very effective, but do not expect them to bring about a permanent cure. If you stop doing them, your symptoms will probably return.

Occasionally, some people try the exercises and still obtain no relief. In such cases, we may have to prescribe prisms in reading glasses. Prisms are special lenses that change the direction of the light rays entering the eyes. Prisms do not strengthen the eye muscles, but they do reduce the degree to which the eyes need to converge at the reading distance. As a last resort, this can be quite effective as well.

Exophoria and Esophoria

A tendency for the eyes to turn in or out can be quite tiring, even if the eyes maintain their straightness all the time. A tendency for the eyes to turn out, as detected by a turning out of an eye when it is covered up, is called an *exophoria,* while a tendency to turn in is called an *esophoria.* Very small degrees of exophoria or esophoria are considered normal. Even if larger degrees

Headaches, tired eyes, blurring, or double vision may be present.

exist, the esophoria or exophoria requires no treatment if it is not causing any symptoms. But if headaches, tiredness in the eyes, or occasional blurring or double vision is present, then something should be done.

As we examine the patient with an exophoria or esophoria that is detected on a routine examination, we proceed with additional testing if symptoms are present. In particular, we measure what are called *divergence amplitudes* and *convergence amplitudes.* These are done while the person is focusing on something in the distance and also at near. This testing, which is accomplished by placing special lenses called *prisms* in front of the eyes, measures the strength of the muscles that turn the eyes out *(divergence amplitudes),* as well as the strength of the muscles the turn the eyes in *(convergence amplitudes).* Depending on the results obtained, special eye exercises, often using prisms, can be prescribed to help strengthen the muscles and thereby alleviate the symptoms.

Double Vision

Double vision is a troublesome symptom that cannot be ignored. People can generally function quite well with reduced vision in one eye and may, in fact, not even notice it for some time. Not so with double vision, which makes life difficult. There are many causes of double vision, so when someone has this complaint, we need to obtain more specific information.

Determining the Cause of Double Vision

We start by asking questions. Is it a true double vision—seeing two equally clear images of everything—or is it merely a "ghost image" type of double vision? With a ghost image, the two (or more) images overlap, and usually one of the images is clearer than the other. What happens if you cover up one eye (either eye)? Does the double vision go away, or does it remain? Are the two images side by side, or is one on top of the other? If there's some of each, are they *mostly* side by side or *mostly* one on top of the other? Does the double vision go away when you move your head in any particular position? If the double vision has been present a while, have the two images been moving farther apart? If the double vision is intermittent, has it been becoming more frequent or staying about the same? Have you been having a headache or pain around either eye? Do you have any other symptoms, such as dizziness, when the double vision is present? Has either eyelid become droopy? Is the double vision present only when you are reading or only when you are looking into the distance? Does the double vision become worse toward the end of the day or when you are tired? You should try to determine the answers to all of these questions before you see your physician. As we discuss the different causes of double vision, you will see why these questions are important.

If the double vision remains even after you cover one eye, you know the double vision is not caused by an eye misalignment. The double vision, then, must be coming from just one eye or from each eye individually. Double vision from one eye does not usually signify a serious problem. It is generally a ghost image type of double vision rather than a true double vision. One of the causes we look for in this situation is a mild cataract in one or both eyes. Cataracts can present as a small opacity or cloudy spot in the lens of the eye, and this opacity can split the light rays entering the eye. Another possible cause is the line in bifocal glasses. If the glasses are out of adjustment, you may be looking through the bifocal line without knowing it, and this can create a split or double image. Astigmatism can cause a ghost image type of double vision if the astigmatism is not or cannot be adequately corrected. This may occur with either glasses or contact lenses.

If the double vision goes away when you cover either eye, then you know that it is caused by a lack of coordination between the two eyes. Let us now look at some examples.

Muscle Problems

In some cases, double vision associated with a lack of coordination between the eyes may be caused by a muscle problem. People who have an overactive thyroid gland, for example, often develop problems with their eyes. Inflammation and thickening of some of the eye muscles may occur, and these thickened muscles can tether the eye so that it cannot move freely in all directions. Rarely, a cancer from elsewhere in the body, for example, breast cancer, may spread to a muscle and have a similar tethering effect on the eye.

Myasthenia gravis is a disease that causes weakness of the body muscles, and the weakness is often most apparent after repeated use of a muscle or toward the end of the day. One form of myasthenia gravis affects primarily the eye muscles. When myasthenia gravis affects the eyes, the upper eyelid muscle is usually involved and causes a droopiness of the eyelids. Myasthenia gravis is therefore a disease that is always kept in mind when someone has what appears to be an eye muscle problem.

Direct injuries to the eye area can damage eye muscles and cause double vision. One type of injury called a *blowout fracture* occurs when a large, blunt object such as a softball strikes the eye. The eye itself may be spared, but fractures may occur in the bones of the orbit, especially below or on the nose side of the eye. One or more of the eye muscles may then become entrapped in the area of bone fracture, and this may tether the eye down and cause double vision.

Nerve Palsies

Nerve palsies may also cause double vision. Three separate nerves that come from the brain control the various eye muscles and hence the movement and alignment of the eyes. These are called the *third (oculomotor), fourth (trochlear),* and *sixth (abducens) cranial nerves*. They may become palsied either individually or in combination. The double vision may come on suddenly or gradually, depending on the cause.

One of the most frequent causes of double vision from nerve palsies is diabetes. Any of the three nerves that control eye movement may be affected. The double vision is usually of fairly sudden onset and may be accompanied by pain around one eye. With a third nerve palsy, the upper lid over one eye usually droops, and the eye turns in a somewhat outward direction. Although third nerve palsies from other causes may result in a dilated pupil in the affected eye, the pupil generally retains its normal size with a diabetic third nerve palsy. With a fourth nerve palsy, the double vision is usually primarily vertical—that is, one image is higher than the other one. One of the images may also appear to be somewhat rotated. With a sixth nerve palsy, the affected eye may turn in, and the double vision is primarily horizontal, with the two images side by side.

Diabetes is a frequent cause of double vision.

These diabetic nerve palsies are usually seen in older individuals and are caused by a shutdown of the tiny blood vessels that nourish the affected nerve. However, a large percentage of elderly people suffer exactly this type of nerve palsy but are not diabetic. They simply have hardening of the arteries affecting their small blood vessels just as people with diabetes do. Hence, we sometimes use the term *vasculopathic nerve palsy* rather than *diabetic nerve palsy*. This indicates that there is a problem with the small blood vessels that can occur in anyone, not just in diabetics. The good news is that these nerve palsies almost always get back to normal, although it may take two to three months. In the meantime, either eye can be occluded (covered) to get rid of the double vision. An occluder can be a patch over one eye or a cover over one of the lenses in a pair of eyeglasses. Clear nail polish over one of the lenses often accomplishes the same thing.

Sometimes further testing, such as a brain scan, must be done.

If it appears obvious that a person's nerve palsy is of the diabetic or vasculopathic type, additional testing may not be necessary. However, if the double vision becomes worse, or if any other symptoms are present or develop that suggest something more may be going on, a brain scan such as an MRI (magnetic resonance imaging) should be done. An *aneurysm,* a dangerous ballooning out of a weakened wall of an artery in the brain, could be bleeding or pressing on one of the cranial nerves. An aneurysm would require urgent surgery. Brain tumors may also cause nerve palsies, although generally these palsies and the double vision they cause are more insidious in onset, gradually becoming worse over time. These may be tumors that originate in the brain or have spread to the brain from elsewhere. An elevated fluid pressure around the brain from any cause may result in a sixth nerve palsy in one or both eyes, so we always keep that in mind as well.

Herpes zoster, or shingles, can occasionally cause nerve palsies as part of an attack that affects the head. Because of the other symptoms caused by herpes zoster, such as the characteristic rash, it is usually obvious that shingles is the cause of the problem.

Multiple sclerosis (MS) can cause double vision, either by causing nerve palsies or by affecting eye coordination centers in the brain. Eye movement disorders are very common in people who have MS, so if a person with MS develops double vision, the MS itself is the most likely cause.

When you go to the ophthalmologist because of a double vision problem, be sure you go to one who is conscientious enough to take the time needed to get to the root of the problem. A high-volume operator who spends two minutes per patient and is mainly interested in screening for potential eye surgeries is not going to do justice to your problem. Determining the nature of the double vision problem and which nerves, if any, are affected can take time.

Determining the cause of double vision can take time and effort.

When you see an ophthalmologist because of double vision and a nerve palsy is suspected, careful measurements of the eyes must be taken. As you fix your gaze at objects both at distance and at near, the amount of deviation of the eyes is measured by holding special lenses called prisms in front of one of the eyes. Measurements may also be taken while the head is turned toward the left or right, while the chin is down or up, and while the head is tilted toward one side or the other. These measurements can not only help differentiate one type of nerve palsy from another but may also indicate whether a problem other than a nerve palsy may be causing the double vision.

Transient Ischemic Attacks (TIAs)

An example of a brain problem that causes double vision without affecting the cranial nerves is a transient ischemic attack (TIA). A TIA represents a warning that a stroke may occur in the near future. It represents a temporary cutting off of the circulation to one part of the brain. If the back part of the brain is involved in a TIA, *skew deviation,* a vertical separation of the eyes, may occur even though the cranial nerves are functioning properly. Besides double vision, a TIA frequently causes dizziness. It is important to diagnose a TIA so that action can be taken to prevent a full-fledged stroke.

An attack of double vision can warn of an impending stroke.

Long-Standing Muscle Imbalances

Some eye muscle imbalances may have always been present but only produce symptoms when a person reaches middle age or at least adulthood. For example, a convergence insufficiency may cause occasional double vision after you have been reading for a while, and this can be easily detected on examination. In someone who complains of occasional slight, vertical double vision, we may notice that the head is kept tilted a little toward one side. A fourth nerve palsy can make people do this because the head tilt can eliminate the double vision. The question, though, is whether the person just developed this fourth nerve palsy, indicating a possibly serious problem, or whether it has been long-standing. The solution to this dilemma is to look at old photos or even a driver's license photo. If the head tilt is long-standing or even lifelong, we can breathe a little easier and be less worried that anything serious is going on. Prescription of some prisms in eyeglasses may eliminate the symptoms. Other long-standing muscle weaknesses or imbalances may similarly present later in life.

CHAPTER NINE

Cataract

*C*ATARACT IS A CLOUDINESS OF THE LENS OF THE EYE. IT IS neither a growth nor a film, but rather a condition in which the formerly clear lens has lost some of its transparency. A gradual loss of lens clarity is a normal and expected part of the aging process, but in some people, the effect on vision becomes noticeable and starts to interfere with their daily activities.

Cataract can affect vision in many ways. Some people experience a general blurriness and may have more difficulty seeing under dim lighting conditions. It may become more difficult to read signs unless there is a great deal of contrast between the sign's letters and the background. Glare is also a frequent complaint. Some people may say that they can barely see outside when it's sunny. They may have a great deal of difficulty driving at night because of the glare from the headlights of oncoming cars. These headlights, as well as streetlights, may produce a starburst kind of effect, with halos and sparklers appearing around the lights. Some types of cataract may cause things to look double or triple. Unlike the double vision caused by an eye turning in or out, this is a "ghost image" kind of double vision that remains even when one eye is covered up.

Generally, cataract affects distance vision more than reading vision. If difficulty reading is the main problem, one must make sure that some other eye problem, such as age-related macular degeneration or dry eye syndrome, is not the cause. The hallmark of dry eye syndrome is a blurring of reading vision that is not present at first but appears shortly after one begins reading.

Cataract itself rarely causes any problems other than difficulty seeing. If, however, a cataract has become *hypermature,* meaning that the lens has become totally white and has partially liquefied, a complication called *phacolytic glaucoma* can occur. This problem is marked by inflammation and high pressure in the eye. If that occurs, emergency cataract surgery must be performed. People who have a hypermature cataract have a white-appearing pupil and cannot even see a hand waving in

If we could delay the development of cataract by ten years, most people would probably never need surgery.

front of the eye. They can tell light from darkness, however. Recent studies have yielded important insights as to how cataract may be prevented or at least slowed. This is important, because if we could just delay the onset of visually disabling cataract by ten years, most people would be able to live out their lives without needing cataract surgery. To understand how to do this, you first need to know more about the structure and function of the lens of the eye.

The Crystalline Lens

The lens of the eye, often called the *crystalline lens,* is a clear disk located just behind the iris (see figure 3.1, page 10). It is suspended in place by spiderweb-like threads called *zonules.* All light traveling through the pupil of the eye, the black circle in the center of the iris, passes through the lens, which refracts or bends the light rays so that they come to a focus on the retina in the back of the eye. In this respect, the eye is very similar to a camera, with the crystalline lens corresponding to the camera lens and the retina corresponding to the film in the camera. However, the eye's lens is even more sophisticated than that. When a person's focus changes from an object in the distance

The crystalline lens can be compared to the layers of an onion.

to one at near, a muscle in the eye contracts, changing the shape of the lens and allowing the eye to see clearly at whatever point the person's attention is directed. This process, called *accommodation,* gradually declines as a person ages, eventually resulting in the need for reading glasses even for people with normal distance vision.

The lens is a true marvel of nature. It is made up of cells whose unique arrangement and composition allow it to maintain a transparent state, at least until something goes awry and cataract develop. The entire lens is enveloped by a thin membrane called the *capsule*. The anterior capsule is the portion in the front of the lens, while the posterior capsule is in back. Along the inside of the anterior capsule is a single layer of cells called *epithelial cells*. These cells help regulate the transport of minerals and nutrients into the lens and produce energy to meet the needs of the lens. They also divide to produce the fiber cells that compose most of the lens. The fiber cells spread out and, beginning at a central core, form multiple shells, much like the layers of skin in an onion. This process begins before birth and continues throughout life. Thus, the oldest fiber cells are located near the center of the lens, while the ones laid down most recently are toward its outer portion.

The fiber cells produce proteins called *crystallins*. These proteins are laid down to produce a crystal-like arrangement that results in the transparency and other special properties of the lens. All told, protein constitutes about 98 percent of the weight of the lens, and the crystallins constitute about 90 percent of this protein. Each fiber cell is responsible for producing its own protein, and aging takes its toll on the oldest cells, which lose their ability to produce new proteins. This is important, because it means that proteins that have become damaged or altered in some way can no longer be replaced.

Types of Cataract

As the lens ages, the oldest fiber cells, the ones located closer to the center of the lens, change in such a way that the appearance of the lens, as viewed by an examining physician, changes. This center portion of the lens, called the *nucleus,* becomes a little less transparent. When a person develops cataract, we usually classify it in terms of the part of the lens that has become opacified. Therefore, when the nucleus becomes cloudy or even yellowed, we call that *nuclear sclerosis* or *nuclear sclerotic cataract.* When the outer layers of the lens, called the *cortex,* develop cloudy areas, we call that *cortical cataract.* Still another type of cataract develops just inside the posterior capsule, the part that covers the back surface of the lens. This is called *posterior subcapsular cataract,* a type often more rapidly progressive and more visually disabling than the other types. It is useful to use this classification system, because the causes of one type of cataract may be different from those of another type. In reality, however, many people have the mixed type of cataract—that is, the cloudy areas are in more than one region of the lens.

How Cataract Occurs

Cortical cataract can occur following a change in permeability of the lens. Recall that the epithelial cells along the inside surface of the anterior capsule of the lens help maintain the chemical balance of the lens. The lens tries to maintain a very low concentration of the mineral sodium and a high concentration of potassium inside itself. This is accomplished by a "pump" mechanism in the epithelial cells. When the system malfunctions, however, potassium can leave the lens, and sodium accompanied by chloride can stream in. The buildup of sodium and chloride (salt) in the lens pulls water into the lens. This excess water can liquefy the lens fiber cells and create spoke-like cloudy areas in the lens's outer layers.

In diabetics, who are prone to cataract, sugar gets into the lens of the eye.

The entrance of large amounts of sugars into the lens can cause similar problems. In diabetics, for example, sugars and related substances called *sugar alcohols* can build up in the lens, drawing water in with them and causing cataract. It is well known that diabetics develop cataract at a much younger age than do non-diabetics. A sugar called *galactose,* which is derived from milk sugar, can do the same thing. Cataract of this type occurs in infants who lack an enzyme to break down galactose. They may also occur in adults who have relatively low levels of one of these enzymes and who consume dairy products. More about this later.

Another way that cataract can form, typified by the nuclear sclerosis type, involves damaging alterations to the crystallin proteins in the lens fiber cells. Oxidation and other chemical reactions cause linkages to occur among individual crystallin molecules. Eventually, huge clumps of crystallin proteins, called *aggregates,* form. These protein clumps are very different from the original crystallins, which have to assume a very precise configuration to maintain the clarity of the lens. These chemical changes in the proteins can also result in the formation of colored substances. Thus, the typical nuclear sclerotic cataract appears as a diffuse cloudiness of the entire nucleus of the lens, often with a yellow or brownish color.

Whatever process is involved in the formation of cataract, oxidation is probably the main underlying mechanism. Oxidation is a common type of chemical reaction. A good example of oxidation is the rust that forms on things made of iron. To a chemist, oxidation means that the molecules of a substance lose electrons. When one substance becomes oxidized, another substance becomes reduced— that is, it gains electrons. Antioxidants are substances that help prevent other substances from becoming oxidized. They do this by becoming oxidized themselves. Although we think of rust as something undesirable, oxidation in the body is not all bad. It does have some beneficial functions, helping the body store energy and supporting the immune system. However, excessive or uncontrolled oxidation in the body can be bad.

Cataract is caused by the oxidation of lens proteins.

Oxidation results in the formation of free radicals, unstable, highly reactive molecules that can trigger damaging chain reactions and attack the DNA, protein, and essential fatty acids in cell membranes. We think this damage can trigger a number of diseases, not only cancer, but also certain eye diseases like cataract.

Oxidative chemical reactions could damage the membranes of cells near the surface of the lens, altering their permeability, and could bring about changes in the crystallin proteins of the lens, causing their clumping. Hydrogen peroxide, a powerful oxidant, is naturally present in the aqueous humor, the fluid surrounding the lens. Oxygen itself under the right conditions can promote oxidation, as can ultraviolet light, a component of sunlight. To protect itself from oxidation and eventual cataract formation, the lens utilizes a number of protective mechanisms.

How the Lens Protects Itself from Oxidation

The aqueous humor and the lens itself are extremely rich in ascorbic acid (vitamin C). Vitamin C has a number of important functions in the body, including its ability to be a powerful antioxidant and scavenger of free radicals. It helps regenerate vitamin E to its active, reduced form. Another antioxidant in the eye is glutathione. Glutathione not only helps eliminate linkages between proteins caused by oxidation; it can also detoxify hydrogen peroxide with the help of the enzyme glutathione peroxidase. This enzyme contains an unusual amino acid, selenocysteine, in which the sulfur in the amino acid cysteine has been replaced by the mineral selenium. Although glutathione itself becomes oxidized, its active form is quickly regenerated by the enzyme glutathione reductase. This enzyme is a flavoprotein, meaning that it contains a chemical called FAD (flavine adenine dinucleotide), one of whose precursors is the vitamin riboflavin. It is aided in its action by the coenzyme NADPH (nicotinamide adenine dinucleotide phosphate), which is derived from the vitamin niacin.

The eye has a strong antioxi-dant defense system, derived from the foods we eat.

All this sounds very complicated, but the point is that many substances derived from the diet help make up the lens's oxidation defense mechanisms. This suggests to us that dietary intervention might be useful in preventing or at least retarding the progression of cataract.

Preventing Cataract

As most people realize, surgery (removal of the eye's lens) can be performed if the cataract becomes debilitating. People are bound to ask, "If cataract surgery is so simple and successful, why bother trying to prevent cataract?" The answer is that although most cataract surgery is successful, any surgery takes its toll on the eye and can result in complications. As we shall see, loss of vision or even the entire eye from infection or from other problems is a small but ever-present risk. Other complications can develop as well, sometimes years later. For example, any cataract operation, no matter how smoothly performed, increases the risk of retinal detachment, a serious, vision-threatening problem requiring major surgery. It could occur a month, a year, or ten years after the operation. The eye is never quite the same after cataract surgery. Therefore, prevention is the best policy.

Cataract surgery takes its toll on the eye.

Many studies have examined people's food intakes and supplement use to see whether any specific nutrients or dietary patterns might help prevent cataract. Most of these have been what we call *retrospective studies*: obtaining dietary histories on people who already have cataract and comparing the findings with a group of similar people who don't have cataract. This assumes that the answers people give on these questionnaires accurately reflect what they eat and have eaten for many years in the past. Clearly, such an assumption is not always valid. Another type of retrospective study involves measuring the levels of various nutrients in the blood. However, the blood levels today may not be what they were years ago when the cataract was developing, and blood levels of a given substance do not necessarily correlate with the levels of that substance in the eye. Furthermore, even if we find that people with cataract have a lower level of a certain nutrient than do people without cataract, it doesn't necessarily mean that the lower level of that nutrient caused the cataract. To really determine whether consuming more of certain foods or taking certain supplements decreases the risk of cataract, long-term prospective studies need to be done. In this type of study, people are randomly assigned to two groups, each of which is placed on a different dietary or supplement regimen. Obviously, it is easier to get people to take a supplement than it is to get them to change their dietary habits.

Eating a poor, unbalanced diet has long been recognized as a risk factor for cataract. The fact that people of low educational or socioeconomic status are at much higher risk of cataract may well reflect inadequate nutrition. India is a country in which cataract is a major cause of blindness, and the incidence of cataract there is much higher than in the United States. Studies in India have suggested that deficiencies of protein, B vitamins, and other nutrients greatly increase the risk of developing cataract. However, overt deficiencies of this nature are relatively uncommon in Western countries, where people generally have plenty to eat.

Daily Vitamins: Panacea or Placebo?

Would simply taking a daily multivitamin/multimineral supplement reduce the risk of cataract? If people did have any vitamin or mineral deficiencies that put them at higher risk for cataract, we might expect that such a supplement would be beneficial. Many studies have looked at this question, and the results have been mixed. Some groups of people studied seemed to benefit from this type of supplement, whereas others did not. In some cases, a protective effect was seen for one type of cataract but not for another. In other

It is questionable whether multivitamin supplements can help prevent cataract.

studies, the effect depended on whether the people taking the supplement were diabetic or not.

If these results seem confusing, that's because they are. They illustrate the limitations of studies of this type. How can we explain such conflicting results? One possible explanation is that people who choose to take supplements on their own are often different in many respects from people who do not. For example, they may be more health conscious and consume a healthier diet. Therefore, although there seems to be at least some indication of a protective effect from multivitamin use, we cannot reach any definite conclusions. Only with good, controlled prospective studies will we know for sure. In fact, there has been one such prospective study, in China. It did show a decrease in the risk for nuclear sclerotic cataract with multivitamin use, although not for other cataract types. However, this study was conducted in an area known for nutritional deficiencies, so the results are not necessarily applicable to Western populations. We await the results of similar trials in the United States.

Should you take a multivitamin/multimineral supplement? In general, I don't think it is necessary or desirable for young or middle-aged people who follow a balanced diet. However, as we age, our immune systems tend to become weaker, and we don't absorb certain minerals as well. The evidence is that most people over age sixty-five would benefit from a daily supplement.

Antioxidants

Since it is generally believed that oxidative damage to the lens initiates the sequence of events that leads to cataract formation, a number of researchers have tried to determine whether antioxidant vitamin intake, either from the diet or from supplements, might help protect the lens and prevent cataract development. It is important to differentiate between supplements and dietary intake, since the form vitamins assume in food is sometimes different from that in supplements.

People who consume more antioxidant-rich foods are less likely to develop cataract.

A number of early studies explored the possible role played by antioxidants like vitamin C, vitamin E, and carotenoids in preventing cataract. Carotenoids are the vitamin A–like compounds in foods, of which beta-carotene is the best known, although not necessarily the most important. These studies showed that all of these antioxidants could be considered promising candidates as cataract preventives. Some of these studies measured the amount of these antioxidants people obtained from foods or from supplements; in other studies, blood levels of these antioxidants were measured. However, just as with the multivitamin studies, enough uncertainty was caused by conflicting results to make us unsure as to which of the antioxidants, if any, were the most important for cataract prevention. Fortunately, more recent studies have shed a great deal of light on the subject.

Vitamin C

Vitamin C, also known as *ascorbic acid,* is well known as an antioxidant. Its importance goes well beyond preventing the deficiency disease known as *scurvy.* Although the recommended dietary allowance is only 75 milligrams a day for women and 90 milligrams a day for men, we should probably be consuming at least 200 milligrams a day, an amount easy to obtain on a healthy, plant-based diet. As noted before, the role that vitamin C may play in preventing cataract becomes even more plausible when we consider that the aqueous humor is extremely rich in vitamin C. Increasing one's intake of vitamin C up to 250 milligrams a day increases its concentration in the aqueous humor. The lens itself absorbs the vitamin C, and the more vitamin C you ingest, the more is present in the lens.[1] If you consume some of the good dietary sources of vitamin C, such as citrus fruits, melons, strawberries, kiwifruits, leafy green vegetables, red and green peppers, tomatoes, potatoes, and sweet potatoes, you should not need to supplement.

With a healthy diet you should not have to supplement with vitamin C.

If you do supplement with vitamin C, some caveats exist. Although we often speak of vitamin C as an antioxidant, some have expressed concern that it could act as a prooxidant (promoting oxidation) under certain conditions. For example, some laboratory studies have shown that vitamin C, in the presence of oxygen and iron, can become oxidized and lead to the formation of hydrogen peroxide, which can in turn generate free radicals that trigger a chain of oxidation reactions. Such oxidation reactions could theoretically promote cataract development. Furthermore, other test tube studies have shown that when vitamin C becomes oxidized, some highly reactive forms of the vitamin C molecule

are transiently produced that can form linkages with the crystallin lens proteins and lead to their clumping. This process would also promote cataract
formation. The degree to which these prooxidant effects of vitamin C actually
occur in the eye, and the question as to whether megadose vitamin C supplementation could augment such reactions, are big unknowns and the subject
of much controversy. My feeling is that vitamin C supplementation is unlikely
to produce any prooxidant effects and, in fact, probably enhances the antioxidant status of the eye, but I remain cautious about megadose therapy. If
you do supplement, I recommend taking no more than 300 milligrams a day.

Vitamin E

Vitamin E, another antioxidant vitamin with great potential, actually exists in
nature in eight different forms: alpha-, beta-, gamma-, and delta-tocopherol;
and alpha-, beta-, gamma-, and delta-tocotrienol. The alpha-tocopherol form is
the one most recognizable by the average per-
son, because that is the form present in most
supplements. However, the average American
diet contains more gamma-tocopherol than
alpha-tocopherol. In its neutralization of

*Only from foods will you
obtain the full spectrum
of vitamin E.*

some oxidants, the gamma form appears to be a more potent antioxidant than
alpha-tocopherol. It is also taken up strongly by many tissues of the body. The
tocotrienol form, much less abundant in nature than the tocopherol form,
appears to be a stronger antioxidant than the latter. Even naturally derived vitamin E supplements (greatly preferable over the synthetic form) generally
contain only alpha-tocopherol. What's more, if you take megadoses of alpha-
tocopherol, say, 400 international units (IU) twice a day or 1,200 IU once a
day, it may cause the levels of gamma-tocopherol in your bloodstream to
plunge, a most undesirable side effect.

What bearing does this have on the eye? Just as with vitamin C, the plausi-
bility of a possible protective effect from vitamin E is increased by the finding
that vitamin E is present in the lens, more in the newer, outer layers of the lens
than in the older, central nucleus.[2] Although there is more alpha-tocopherol
than gamma-tocopherol in the lens, at least one study has shown that the proportion of gamma-tocopherol compared with alpha-tocopherol in the lens is
greater than that in the bloodstream.[3] Thus, the gamma form of tocopherol

may also play an important role in cataract prevention. Take a supplement of natural alpha-tocopherol up to 200 IU a day if you wish, but don't ignore the foods that contain the other important forms of vitamin E. The best food sources of gamma-tocopherol include soy products (except the fat-free variety) and peanuts and nuts, especially pecans and pistachios (the latter is also a good source of the tocotrienols). Dark, leafy green vegetables and whole grains are also good sources of vitamin E in general (but 95 percent is removed when grains are refined).

Lutein

The early studies showed that carotenoids appear to help protect the eye from cataract, but in general the researchers just studied carotenoids in general without narrowing them down to any specific one. This is very important, because numerous carotenoids (to date, about 700) besides beta-carotene have been discovered in nature, of which at least forty can be absorbed by the human body. Some may be stronger antioxidants than beta-carotene and may help prevent diseases unaffected by beta-carotene. Other important carotenoids include lycopene (from tomatoes, watermelon, pink grapefruit, and guava), alpha-carotene, beta-cryptoxanthin, lutein, and zeaxanthin.

Lutein, which comes from dark, leafy green vegetables, may prevent cataract.

Recent studies have shown that people who consume above average amounts of dark, leafy green vegetables seem to be protected from both age-related macular degeneration and cataract.[4,5] Although we are not absolutely sure right now as to the nature of the protective effect, the common thread seems to be the carotenoid lutein, a yellowish pigment found in abundance in many leafy green vegetables, including kale, collard greens, spinach, parsley, mustard greens, and turnip greens. It turns out that lutein (along with its close relative zeaxanthin) is the dominant pigment in the macula (central area of the retina) and is also the only carotenoid in the lens! It would be logical to assume, then, that the lutein is there for a purpose, and that purpose is probably to protect these delicate structures from oxidation, which, in the case of the lens, results in cataract formation.

Should you take a lutein supplement? I would recommend lutein supplementation only as a last resort for people who don't listen to their mothers' advice and refuse to eat their vegetables! We don't know for certain that it is the lutein in these vegetables that is protective, and even if the lutein is playing a role, it may be working in concert with other substances in these vegetables. My advice is to consume at least one serving a day (half a cup, either cooked or raw) of any of the lutein-rich green vegetables mentioned earlier, if possible.

Other Antioxidants

Supplementation with other vitamins and minerals that participate in oxidation reactions, either directly or indirectly, is also being studied. *Riboflavin (vitamin B_2)* is one of the dietary precursors of flavin adenine dinucleotide (FAD), a chemical that has antioxidant properties in the eye. One study showed that about one-third of elderly people with cataract were deficient in riboflavin, whereas in a small group of elderly people who did not have cataract, no deficiency was noted.[6] A major study involving nurses, in contrast, found no association between the amount of riboflavin in the diet and cataract.[7] It is possible that people deficient in riboflavin are also deficient in other nutrients, so we cannot be sure about the importance of riboflavin with respect to cataract, but it would certainly seem prudent to avoid riboflavin deficiency. Megadoses should be avoided as well, because it is conceivable that such large doses of riboflavin might even trigger cataract formation. The structures of the eye contain small amounts of riboflavin itself, and riboflavin is the type of substance we call a *photosensitizer*. When riboflavin absorbs light, it becomes chemically changed and can trigger the formation of oxygen free radicals that can then precipitate a chain of oxidation reactions. Whether high-dose riboflavin supplementation would increase the levels of riboflavin in the eye is unknown, but if it did, there could certainly be undesirable consequences.

Niacin, or *vitamin B_3,* is a precursor of nicotinamide adenine dinucleotide (NAD), another substance that aids in the antioxidant functions of the eye. A major Chinese study, conducted in an area where nutritional deficiencies are known to exist, found that a supplement containing both riboflavin and niacin appeared to protect from some forms of cataract. Again, there is probably no reason to supplement in people from Western countries consuming a balanced diet. The tendency for B vitamin deficiency in some areas of China is related to the refining of rice, which removes important nutrients. Brown rice is looked on as inferior because of its association with the poor, whereas refined white rice is regarded as the food of the rich.

An interesting source of antioxidants is tea. One early study found that drinking over four cups of tea per day was associated with a lower risk of cataract.[8] If a true cause-and-effect relationship exists, one explanation might be that tea is a rich source of *polyphenols,* phytochemicals (plant-derived chemicals) that have significant antioxidant activity. Some researchers have speculated that polyphenols

Tea, like red grapes, is rich in antioxidants.

may offer protective benefits with regard to other diseases, such as cancer and heart disease. These polyphenols are in many foods of plant origin, most notably tea (especially green tea) and red wine and grape juice.

It may not even be necessary to look for specific foods and nutrients to lower your risk for cataract. It is well established that simply eating a good variety of fruits and vegetables in abundance has a strong protective effect. In one study, a low intake of both fruits and vegetables increased the risk of cataract almost sixfold![9] All of the nutrients, both known and unknown, are there, packaged by nature in their most effective forms and combinations. Nature's cornucopia remains more effective than mankind's pharmacopeia.

The Dairy Connection

There has been much speculation in recent years that dairy product consumption might increase the risk of cataract in susceptible individuals. Dairy products contain a form of sugar called *lactose,* which is a double sugar. This sugar is broken down in the small intestine to two simple sugars, glucose and galactose. These simple sugars can then be absorbed into the bloodstream and used by the body for energy. However, there is a genetic disease called *galactosemia* that is characterized by the lack of one of two enzymes that help convert galactose to other substances. Galactose then builds up in the bloodstream and has toxic effects, including cataract formation. Babies lacking one of these enzymes, galactose-1-phosphate uridyl transferase, become very sick from the disease and sometimes die. People who are missing the other enzyme, galactokinase, are usually healthy except for the cataract. If galactosemia is detected early, elimination of milk from the diet can prevent progression of the disease.

Galactose itself may not be toxic to the lens, but it can be converted in the lens to galactitol, a type of sugar alcohol. The galactitol is trapped inside the lens and builds up, creating what we call *osmotic pressure,* which draws water into the lens. This excess water can disrupt the fiber cells of the lens and cause the opacification that we call *cataract.* Sugars such as galactose can also trigger oxidation of the crystallins, the proteins in the lens. This ultimately results in clumping of these proteins and cataract progression.

Some researchers have suggested that people who are simply carriers for one of the forms of galactosemia, meaning that their enzyme levels are reduced but not absent, may be at risk for developing cataract later in life, say, in their thirties or forties. Dr. Harold Skalka and Dr. Josef Prchal examined 147 people with cataract, 94 of whom were fifty years old or younger. In those younger patients who had cataract in both eyes for no apparent rea-

Galactose, derived from milk sugar, may cause cataract in susceptible people.

son, there was a greatly increased incidence of low levels of one of the two galactosemia-related enzymes (primarily galactokinase) as compared with the older patients with "age-related" cataract. The most common cataract type in the younger patients was posterior subcapsular. They estimated that 1 percent of the population may be carriers for one of these enzyme defects.[10] In a follow-up study on 87 additional patients below the age of fifty who had cataracts, they found that 7 percent had low levels of galactokinase.

Although only 1 percent of the population may be carriers for galacto-semia, there is a wide range of levels of enzyme activity in people who are not carriers. Galactokinase levels were measured in 94 people undergoing cataract surgery in Chicago. People below the age of fifty had, on average, significantly lower galactokinase levels than the patients over the age of fifty.[11] This supports the notion that lower enzyme levels may be a risk factor for people who develop cataract prematurely. Another study in patients who were forty to seventy years old showed that in people whose galactokinase levels were below the median level, people whose dairy consumption was high had a fourfold higher risk of cataract than people with low dairy consumption.[12] Both of these studies indicate that high dairy product consumption might increase the risk of cataract formation for much more than 1 percent of the population. Multiple, small galactose challenges during life in people with normal but below average levels of the enzymes could conceivably exert a harmful effect on the lens, but no definite conclusions can be reached at present.

Other Risk Factors for Cataract

Smoking has been identified as a major risk factor for both the nuclear sclerotic and posterior subcapsular forms of cataract. The effect may well be related to oxidative damage. Cigarette smoke is known to contain powerful prooxidants, and some studies have shown evidence of increased oxidation of the fatty acids in smokers. Lower blood levels of antioxidants such as vitamin C and the carotenoids have also been observed in smokers. In short, smoking takes its toll on the eye, just as it does on the rest of the body.

Add cataract to the list of smoking-caused illnesses.

Diabetes has already been mentioned as a major risk factor for cataract. Most people with the adult-onset form of diabetes also happen to be overweight. However, even overweight people who are not diabetic are at increased risk for cataract. The risk may be greatest in people in whom the excess fat is located around the waist.

Chronic use of corticosteroid (cortisone-related) medication such as prednisone can cause posterior subcapsular cataract. The rate of development depends on the dose, the length of time it has been taken, and an individual's own susceptibility. Although unusual, even inhaled steroids, which are prescribed for asthma and related conditions, can cause cataract in the long term. Everyone who must take this type of medication on a chronic basis should be aware of the many possible side effects. The best approach is to take the minimum effective dose under the supervision of a physician. Cataract of this type, which begins while one is on steroid therapy, usually stops progressing (but does not reverse) if the medication can be discontinued. Never stop steroid medication suddenly on your own, however, because the results can be disastrous. The longer you have been taking it, the more slowly it needs to be tapered, and that is the job of the prescribing physician.

Cortisone pills, eyedrops, shots, and even inhalers can cause cataract.

Alcoholism is also a cause of cataract, especially those of the posterior subcapsular type. A toxic effect of the alcohol is a possible reason, as is the nutritional deprivation that often accompanies the disease. There is no evidence that alcohol in moderation should be a problem; it may even be slightly beneficial.

Exposure to the ultraviolet rays of sunlight appears to increase the risk of cortical and possibly posterior subcapsular cataract. People who spend much of their time outdoors as a result of their occupation or avocation would naturally be at the highest risk. Such individuals should consider wearing ultraviolet-absorbing glasses when they are in the sun. Interestingly, people with brown eyes may be at higher risk for cataract than people with blue eyes, although the explanation for this finding is not entirely clear.

Too much sunlight can increase your risk of cataract.

Trauma to an eye can cause cataract, either immediately or years later. The risk of glaucoma and other problems is increased by trauma as well. Again, the best advice is prevention. Many people take their eyes for granted and fail to protect them in dangerous situations. Playing racketball or using a weed whip without eye protection is just asking for trouble.

In many people who develop cataract at a young age, some genetic factor is clearly at work. In most of these cases, we do not know exactly what enzyme or factor is missing. The best we can do now is to follow the commonsense guidelines discussed in this chapter and hope that they make a difference.

Cataract Surgery

Except for the rarest circumstances, no harm comes to an eye from cataract. Although the lens can be removed surgically, the operation can be safely performed at any time, whether the cataract is mild or advanced. Thus, there is usually no medical necessity for the operation. Nevertheless, cataract surgery has become of the most widely performed operations, and one of the costliest to our society.

Why did this cataract surgery epidemic occur? The problem can be attributed to the lack of ethics in medicine today and to the gullibility of the public. Ethical physicians always do what is in the best interests of their patients. They do not advertise but build their practices through referrals from other physicians and from their patients as their reputations grow. In 1982, however, the Federal Trade Commission ruled that medicine is a trade and that there should be no restraint on advertising. A plethora of advertising followed, initiated by the most unscrupulous doctors, who saw the

Many of the cataract operations performed have been unnecessary.

opportunity to make a fortune from cataract surgery. They labeled themselves "cataract specialists," even though it is absurd to regard a single operation as a specialty in itself. With total abandonment of reason, people who would normally shy away from free brake lining checks have flocked to these clinics, which often label themselves as "institutes." There they are greeted by public relations experts in the guise of medical personnel, who try to persuade them to have cataract surgery as soon as possible. Needless to say, this has resulted in a huge volume of unnecessary surgery.

Cataract surgery is indicated only when a person is no longer able to carry out everyday functions in a satisfactory manner. Therefore, the decision to have surgery should be primarily that of the patient, who is the only person who knows the degree of disability the cataract causes. Some people have expressed concern that poor vision may increase the risk of falling and breaking a hip, especially in elderly women. That may be a factor in people who have moderately reduced vision in both eyes or who have poor vision, say, 20/100 or worse, in just one eye, but ultimately it is the patients who should decide just how impaired they feel.

As part of a complete eye examination, a very careful refraction (check for glasses prescription) needs to be done, because cataract can often result in a change in the prescription. Simply changing the glasses will often result in the restoration of satisfactory vision. If difficulty reading is a problem, the cause should be determined. If a person can read easily at first, but the words start to blur and run together after a short while, we would suspect a form of dry eye problem as the cause of the symptoms rather than cataract. Even if decreased reading vision can be attributed to cataract, the bifocal portion of the glasses can often be strengthened to provide satisfactory vision. I have seen the records of many patients for whom cataract surgery had been recommended because they had complained of difficulty reading, and I have found that in many cases, the reading vision was never even checked as part of the examination.

The examination must also determine whether any other eye problems are present that might account for the vision problem. Of these, the most common would be age-related macular degeneration. This affliction of older people can cause blurring or distortion in straight-ahead vision. In a patient who has both cataract and macular degeneration, it can sometimes be difficult to determine how much each one is contributing to the decrease in vision. Nevertheless, it is important to attempt to make such an assessment, because the condition of the retina is usually the limiting factor that determines how well the eye sees after cataract surgery. In some cases, this may mean that no improvement in vision occurs after cataract surgery, and any surgery performed in such a situation will have been in vain.

Cataract surgery is indicated only when the blurring becomes disabling.

To determine whether improvement in vision is likely after cataract surgery, the physician must carefully evaluate the cataractous lens to determine whether the cloudiness is sufficient to cause the patient's complaints. One way to do this is to look into the eye through an undilated pupil with an *ophthalmoscope,* the instrument used for examining the retina. If what a person sees through an eye seems blurred, then what the physician sees looking into the eye should be blurred as well. The macula must also be carefully checked for changes in its appearance that would signify the presence of macular degeneration.

In short, cataract surgery is indicated if a person, even with the best possible glasses, is unable to see well enough to perform everyday activities, and only if the cataract is severe enough to explain the poor vision, with no other disorder in the eye that would prevent improvement of vision. Clearly, if these criteria were followed, the number of cataract surgeries performed would be a fraction of what they are today.

My recommendation is that when your doctor discusses the possibility of cataract surgery, get a second opinion. From whom? From yourself! Because only you can decide when you should have the surgery. Remember, any surgery can have complications. If you are functioning well with the vision you have and the cataract

Always get a second opinion. From yourself!

symptoms are only a mild annoyance or minor inconvenience, surgery is inadvisable. However, if the vision problems are interfering significantly with your work, driving, reading, or ability to function in general, then you should consider the surgery. Except in rare situations (such as mature or totally opaque cataracts), there is no medical necessity or urgency for the surgery.

Alternatives to Surgery

No medication can reverse the cloudiness caused by cataract. However, with the posterior subcapsular type of cataract, which often begins with a small, cloudy spot located centrally, a mild dilating type of eyedrop can often produce a nice improvement in vision. Enlarging the pupil in this way often allows the light rays entering the eye to bypass the central cloudy spot. Of course, this is only a temporary solution that will no longer work when the cataract becomes more advanced. It may also be less practical for people who live in very sunny climates. But it is useful when the patient would like to "buy some time" before undergoing surgery.

Glare problems caused by cataract can sometimes be mitigated by wearing sunglasses, or at least tinted glasses that block out the blue wavelengths of light. Some people object to the yellowish tint that these glasses

If your main problem is with reading, simply strengthening the reading glasses or bifocals may help.

impart. And since cataract often reduces the amount of light entering the eye, tinted glasses may aggravate the vision problem under some circumstances, e.g., at night.

Finally, remember that if the vision problem is mainly at the reading distance, the reading glasses or the reading portion of the bifocals can often be strengthened. This will make you hold your reading material closer to your face, but many people do not mind doing that if it allows them to avoid surgery.

How Cataract Surgery Is Done

Cataract surgery means removal of the lens. It is a surgical technique and is not performed using a laser, although that is a common misconception. Don't make the mistake of choosing a surgeon on the basis of the method of cataract removal. All current methods of removal are highly effective. All that matters are the conscientiousness, skill, and dedication of the ophthalmologist in whose care you have entrusted yourself. Does it really matter whether one stitch, two, or none at all is used? What matters are that the surgery is well done and there is no leakage from the incision afterward. Does it matter how the surgeon numbs the

Laser is not used in cataract surgery.

eye? Avoid individuals who advertise that they perform this or that technique with the implication that it is superior to the techniques used by other surgeons. These are just marketing gimmicks employed to lure in the gullible.

Cataract surgery is usually performed by what we call an *extracapsular technique*. This means that rather than removing the entire lens intact in one piece, as was usually done prior to 1980, the surgeon removes the lens piecemeal. A small incision is made in the eye, and an opening is then created in the anterior capsule, the front part of the envelope that surrounds the lens. The nucleus, or central portion of the lens, can then be removed in one piece, or, more commonly today, a technique called *phacoemulsification* is used to pulverize the lens using an instrument that employs ultrasound (high-frequency inaudible sound waves). The nucleus remains in its normal position in this eye as it is pulverized, and the fragments are removed from the eye by a suction-producing vacuum-like instrument. After removal of the nucleus, the remaining cortex of the lens is then removed with suction, with care being taken not to cause any rents in the portion of the lens capsule that remains. This back portion of the lens capsule is left intact because it is safer for the eye, especially the retina, that way.

Remember that the function of the lens is to focus incoming light rays onto the retina. Removal of the lens makes the eye extremely hyperopic (farsighted). A lens in eyeglasses that would correct this hyperopia is quite thick, has a magnifying effect (about 25 percent), and tends to distort things in your peripheral vision. Because of the magnification, it cannot be used together with an eye that has not undergone cataract surgery. Although glasses can be used to correct vision in people who have had cataractous lenses removed from both eyes, many people do not like the quality of vision they obtain with "cataract glasses."

Contact lenses after cataract surgery only magnify what you see about 10 percent, and there is no distorting effect. However, many older people cannot or do not want to deal with contact lenses. Therefore, the lens implant was developed.

An intraocular lens implant, which is an artificial lens with flexible loops that wedge the lens in place, is inserted at the time of cataract surgery into the remaining portion of the lens capsule inside the eye, where it can focus incoming light rays just as the eye's natural lens did. Prior to the surgery, special measurements of the eye are done to estimate what power of lens to insert in the eye. But it is only an estimate, and glasses may be needed afterward to "fine-tune" the vision. Generally, these are bifocals.

Even in people with a lens implant, glasses may "fine-tune" the vision.

Significance of the Incision Size

In the long run, the incision size does not matter much. In the short run, a shorter incision allows the eye to achieve stable, clear vision much more quickly than a larger incision does. However, the end result is usually excellent in either case. One reason for using a larger incision would be an eye with a small pupil that dilates poorly. A larger incision would allow more room in which to operate and may be safer for the eye.

Cataract surgery often lowers the eye pressure, a boon to people with glaucoma.

Cataract surgery with both large and small incisions has been associated with long-term lowering of the intraocular pressure, a definite boon to people who have glaucoma or might develop it in the future. However, in my hands, extracapsular cataract surgery with the larger incision has resulted in a greater lowering of the pressure than is generally seen in patients who have undergone phacoemulsification with the smaller incision.

Complications of Cataract Surgery

Cataract surgery is one of the most successful types of surgery, and at least 95 percent of the time, improvement in vision is achieved. But, as with any surgery, there can be complications, even total loss of vision or of the eye. Occasionally, additional operations are required. That is why you should not have the surgery unless you really need it.

One major complication is infection inside the eye, which occurs in 1 out of every 500 operations and results in loss of the eye about half the time. About 1 percent of the time, clouding of the cornea occurs, a complication that requires another major operation, a corneal transplant. Retinal detachment, also with a 1 percent incidence, requires surgery that is successful 90 percent of the time. It can occur right away or

Clouding of the cornea and retinal detachment may occur even years down the road.

many years after a cataract operation. Bleeding in the eye, continued inflammation, glaucoma, double vision, dislocation of lens implants, and cystoid macular edema (fluid buildup in the center of the retina that blurs and distorts the vision) are other possible complications.

Recall that the surgery is performed in such a way as to leave the back portion of the capsule that surrounds the lens intact. However, should a tear in this part of the capsule occur during the operation, the vitreous (gel-like substance) that fills the inside of the back part of the eye may come forward. This problem, called *vitreous loss,* greatly increases the risk of many of the complications just mentioned. To minimize the risk, this extruded vitreous must be removed very carefully from the front of the eye, and if insufficient support from the remaining lens capsule is left, sometimes a different style of lens implant must be inserted. An even more challenging problem arises if parts of the central core of the lens, the nucleus, fall back through the tear in the capsule. They must then be carefully recovered using special techniques.

> *Any surgery, even the most minor, can have complications.*

Although not a true complication, clouding of the posterior capsule, the portion of the lens capsule that remains in place behind the lens implant, occurs in up to 50 percent of people within a few years of the cataract surgery. This is called *secondary cataract,* and it causes blurring very similar to that caused by the original cataract. The blurring can be eliminated by creating a hole in the center of the cloudy capsule with a special laser called a *neodymium: YAG laser.* Such a treatment will slightly increase the risk of developing a retinal detachment or macular edema, two of the complications mentioned earlier.

This discussion of possible complications is not meant to scare you. It is simply to let you know that any surgery, from the most minor on up, can have complications.

Summary and Recommendations

When chemical changes occur in the proteins of the eye's crystalline lens, the lens loses its clarity, a condition we call *cataract.* These changes appear to be triggered by a series of oxidation reactions. The lens and the fluid surrounding it maintain high levels of antioxidants, which can help keep the lens healthy. Over time, however, the oxidative stresses in the lens's environment can overcome the eye's defense mechanisms. Preventing cataract may be a matter of keeping the antioxidant systems finely tuned and in top working condition. Since antioxidants are derived from the diet, a nutritional approach seems the most natural and may prove effective.

Lutein, a yellow antioxidant pigment in many dark, leafy green vegetables, may help prevent cataract. Consuming at least one serving a day of these vegetables is recommended. Vitamins C and E and other antioxidants in vegetables and fruits are felt to play an important role as well. People who consume more vegetables and fruits are at lower risk for cataract and other degenerative problems. Consuming at least eight servings a day is recommended. For people over age sixty-five, a daily multivitamin/multimineral supplement may also be helpful.

Cataract surgery is highly successful but should be considered only when you feel it is necessary to improve your vision. Even with perfectly performed surgery, the eye is never quite the same as it was before the cataract developed.

CHAPTER TEN

Glaucoma

*G*LAUCOMA IS A DETERIORATION OF THE OPTIC NERVE THAT progresses slowly over time. The optic nerve, which carries messages from the eye to the brain so that you can "picture" what is around you, consists of over one million nerve fibers. In glaucoma, these nerve fibers gradually die off, resulting in blind spots in the field of vision (area of seeing) and, in the final stage, blindness. A great deal of damage must occur before the blind spots appear. Even when they do, you usually do not notice them until they become severe. At this point, most of the optic nerve is already gone, irreversibly so. You might compare it to the invasion of a wood frame house by termites. A great deal of destruction can occur without being detected by the untrained observer. By the time the damage is noticeable, the house is on the verge of collapse. Some people have also compared glaucoma to jumping out of a ten-story window. Everything feels fine—until you hit bottom.

Many people mistakenly believe that having their eye pressure checked will tell them whether they have glaucoma. Although a high pressure of the fluid inside the eye is

A pressure check is not a glaucoma test.

the main risk factor for glaucoma, about 25 percent of glaucoma patients have what we call *low-tension glaucoma*. In these people, the pressure in the eye, no matter when it is checked, is always in what we consider the normal range. Therefore, a pressure check is most certainly not a glaucoma test, that is, a test that tells whether you have glaucoma. Not only are there many people with glaucoma who have normal eye pressures, there are also many people who have high eye pressures but who do not show any evidence of damage to the optic nerve. These individuals are said to be *ocular hypertensives* or *glaucoma suspects*. Clearly, there is much more to diagnosing glaucoma than simply checking the pressure. If that were the only test done, many cases of glaucoma would be overlooked. In practice, that is exactly what happens to many people who undergo inadequate eye examinations. Their glaucoma may become far advanced before it is diagnosed and treatment is begun.

A Careful Examination: The Key to Diagnosis

The most crucial part of the eye examination for diagnosing glaucoma is not a pressure check but a very careful examination of the optic nerve where it enters the back of the eye. In this area, the optic nerve appears as a disk, oval in shape, pinkish in color, and surrounded by the retina. This portion of the optic nerve is called the *optic disk*. All of the nerve fibers on the surface of the retina come together at the optic disk and then follow the optic nerve to the brain. The center of the optic disk usually contains a craterlike area that we call the *cup*, which can vary greatly in size from one person to another. The first sign of glaucoma is often a change in the appearance of this cup. It enlarges and sometimes extends close to the rim of the optic disk in one area. If the glaucoma is developing at a different rate in the two eyes, there may be a marked difference in the size of the cups in the two eyes.

The appearance of the optic nerve, not the pressure, is the most important part of the eye exam for glaucoma.

The physician examining the eye notes what we call the *cup/disk ratio*. This is simply the distance across the cup divided by the distance across the whole optic disk. The average cup/disk ratio for normal eyes is about 0.3, which means that the distance across the cup is 30 percent (almost one-third) of the distance across the optic disk. The important thing, though, is whether a change in the size of the cup occurs over time. For this reason, we sometimes take photographs of the optic disks in people who are glaucoma suspects so that we will be able to detect any changes in the size of the cups. Changes in the appearance of the optic nerve often occur before any blind spots appear in a person's field of vision.

A less common finding in glaucoma patients is a small hemorrhage (blood spot) on the surface of the optic disk. This is a strong sign that damage is occurring to the disk. Therefore, it can aid in diagnosing glaucoma as well as in determining whether the treatment being given is adequate.

It should now be apparent why careful examination of the optic nerve is the most important part of the eye examination for glaucoma. A very slight change in the appearance of the optic disk can arouse the physician's suspicion that glaucoma might be present, regardless of what the pressure is in the eye. Further testing and follow-up checks can then be arranged.

A visual field test measures the amount of vision that has been lost.

Visual field testing, also called *perimetry,* is a way of measuring the completeness of the field of vision. When we speak of the visual field, we are talking about the entire area in a person's vision, both centrally (straight ahead) and peripherally (to the side). We often compare the visual field to a mountainous island of vision in a sea of darkness. In the periphery (side) of our visual field, corresponding to the outlying, low areas of the mountain slope, we can make out basic forms and shapes but cannot discern fine details. As we move toward the center of our visual field, climbing up the slope of the mountain toward its peak, our sharpness of vision increases, and we can soon make out every detail in the object at which we're looking. If a trench or a crater occurs in one part of the mountain (loss of optic nerve fibers), we may not be able to see quite as well in one area, and this is what visual field testing measures.

There are two main types of perimeters (visual field testing machines). The first is the *Goldmann perimeter,* which has been the standard for many years. In this type of examination, the patient sits in front of a large white bowl and with his or her gaze fixed on a spot in the center of the bowl. The physician or an assistant causes a white circle of light, the size and brightness of which can be changed, to move along the bowl until the patient signals that it is visible. This process is repeated many times until the field of vision is mapped out. Goldmann perimetry (visual field testing) depends greatly on the skill and knowledge of the examiner. The perimeter is merely a tool in the examiner's hands, much as a scalpel is a tool in the hands of a surgeon.

The newer *computerized perimeters* are now widely used. Rather than using a moving target of light, these machines present the light targets at individual locations on the bowl, varying the brightness to determine how dim the light can be made yet still be seen at each tested point in the field of vision. Computerized perimeters provide important information that has aided in the evaluation and treatment of glaucoma patients. Since they provide somewhat differ-ent information from that of the Goldmann perimeters, we sometimes like to perform

Computerized perimetry has supplanted rather than supplemented Goldmann perimetry.

both types of perimetry on a patient to obtain the most information possible about the patient's condition. Computerized perimetry is usually a more time-consuming examination than Goldmann perimetry and can be harder on people with limited endurance for such testing. Goldmann perimetry can be tailored more easily to the needs of an individual patient since the testing is controlled by a person rather than by a machine. However, most physicians do not want to spend the time performing visual field examinations themselves, and skilled technicians are extremely difficult to find. Therefore, computer-ized perimetry has supplanted rather than supplemented Goldmann perime-try in most medical offices.

The main limitation of perimetry is that a considerable amount of dam-age must occur to the optic nerve before abnormalities of the visual field can be detected. However, perimetry is a sensitive way of following the condition of people who already have blind spots or other defects in their field of vision to make sure that they are not getting worse. In people with elevated eye pres-sures or established glaucoma, regular visual field testing is necessary.

Measurement of the intraocular pressure (IOP), that is, the pressure of the fluid inside the eye, is important for detecting people who are at risk for glaucoma. Since glaucoma treat-ment involves the lowering of IOP, pressure

Goldmann tonometry is the most accurate way to check IOP.

checks at regular intervals are performed to make sure that the IOP is staying low enough. The most accurate method in the doctor's office for determining the IOP is called *Goldmann tonometry*. In this method, a small plastic device is pressed against the cornea and measures just how much pressure it takes to flat-ten the cornea against it. Other methods, such as *noncontact tonometry* (air puff), are not as accurate but are sometimes used to screen people for glaucoma. The IOP ranges from 10 to 21 millimeters of mercury in most normal eyes.

Still another important part of the glaucoma examination is a technique called *gonioscopy*. A special type of lens that allows the physician to look into the part of the eye we call the *angle* is placed over the patient's cornea. This area is the entranceway to the drainage channels (trabecular meshwork) of the eye. Since fluid (aqueous humor) is constantly being pumped into the eye, these drainage channels are important, because they allow the fluid to drain out. If the fluid cannot get to the drainage channels, or if there is a blockage or other form of resistance in those channels, then a buildup

An eye with high pressure is like a sink with a clogged drain and the faucet turned on.

in the fluid pressure of the eye can occur. You can compare it to a sink. If the faucet is turned on but the drain becomes clogged, then the water builds up in the sink. In the case of the sink, the water can simply overflow. However, in the case of the eye, the water has no place to go, so the pressure in the eye rises.

In most people, including those with glaucoma, the angle of the eye is open, and fluid can easily reach the drainage channels. People with glaucoma who have open angles are said to have *chronic open angle glaucoma*. The main risk factors for this type of glaucoma are (1) high intraocular pressure, (2) age (the older you are, the greater the risk), (3) family history of glaucoma, and (4) African American race. Myopic individuals are at slightly higher risk.

In a small percentage of people the angle can be very narrow and can even close down. When that happens, the pressure in the eye rises, resulting in what we call *angle-closure glaucoma*.

There are several types of angle-closure glaucoma. In *acute angle-closure glaucoma*, the angle, which had been open, becomes closed. The pressure, which had been normal, can shoot up to very high levels. Symptoms include pain, redness of the eye, and blurred vision, with halos seen around lights. In *chronic angle-closure glaucoma*, the angle remains partly closed on a continuing basis, resulting in a persistent elevated pressure, although not to the degree seen in acute angle-closure glaucoma. There are usually no symptoms. In *subacute angle-closure glaucoma*, there may be intermittent symptoms resembling those in the acute form. These symptoms may be triggered by certain events, such as sitting in a dark room, which causes the pupil to dilate slightly, and this in turn can cause the angle to close.

The people who are prone to angle-closure glaucoma are those whose eyes have narrow angles to begin with. These are typically hyperopic individuals, who have shorter eyes. Nevertheless, they usually do not get angle-closure glaucoma until middle age or later in life. The reason is that the lens of the eye swells a bit with age and presses on the iris from behind, thereby creating a configuration more prone to closure.

In people with chronic open angle glaucoma the pressure in the eye is high because a form of resistance to flow develops in the

Chronic glaucoma generally causes no symptoms at all.

drainage channels themselves. It is important to distinguish between the closed and open angle forms of glaucoma, because the closed angle variety should be treated surgically (usually with a laser), whereas the open angle variety is treated with medication whenever possible.

Other less common forms of glaucoma exist. These include *congenital* or *infantile glaucoma,* which is diagnosed soon after birth. It is due to certain malformations in the eye and is treated surgically. Another major category of glaucoma is what we call *secondary glaucoma.* This means that the high pressure is the result of some other problem in the eye. Previous injuries to the eye, uveitis, bleeding in the eye, and tumors in the eye are just some possible causes. Treatment is often directed at the underlying condition as well as at the pressure.

Glaucoma Treatment: Control Is the Goal

A high IOP is the main risk factor for glaucoma, and the higher the pressure, the greater the risk. Therefore, lowering the IOP has become the mainstay of glaucoma treatment. If the IOP can be sufficiently lowered, then progression of optic nerve damage can usually be halted. Even in cases of low-tension glaucoma, where the pressures are in the normal range to begin with, lowering the IOP can help. How much the pressure must be lowered is not the same for all individuals. It depends on the level of IOP before treatment and the extent of optic nerve damage. Often, we can only determine what a safe IOP is for a given patient by closely following that patient's condition with optic nerve examinations and visual field tests and making sure that no further damage is occurring at a given level of pressure.

Since optic nerve damage from glaucoma occurs at different pressures in different people, and since many people with glaucoma don't even have truly elevated IOPs, it is clear that many other factors are at play. One of these is blood circulation. People with chronic open angle glaucoma tend to have somewhat poor circulation to certain areas around the optic nerve. Another factor may be the effect of toxic substances, including those produced by the body, on the optic nerve. Researchers are currently trying to find medications that protect the optic nerves from damage—medications that work not by lowering IOP but by other mechanisms. Many drugs and similar substances are being investigated, including nerve regeneration and growth factors, antioxidants and free radical scavengers, calcium channel–blocking agents (currently used for high blood pressure and heart problems), and inhibitors of excitotoxins—chemicals in the nervous system that can have toxic effects. I predict that in ten years, one or more of these medicines will have been shown to be effective and will be on the market.

A given intraocular pressure may cause damage in some people but not in others.

The drugs used to lower IOP in glaucoma patients generally take the form of eyedrops. Several classes of effective drugs are now available. As a result, it is now easier to control IOP. The number of patients requiring laser or surgical treatment has been declining. But all drugs, even eyedrops, can have side effects, both on the eye itself and on the body as a whole. Several studies have now shown that use of glaucoma eyedrops has a negative effect on the front surface of the eye. Some of the cells that produce components of the tear layer are reduced in number by the glaucoma treatment. This can cause a drying out of the front of the eye. The tissues on the eye often show signs of low-grade inflammation (irritation) in people who have been treated for glaucoma for a long time. These effects could possibly lower the chance of success of glaucoma surgery should that ever become necessary, although the effects do tend to wear off after the medication is discontinued. Although the glaucoma drug itself may be contributing to the problem, chemical preservatives such as benzalkonium chloride in the eyedrops are probably the main culprits.

Beta Blockers

The beta blocker class of medications includes timolol (Timoptic), levobunolol (Betagan), betaxolol (Betoptic), carteolol (Ocupress), and metipranolol (Optipranolol). They are often among the first eyedrops to be tried in glaucoma treatment. These drugs lower IOP by reducing the secretion of fluid into the eye. Most of them can trigger asthmatic attacks in susceptible people. Betaxolol is less likely than the others to affect breathing in this way, although its IOP-lowering effect is not quite as great as those of the others.

Beta blockers can also affect the heartbeat, especially in people who have a slowing of the electrical impulses in the heart, a condition called *heart block*. When dealing with elderly individuals, I often call their internist or other primary care physician to make sure that their last electrocardiogram showed no evidence of heart block. Beta blockers can also lower blood levels of HDL cholesterol, the "good" form of cholesterol that reduces the risk of heart disease. Thus, it may be prudent to recheck the cholesterol profile after using a beta blocker for a few months. Carteolol has less effect on HDL cholesterol than the other beta blockers.

Eyedrops, like all drugs, can have side effects.

Other side effects associated with beta blockers include depression, tiredness, weakness, impaired thinking ability, impotence, and periods of lower blood pressure. If you think you are experiencing any of these side effects, report your symptoms to your doctor.

If you already take a beta blocker drug orally for high blood pressure, as some people do, you may not get as much IOP-lowering effect by adding a beta blocker eyedrop as you might obtain otherwise. In such a case, another type of glaucoma eyedrop might be preferable to avoid adding to the quantity of beta blocker in your system.

Epinephrine Compounds

Another class of glaucoma medication is related to the natural hormone adrenaline, also known as *epinephrine*. However, epinephrine eyedrops tend to be quite irritating to the eye, and they could be harmful to people with irregular heartbeats. Dipivifrin (Propine) is an improved form that is better tolerated by the eye and has less of an effect on the rest of the body. My experience has been that it does not lower IOP as well as the beta blockers do, and adding this drop to someone already on a beta blocker does not always provide any additional pressure-lowering effect. Finally, I have found that a significant percentage of people develop an allergy-like sensitivity to this drug after a while and can no longer use it.

Pilocarpine and Related Drugs

Pilocarpine is a drug derived from South American plants and has long been used to treat glaucoma. It belongs to a class of substances that make the pupil of the eye become small. They lower IOP by making it easier for the fluid in the eye to drain out through the drainage channels, perhaps by stretching them open a bit. Blurred vision, poor night vision, and ache around the eye are common side effects. Occasionally, people can develop a sensitivity to pilocarpine, resulting in an inflammatory reaction that in rare cases can even scar shut the channels that drain tears out of the eye. A disadvantage of pilocarpine eyedrops is that they normally have to be instilled four times a day. However, pilocarpine also comes in the form of a gel, which is instilled at bedtime only. Ocusert is a brand that uses an innovative drug delivery system—a thin wafer placed between the eyelid and the eye that gradually releases pilocarpine over a one-week period. The side effects usually seen with pilocarpine are often reduced with this method. It is a good alternative for younger people whose fingers are nimble enough to insert the wafer, but with a little practice, most people can do it. Carbachol is another drug in this class that is less commonly used, and it usually requires instillation three times a day. Rarely used is echothiophate phosphate, a potent twice-a-day eyedrop that can cause cataracts with long-term use.

Apraclonidine and Brimonidine

Apraclonidine (Iopidine) is a newer agent that has been very effective in blunting acute rises of IOP in people undergoing laser treatments and surgery. It is also available to treat open angle glaucoma. Some studies have shown a high incidence of allergic reactions with long-term use. A newer drug in this class is brimonidine (Alphagan), which seems to be much better tolerated over time. Nevertheless, allergic-like sensitivity reactions occur in 5 to 10 percent of people using brimonidine. Feeling tired is an occasional symptom, and development of low blood pressure may occur infrequently. Iritis, an inflammation inside the eye, was recently reported in several patients who had been taking brimonidine.

Carbonic Anhydrase Inhibitors

The orally administered drugs we call *carbonic anhydrase inhibitors* include acetazolamide (Diamox), methazolamide (Neptazane), and one or two lesser used agents. Carbonic anhydrase is an enzyme that helps promote a certain chemical reaction in the body, and these drugs interfere with its action. In the eye, the effect is to decrease the secretion of fluid into the eye. Since they are taken by mouth, they can be associated with many side effects, including lethargy, fatigue, depression, poor appetite, impotence, nausea, diarrhea, and kidney stones. These side effects can make these drugs intolerable to many individuals. Rarely, serious bone marrow problems may also develop, so checking a complete blood count every month or two during the first six months of treatment and every six months thereafter may be advisable. Recently carbonic anhydrase inhibitors called dorzolamide (Trusopt) and brinzolamide (Azopt) were developed. They are used in eyedrop form, thereby reducing the side effects seen with the other drugs. They do not lower IOP quite as much as the oral forms do, however. In one study, dorzolamide appeared to increase blood flow to the eye, a possible benefit.

Prostaglandin Analogues and Related Compounds

For many years, researchers have worked on developing a form of prostaglandin that could be used to treat glaucoma. Prostaglandins are fat-derived chemicals in the body that are important regulators, especially with regard to inflammation and the immune system. Their effects vary, depending on the type of prostaglandin and how much is present in a given tissue of the body. One favorable effect of certain prostaglandins is their ability to lower IOP, which they accomplish by increasing uveoscleral flow, a passive transfer of fluid out of the eye that does not use the drainage channels described earlier. Latanoprost (Xalatan), which is similar to a natural prostaglandin called PGF_{2alpha}, is the first such medication on the market. It can cause some irritability in the eye and increase pigmentation of the iris, turning blue eyes brown. The eyelashes around the treated eye may become darker, thicker, and longer, and more of them may grow in. The skin around the eye can sometimes become darkened as well. So far, this darkening effect on the iris and other tissues does not seem to lead to any more serious problems later on, although time will tell. Latanoprost may have a bit of an inflammatory effect in some people, so that also must be monitored by the ophthalmologist. Latanoprost needs to be instilled only once a day (at bedtime). It appears to be very effective and may even increase blood flow to the eye. Two new drugs in this class, unoprostone (Rescula) and bimatoprost (Lumigam), are now available as well.

Using Glaucoma Medications Effectively

The eyedrop medications used for glaucoma can be used alone or in combination if necessary. If you are scheduled to use more than one eyedrop around the same time, try to separate them by at least five to ten minutes so that the second drop does not wash the first one out. If you are uncertain whether you are getting the drops in your eyes, try keeping the bottles in the refrigerator. You can usually tell when you get a cold drop in your eye.

There are a number of ways to minimize the side effects and maximize the effectiveness of glaucoma eyedrops.

There are a number of useful ways of reducing the amount of eye drop medication absorbed into the circulation, thereby minimizing side effects. First, if a particular medication comes in more than one strength, the weaker strength can often be tried first. In many individuals, it may be just as effective as the stronger strength. Second, although beta blocker eye drops are often prescribed for twice-daily use, once a day use may provide adequate pressure-lowering effect for many people, especially when combined with techniques for maximizing the effect on the eye. One such technique is to simply close your eyes immediately after instilling your eye drops. An even better way is to press with the tip of your finger over the area between the bridge of the nose and the inner corner of your eye. Do this immediately after instilling the eyedrop. These maneuvers keep the eyedrop from entering the tear sac, thereby keeping more of the drop in your eye and allowing less of it to enter your circulation.

Medical treatment controls glaucoma but does not cure it.

In summary, many glaucoma medications are available that, alone or in combination, can lower IOP and help prevent further optic nerve damage and visual field loss. Could we ask for anything more? Well, how about prevention?

Medical treatment does not cure glaucoma; it only controls it. Optic nerve damage sometimes progresses despite apparently successful control of IOP.

Unfortunately, we don't know how to prevent open angle glaucoma; we're not even sure of its cause. Frankly, I can't foresee a preventive measure for glaucoma in the near future. But even if we can't prevent glaucoma, it would be nice to be able to control it more easily, preventing large swings in IOP and using the least medication possible. After all, all drugs have side effects, and glaucoma eyedrops are no exception, as discussed before. Let us take a look, then, at the effects of food and other natural modalities on intraocular pressure and glaucoma.

The Effects of Lifestyle Choices on Glaucoma

The vast majority of the glaucoma research being done revolves around the use of drugs. This is to be expected, since drug companies are motivated by financial considerations to fund research involving the development of new drugs. More governmental support of research would allow other approaches to be tested. Nevertheless, a number of studies over the years provide important clues as to the potential benefits to be derived from certain lifestyle factors.

Exercise

Aerobic exercise (the kind that makes your heart beat more rapidly) can be an important part of healthy living, reducing the risk of heart disease, cancer, and other degenerative ailments. Now, findings from one study point to a beneficial role that such exercise can play in the control of IOP. A small group of sedentary, middle-aged men and women with elevated IOP underwent a program of exercise conditioning using an exercise bike. After three months of such exercise, their average IOP fell by four and one-half points.[1] This is a very significant decrease, almost as much as one might expect from a typical glaucoma eyedrop. These people then stopped exercising and returned to their sedentary lifestyles. Three weeks later, their IOPs had returned to previous levels. A more recent study confirmed these findings. This demonstrates that exercise is an effective means of lowering IOP and can add to the effect of medication or even substitute for medication in mild cases.

I would caution that exercise such as running may cause a temporary rise in pressure in some people who have a less common form of glaucoma known as *pigmentary glaucoma*. The typical patient with this condition is a young, nearsighted male who develops an elevated IOP because of the structure or shape of his eye. Pigment becomes knocked off the back surface of the iris because of friction with the zonules. These dispersed granules of pigment can then clog up the drainage channels of the eye and damage them, resulting in a high IOP. Therefore, check with your physician before embarking on a vigorous exercise program.

Smoking

People with glaucoma sometimes ask whether smoking has any effect on the disease process. Cigarette smoke contains nicotine, a stimulant that can affect blood flow. A recent study has shown, in fact, that blood flow to the eye is reduced in smokers. Further, long-term smoking is known to damage both small and large blood vessels. Therefore, if poor blood circulation to the optic nerve speeds up the optic nerve damage in people who have glaucoma, then smoking could have a negative effect. Studies in this area have yielded conflicting results, however, so we can't draw any definite conclusions. My own feeling is that we will eventually find that smoking increases the risk of glaucoma in one way or another. Since the final word is not yet in, should we advise people with glaucoma not to smoke? Absolutely. Everyone should be advised not to smoke. With a mile-long list of reasons not to smoke, we don't really need another reason to recommend quitting.

Coffee

How about that common but questionably harmful addiction, caffeine consumption? Ever since the early part of the twentieth century, caffeine has been suspected of raising IOP. Some people have even recommended that it be used as a test for glaucoma, the idea being that a greater pressure rise would be seen in eyes susceptible to glaucoma than in normal eyes. The test did not prove to be of value. In one study, a large pressure rise was seen in only a small proportion of eyes in people known to have glaucoma.[2] Coffee drinking would be expected to provide even less caffeine than the amount used in these studies. In another study of glaucoma patients who drank either coffee or herbal tea, the pressure rise in the coffee drinkers was so slight as to be insignificant. In other words, it was not enough to cause any acceleration of optic nerve damage. It does not appear, then, that caffeine causes any significant change in IOP.

What, then, should we advise glaucoma patients about drinking coffee? I would advise caution for two reasons. First, even if coffee drinking in the average person does not cause much of a rise in IOP, it is possible that a few individuals might respond with a larger than average rise, and you never know whether you might be one of those individuals. This could indeed be harmful, because in the treatment of glaucoma, we always try to keep the pressure under control twenty-four hours a day. Even a temporary rise in pressure could be harmful. Therefore, it might be useful for glaucoma patients who drink coffee to have their IOP checked within an hour after drinking a cup or two. Only then will they know whether it makes any real difference in their own cases.

Caffeine reduces circulation to the areas around the optic nerve.

Second, whether coffee drinking affects IOP or not, we might also want to consider its effects on the optic nerve. At a given level of pressure control, does caffeine consumption in the form of coffee drinking increase the risk of progressive optic nerve damage and visual field loss? The answer to this question is not known, but one study did evaluate the effect of caffeine on the circulation of the macula. As mentioned before, some glaucoma patients tend to have reduced circulation to certain areas around the optic nerve, including the macula. This study found that consumption of the amount of caffeine in one cup of coffee caused an average 13 percent reduction in blood flow in the macula.[3] This may have been due to blood vessel constriction induced by the caffeine. Since lessening the circulation around the optic nerve may worsen optic nerve damage in people with glaucoma, this study provides some cause for concern. Because of the uncertainty, my recommendation to glaucoma patients is to avoid caffeine-containing coffee.

Water

Any liquid consumed in quantity can raise IOP. It has been known for almost a hundred years that drinking a quart of water at one sitting can make IOP go up, especially in people who have a tendency toward elevated pressures to begin with. This finding became the basis for the water-loading test, which was supposed to help detect people with high pressures who were most at risk to develop glaucoma. (Recall that not everyone with high IOP has glaucoma.) People would drink a quart of water and then have their pressures checked every fifteen minutes for one to two hours. Unfortunately, the test did not prove to have good predictive value with regard to the likelihood of developing glaucoma and has been abandoned. What we can learn from this is that glaucoma patients should refrain from drinking more than a pint of liquid at one time (unless they live in the desert and need to avoid dehydration!).

Alcohol

People who drink alcohol do not appear to be at increased risk for open angle glaucoma, and people with elevated IOP but no optic nerve damage are not at any increased risk to develop glaucoma-related optic nerve damage as compared with nondrinkers. In fact, alcohol can actually lower IOP. After drinking whiskey or even beer, the fall in IOP can be quite significant, especially in people with open angle glaucoma. Some people have speculated that alcohol might accomplish this by its effect on the pituitary gland, the "master gland" of the brain. However, alcohol was shown to lower IOP in a man whose pituitary gland had previously been surgically removed, so this cannot be the whole story. Alcohol most likely exerts its effect by virtue of what we call an *osmotic effect*. This means that the alcohol molecules cause a drawing out of water from the eye, resulting in a lowered pressure. The effect can last for two to three hours. Obviously, we cannot recommend heavy alcohol consumption as a way to keep IOP low, but it does suggest a way of rapidly lowering IOP at times that it is dangerously elevated, although other methods are also available. It also suggests that if you are about to undergo a pressure check on your eyes, you should refrain from alcohol consumption for the preceding three hours so that a reliable and representative measurement of the IOP can be obtained.

Vitamin C

Another substance that can lower IOP by an osmotic effect is ascorbic acid, better known as vitamin C. Early reports indicated that megadoses of vitamin C, given either intravenously or by mouth, could cause large drops in IOP. Some of these studies used doses by mouth as large as 35 grams. (That's about 400 times the current recommended dietary allowance!) Clearly, such a dose is impractical and likely to have pronounced side effects. More reasonable is the dosage of 500 milligrams four times a day used in a Swedish study of twenty-five patients with ocular hypertension (elevated IOP). An average drop in pressure of only a little over 1 millimeter of mercury was recorded. Such a minimal decrease is meaningless from a practical standpoint. Nevertheless, it is certainly possible that a few individuals might be unusually responsive to the effects of vitamin C and might benefit from treatment. The only way to know is to try it and have the IOP checked about two hours after a dose.

Vitamin B$_1$

The possible role of thiamin (vitamin B$_1$) deficiency in glaucoma was investigated in one study because low body levels of thiamin can cause optic nerve deterioration. A group of glaucoma patients was compared with a similar group of people who did not have glaucoma. Blood levels of thiamin were measured, and dietary histories were taken. The study found no difference between the two groups in terms of the amount of thiamin they obtained from food, but the glaucoma patients did have lower blood levels of thiamin than the controls. It is hard to know what to make of this study, as it suggests that glaucoma patients may have some problem with their body chemistry or some absorption problem that affects the amount of thiamin in their bodies. Unfortunately, no further studies were ever done to confirm these findings. Therefore, no recommendations about thiamin supplementation can be made at this time.

Rutin and Pilocarpine

In the late 1940s, Dr. Frederick Stocker of Duke University began looking for new and unusual approaches to treating glaucoma. He performed studies on what we call the *blood-aqueous barrier* in the eye. The blood-aqueous barrier refers to the finding that as blood travels through the part of the eye called the *ciliary body,* a filtration process occurs. A watery fluid (aqueous humor) is secreted into the eye, but because of the blood-aqueous barrier, many substances from the blood are kept out of the eye. Inflammation and certain chemicals or drugs can cause a breakdown of this blood-aqueous barrier, however. When that happens, protein and other substances from the blood enter the eye, and sometimes the ability of the fluid to drain out of the eye becomes compromised, resulting in a rise of the IOP. Dr. Stocker knew that pilocarpine, one of the medicines used to treat glaucoma, can break down the blood-aqueous barrier somewhat, and he was concerned that this might interfere with the pressure-lowering effect of pilocarpine in some of his patients.

He looked at ways of restoring a broken-down blood-aqueous barrier to its normal state. One group of substances he studied was the flavonoid group. *Flavonoids* are a diverse group of chemicals present in foods, and many of them have antioxidant, anti-inflammatory, and other properties. Unlike vitamins, there is no recognized minimum requirement in the diet for flavonoids, although in the past they have sometimes been referred to as vitamin P. At one time, physicians could prescribe flavonoid preparations. The FDA (Food and Drug Administration) decided that there was no proof that flavonoids were beneficial, so it put an end to that. Not to worry— you can still get them as a supplement over the counter.

Flavonoids are plant-derived chemicals that are not currently recognized as vitamins.

Dr. Stocker did some studies on a flavonoid called *rutin* and found evidence that it could restore the blood-aqueous barrier broken down by medications. He also found other flavonoids to be promising. The next step was to use rutin in a group of glaucoma patients being treated with pilocarpine. He first used 20 milligrams three times a day and, in other studies, increased the dosage to 50 milligrams three times a day. He found a pressure-lowering effect that he attributed to the rutin, and he felt the effect was most marked in patients in whom pilocarpine had produced the least lowering of pressure. Further studies were promised but apparently never done.

My own clinical experience with rutin in pilocarpine users has been limited and inconclusive. If there is a beneficial effect, it might also be seen with other drugs in pilocarpine's class, such as carbachol and echothiophate iodide (Phospholine Iodide). Since the use of a rutin supplement seems harmless enough, it would certainly be worth a try.

Meals and Diurnal Rhythm

The timing of meals may actually play an important role in the fluctuations of IOP during the day. Over eighty-five years ago, Dr. Carlo Pissarello, an Italian physician, performed studies on the different factors that might affect the IOP over the course of a day. It has long been known that people have what is called a *diurnal rhythm* to their IOP, which means that the IOP may be higher or lower at certain times of the day. Experience has shown that IOP is often highest right after awakening in the morning. Dr. Pissarello studied this rhythm in patients with different types of glaucoma.[4]

Your pressure may be lowest right after you eat and highest just before you eat.

He made a very interesting observation. The IOP tended to be higher before meals but lower right after meals. This could certainly help explain why the IOP in many people is highest early in the morning before breakfast, as the overnight period generally represents the longest period of abstention from food over a twenty-four-hour period. This finding also suggests some intriguing possibilities. For example, could a "grazing" type of diet, in which one eats perhaps six small meals a day rather than three large ones, help keep the IOP under better control? Grazing diets may actually be a more natural type of diet, and they have already been found to be beneficial in weight loss and cholesterol-lowering programs.

The concept of the timing of meals and its relation to IOP has not been adequately studied, and there have been conflicting opinions. Sir Stewart Duke-Elder, a renowned English ophthalmologist, stated that he did not feel that the daily rhythm of IOP was related to the intake of food, but he did not cite any studies to bolster his position. Dr. H.-J. Merté, the director of a university eye clinic in Germany, reported that the intake of food could indeed cause a change in the IOP rhythm in eyes without glaucoma, but he did not find a consistent pattern in the eyes of people with glaucoma.

In my own experience, I have had the distinct clinical impression that the timing of meals does influence the IOP. I have often measured patients whom I've suspected of having swings of IOP both before and after lunch, and occasionally early in the morning before breakfast. I want to be sure that their pressures are under good control at all times. Whether you have glaucoma or just ocular hypertension, you might want to have your pressure checked before breakfast while you are "at your worst."

The Rice Diet

Now that we've discussed the timing of meals, how about food choices? Do specific foods have any effect on IOP? Again we must turn to an interesting study performed by Dr. Stocker and his colleagues. At that time, Dr. Walter Kempner, an internal medicine specialist at Duke University, had devised a diet called the "rice diet" for his patients with hard-to-control high blood pressure. The diet was limited to rice (brown or white), sugar, fruit, and fruit juices, and it was supplemented with vitamins and iron. This diet provided much less protein than the recommended dietary allowance. Only 2.5 percent of calories came from fat, and there was minimal sodium and chloride (salt). An impressive lowering of blood pressure was achieved, and, as an added bonus, blood cholesterol levels dropped by an average of 25 percent.

Dr. Stocker decided to see what effect this diet would have on the IOP in a group of people without glaucoma. He reported that right after beginning the rice diet, these people showed a striking reduction in IOP. He

The rice diet, ultralow in fat, produced striking reductions in pressure.

commonly observed long-lasting reductions in pressure in the range of 5 to 7 millimeters of mercury.[5] He was hard pressed to explain the phenomenon, but he guessed that the ultralow salt content (0.2 grams of sodium a day) of the diet might have been the factor responsible for lowering the IOP. Further studies on glaucoma patients were never performed.

There may be a better explanation for the apparent effect of the rice diet on IOP, based on the results of a study reported by two Israeli researchers. They studied twenty-eight patients who, because of various intestinal problems, were placed on intravenous feedings only. For about seven weeks, the intravenous fluids contained no fat, after which the fluids were supplemented with fat as they normally are. Intraocular pressures were checked on a regular basis before treatment and during both phases of the intravenous feedings. The researchers found that the IOP was significantly lower during the fat-free phase than during the fat-supplemented phase (about three and one-half points, on the average).[6] It appears that something about the lack of fat had a lowering effect on IOP.

During the various parts of this study, blood levels of a prostaglandin called PGE$_2$ were also measured. *Prostaglandins* are substances that our bodies produce from certain fats, and they have a wide array of actions, affecting virtually every bodily function. As mentioned earlier, some prostaglandins have been found to lower IOP, and one form of prostaglandin is now being used in eyedrop form to treat glaucoma. These researchers found that the blood levels of PGE_2 during the fat-free phase were just half those seen during the fat-supplemented phase. They felt that this drop in prostaglandin levels might have been responsible for the lower IOPs. How can this be if prostaglandin eyedrops, which raise the levels of prostaglandins in the eye, lower the IOP? We can't say for sure why the IOPs were lowered, but the findings are not necessarily contradictory. Prostaglandins are tricky substances, and their actions can differ depending on their concentration in a given tissue. It is entirely possible that both raising and lowering prostaglandin levels in the eye from their baseline levels could bring the IOP down.

Getting back to the rice diet study, one of the remarkable aspects of that diet was that only about 2.5 percent of the calories it supplied came from fat. This level of fat intake is certainly low enough to create a fatty acid deficiency (there is a requirement for small amounts of fat in the diet), which in turn could lower prostaglandin levels. Therefore, I suggest that the rice diet might lower IOP not because of its low salt content but as a result of its extremely low fat content. Naturally, this is only an educated guess, but further studies in this area could provide some answers. The rice diet does not appear to be nutritionally adequate on a long-term basis, and I definitely don't recommend your trying it on your own. It would be interesting, however, to see whether diets that are not quite so stringent might also have a favorable effect on the IOP. Vegetarian diets deriving about 10 percent of their calories from fat have enjoyed much success in lowering blood cholesterol levels and reversing coronary heart disease, so perhaps we should give them a try in glaucoma patients as well.

Blood Flow, Omega-3 Fatty Acids, and Ginkgo Biloba

Current glaucoma treatment involves lowering the IOP, but trying to preserve the optic nerve by other means, such as improving blood flow (circulation) to the optic nerve and to the area around it, may be the next great advance. Some studies have compared the blood viscosity in patients with glaucoma to that of people without glaucoma. *Viscosity* can be thought of as the "thickness" of the blood. Blood with high viscosity travels more slowly through small blood vessels than does blood of lower viscosity. Thus, circulation might be impaired when blood viscosity is high. These studies

Lowering blood viscosity may promote better circulation to the optic nerve.

have found that patients with glaucoma, including the low-tension variety, have blood with significantly higher viscosity than people with normal eyes or people with elevated IOP but no sign of optic nerve damage.[7,8] This suggests why some people with elevated IOP may develop optic nerve damage while others do not.

The most common reasons why some people have a high blood viscosity are a very high red blood cell count or very high levels of proteins in the blood. However, another factor that can play a role is the flexibility of red blood cells, which we call *erythrocyte deformability*.

When the blood cells are able to "flex" more easily, they are able to flow more easily through tiny blood vessels. Taking dietary supplements of omega-3 polyunsaturated fatty acids (a type of building block of fat) causes a significant lowering of blood viscosity, apparently by increasing the erythrocyte deformability. Flaxseed oil and fish oils are especially rich in these fatty acids. Therefore, consuming these oils may lower blood viscosity and improve circulation to the optic nerve and elsewhere.

Eskimos, whose diets are very rich in these omega-3 fatty acids, have an extremely low incidence of open angle glaucoma, and this fact has led some people to speculate that the omega-3 fatty acids are protective in this respect. However, many other tribes of Native Americans, whose diets are much lower in omega-3 fatty acids than those of Eskimos, also have an extremely low incidence of open angle glaucoma. Therefore, it is likely that the low incidence in Eskimos has a genetic basis.

Omega-3 fatty acids, ginkgo biloba, and a healthy lifestyle (diet and exercise) all lower blood viscosity.

The use of omega-3 fatty acid supplements in patients with glaucoma has never been evaluated in any formal study. Nevertheless, the possibility of protecting the optic nerve in glaucoma patients in this manner is intriguing. Omega-3 fatty acid supplementation for other conditions, such as heart disease and rheumatoid arthritis, has been studied to some degree, but the long-term effects of such supplementation, both good and bad, remain to be determined.

Scientists are now beginning to produce pure preparations of long-chain omega-3 fatty acids, for example, from bacteria or algae, so this type of supplementation may become a reality, allowing people to avoid unwanted fatty acids and other substances present in the fish oils, the most common source of omega-3 fatty acids. Since questions remain about the long-term safety of fish oil and other omega-3 fatty acid supplements, however, I do not recommend their use at present.

Another substance that has been shown in many studies to lower blood viscosity is an herbal extract of the plant ginkgo biloba. This extract, which contains many components, has already been under consideration as a possible aid to glaucoma treatment because of the potent antioxidants in it. (Antioxidants may help protect the optic nerve, although this is unproven.) This extract also contains *bilo-balide,* a substance that may help protect nerve tissue from damage. But the

Ginkgo biloba increases blood flow to the eye.

extract's main value may be its ability to increase circulation to areas that need it. A recent study showed that taking ginkgo biloba causes a significant increase in blood flow through the ophthalmic artery (the artery that supplies blood to the eye).[9] Ginkgo biloba is one of the most frequently prescribed medications in Germany and France, where it has been found effective in improving mental functioning in the elderly, reducing dizziness and tinnitis (ringing in the ears), and lessening the symptoms of claudication (inability to walk more than a short distance because of poor leg circulation).

Ginkgo biloba's lowering of blood viscosity may be the means by which it increases blood flow to the eye and other organs. Ginkgo biloba is remarkably free of side effects, but the effects of long-term use have not been fully evaluated. Because it has a mild effect on platelets, the tiny fragments in the blood that prevent bleeding, it should not be used in people who have bleeding tendencies or in people who take the drug warfarin (Coumadin), which affects blood clotting. Actually, this effect on blood platelets could in itself help improve circulation. Although sold by prescription in Europe, ginkgo biloba (Ginkgold and others) is available as an over-the-counter supplement in the United States. Ginkgo biloba appears to have great promise in the treatment of glaucoma, especially the low-tension variety, in which the amount of blood flow to the optic nerve may be critical.

Finally, there is evidence that both exercise and a high-fiber, low-fat diet can lower blood viscosity. In particular, vegetarians, who abstain from beef, fowl, and fish, have been found to have significantly lower blood viscosities than meat eaters, including people who consume animal flesh less than once a week. Exercise and the rice diet, a form of high-fiber, low-fat vegetarian diet, have already been discussed as ways of lowering IOP, but their effects on blood viscosity represent another mechanism by which they may protect the optic nerve in people with glaucoma. Whether a low-fat vegetarian diet can help keep your pressures down or retard the progression of your glaucoma remains to be seen, but such a diet is certainly associated with benefits from a general health standpoint.

Glaucoma Surgery

Angle-Closure Glaucoma

Normally, we think of surgery as a last resort. However, for angle-closure glaucoma, it is the treatment of choice. When a person presents with the red, painful eye and extremely high pressures of acute angle-closure glaucoma, the first order of business is to "break" the attack. Pilocarpine and other pressure-lowering drops are instilled in the involved eye, and substances called *osmotic agents* are given either by mouth or intravenously. These sub-

An iridotomy is performed to treat or prevent angle-closure glaucoma.

stances enter the bloodstream and tend to draw fluid out of the eye, a process that breaks the attack most of the time. Once the attack is broken, we generally let the eye "cool" down for several days before performing an *iridotomy*, the creation of a small hole in the iris of the eye. This hole is usually created with a laser, either an argon laser, which burns a hole in the iris, or a neodymium: YAG laser, which causes a miniexplosion that results in the tiny hole. This hole allows fluid to travel from the area behind the iris to the area in front, thereby bypassing the pupil and deepening the anterior chamber of the eye and allowing the angle to open up. In addition, an iridotomy is usually performed on the other eye as well. Why? Because both eyes usually have the same shape and structure, and if an attack of acute angle-closure glaucoma has occurred in one eye, there is a good chance it will occur in the other. This type of preventive treatment is important, because an attack of acute glaucoma can sometimes cause irreversible damage to the eye.

Occasionally, we may even perform a laser iridotomy before an attack of glaucoma has ever occurred. For example, if a person who is found to have narrow angles on examination also has a history of occasional eye pain and blurring after sitting in a dark room, we may suspect that intermittent mini-attacks are occurring. In such a situation, we might even instill (very cautiously) a very mild dilating eyedrop in one eye to see whether a pressure rise can be induced. If the person is felt to be at significant risk for the development of angle-closure glaucoma, an iridotomy can be performed. Be forewarned, however: Laser iridotomy, like any surgical procedure, may be recommended inappropriately by some surgery-hungry physicians.

Chronic angle-closure glaucoma does not present with a hot, inflamed eye, so the laser iridotomy can be performed at any time. If, for some reason, a patient cannot sit still to have a laser treatment, the procedure can also be performed by conventional surgery.

Why Not Treat with Medication?

It is true that glaucoma eyedrops may bring the pressure down to an acceptable level, just as they do in people who have chronic open angle glaucoma. However, permanent damage to the drainage channels of the eye may occur in a partially closed angle if steps are not taken to open it back up right away. As a result, laser iridotomy may not be completely successful in restoring the pressure to normal if the angle has remained partially closed for a long time.

Chronic Open Angle Glaucoma

Chronic open angle glaucoma is treated with medication for as long as the medication keeps the pressure under adequate control. However, if the pressure does not hold at a safe level despite all attempts to control it with medication, or if a patient does not take the eyedrops as prescribed, then surgery is necessary. (Some ophthalmologists may perform laser or other surgery before this point is reached, but I don't recommend it.)

The first approach is generally *argon laser trabeculoplasty*. In this simple office procedure, the laser is used to create multiple tiny burn spots all around the trabecular meshwork, the area of the drainage channels inside the eye. The burned areas contract as they heal, and this stretches open the drainage channels, thereby allowing fluid to drain out of the eye more easily. On the average, the pressure is lowered about 7 millimeters of mercury, and the results may be long lasting. Generally, only about half of the trabecular meshwork is treated at a session, so the procedure can be repeated at least once if necessary. The results are usually better in people who have not undergone cataract surgery in the past. Only rarely may the pressure end up worse in the long term. In the short term, a pressure rise is a common complication. If the ophthalmologist checks the intraocular pressure an hour or two after the procedure, a high pressure can be detected right away and treated. Instilling a drop of apraclonidine (Iopidine), a pressure-lowering medication, at the time of the surgery is also helpful in blunting any pressure spikes.

If the pressure cannot be controlled even with laser trabeculoplasty, something more needs to be done. If a significant cataract in the eye is affecting vision and it is clear that cataract surgery would have been required in the not-too-distant future anyway, then doing cataract surgery at this point is a way of lowering the pressure further. When done correctly, cataract surgery alone

Cataract surgery by itself often produces lasting reductions in pressure.

often produces a striking reduction in intraocular pressure, and one or more of the glaucoma medications being used can often be discontinued. In many cases, this is preferable to combining cataract surgery with glaucoma surgery, because the risks associated with the combined procedure are definitely higher.

Conventional surgery for open angle glaucoma is called a *trabeculectomy* or *filtering procedure*. This operation is performed in the operating room, usually under local anesthesia (an injection through the skin below the eye to numb the nerves going to the eye). A very narrow piece of sclera is removed close to the point where the cornea of the eye begins. This creates a passageway through which the fluid inside the eye can bypass the usual drainage channels and exit the eye. The fluid forms under the conjunctiva, forming a shallow, blisterlike elevation called a *bleb*. From there, the fluid is gradually absorbed into the circulation. If the surgery is completely successful, the intraocular pressure remains under good control without medication. If it is partially successful, glaucoma medication may still be needed later on, but the pressure is much lower than it was before the surgery.

As with all surgery, complications can occur. Infection inside the eye is a rare problem but threatens the vision and the eye itself. Sometimes the surgery may not work because a good bleb does not form, and in this situation, the pressure in the eye remains high, just as it was before the surgery. In other cases, fluid may leave the eye too readily, resulting in a pressure that is too low accompanied by a shallowing or even flattening of the anterior chamber of the eye. This problem may be caused by creating a surgical opening that is too large or by a leak through the conjunctiva. Of course, procedures exist for handling these problems, but sometimes additional surgery is necessary. Suffice it to say, filtering procedures should be done only on people who really need it.

When filtering procedures are unsuccessful or cannot be done for one reason or another, procedures that partially destroy the ciliary body, which produces the aqueous humor, can be performed. One of these, *cyclocryotherapy,* involves application of an extremely cold probe to the outside of the eye over the area of the ciliary body. This procedure can cause a fair amount of inflammation in the eye, and there is the danger that too much of the ciliary body will be destroyed, resulting in an eye with little or no pressure, which can cause the demise of the eye.

Summary

Glaucoma is a chronic degeneration of the optic nerve, whose main risk factor is a high IOP. Although the cause of glaucoma is unknown, it can be treated by drugs, usually in the form of eyedrops, which lower the pressure. These drops have an array of possible side effects. Very little research has been done to explore nutritional and other lifestyle factors that can affect IOP or that can prevent damage to the optic nerve more directly.

Engaging in aerobic exercise, the kind that gets you huffing and puffing, on a regular basis can cause a moderate decline in IOP and possibly reduce the need for medication. It may also reduce blood viscosity and thereby improve circulation to the area around the optic nerve. Therefore, exercise is good for your eyes as well as for your heart and lungs.

A few studies have suggested a relationship between smoking and glaucoma, but proof is lacking. Nevertheless, poor blood circulation to the optic nerve may predispose it to damage, so anything that can lead to poor circulation (including smoking) should be discouraged. Although chronic alcoholism is associated with nutritional deficiencies that cause the optic nerve to deteriorate, alcohol consumption in moderation is not considered a risk factor for glaucoma. In fact, drinking an alcoholic beverage can cause a transient lowering of IOP.

Drinking a large quantity (over a pint) of any liquid all at once can raise IOP, especially in people with higher pressures. The need for glaucoma patients to keep their IOP under good control at all times makes this an important consideration. Caffeine consumption in the form of coffee produces only a minimal rise of IOP in the average person, although some people may be more susceptible to its effects than others. Caffeine can also reduce the circulation to the eye, an action that could have a negative impact on the health of the optic nerve.

Vitamin C in moderately high doses causes just a slight lowering of IOP in the average person. As with caffeine, though, we have to consider the possibility that a small percentage of people may show a very good response, so it may be worth trying. One study found that glaucoma patients had lower blood levels of vitamin B_1 than did people without glaucoma, but the significance of this finding is unknown. We do not know whether taking thiamin supplements would be of any benefit. Rutin, which is not a vitamin but a flavonoid found in certain plants, may help lower IOP in some but not all patients taking pilocarpine or related drugs for their glaucoma.

People with glaucoma may have higher blood viscosity (thickness) than people without glaucoma. Therefore, substances that reduce blood viscosity and increase the flow of blood to the optic nerve may be useful. Omega-3 fatty acids (from flaxseed oil, fish oil, and other sources) and the herbal extract ginkgo biloba are both able to lower blood viscosity and may eventually prove useful in protecting the optic nerve from glaucomatous damage. A healthy diet and exercise can do the same. Ginkgo biloba was recently shown to increase blood flow to the eye.

The IOP over the course of a day may be affected by the timing of meals. The pressures are often higher just before meals and lower afterward. This tempts us to speculate that small, frequent meals might be more beneficial than the usual two or three large meals a day. An ultralow-fat diet may lower intraocular pressures, but how restrictive the fat intake needs to be to accomplish this remains to be determined.

Surgery, by either laser or conventional means, is the treatment of choice for angle-closure glaucoma (iridotomy) but is more of a last resort in open angle glaucoma (laser trabeculoplasty and filtering procedures).

Recommendations

Since glaucoma is a silent disease whose incidence increases with age, regular examinations by a competent ophthalmologist are necessary both for detection and for control. Prescribed medications should be used exactly as directed, and any adverse reactions should be reported to your physician. Other recommendations are as follows:

1. Avoid drinking more than two cups of water or other liquid over a short time.
2. Limit or avoid consumption of caffeine-containing coffee.
3. Alcohol consumption is all right in moderation, but try to avoid it for several hours before a pressure check.
4. Don't even think about smoking!
5. Try taking vitamin C, 500 milligrams four times a day, and continue it only if a pressure check shows that the pressure has been significantly lowered. Avoid vitamin C, however, if you have a history of calcium oxalate kidney stones.
6. If you use pilocarpine in any form as treatment for glaucoma, try taking rutin, 50 milligrams three times a day, and continue it if it lowers your pressure.
7. Consider taking ginkgo biloba extract (Ginkgold), 60 milligrams twice a day. Do not take it if you have a bleeding tendency or if you take the drug Coumadin. Aspirin and vitamin E can also increase your bleeding tendency.
8. Begin a program of aerobic exercise, such as stationary bike riding, if your physical condition permits it and your physician approves it.
9. Make the transition to a low-fat (maximum 15 percent of calories), plant-based diet, rich in fresh fruits and vegetables, whole grains, and occasional nuts and seeds. Multiple, small meals over the course of a day are ideal.

CHAPTER ELEVEN

Diabetes

*D*IABETES MELLITUS, A DISEASE MARKED BY HIGH BLOOD SUG-
ars, is caused by either a lack of insulin or resistance to its
action. It takes its toll on the entire body by affecting the blood vessels of the
heart, kidneys, brain, and legs. It can also affect nearly every part of the eye.
Diabetes has become an epidemic in Western countries.

We generally recognize two main types of diabetes. *Insulin-dependent diabetes mellitus* (IDDM) usually begins in childhood and requires insulin injections. In some people, the blood sugar is relatively easy to control, while in
others, so-called *brittle diabetics,* the blood sugars may be wild and unpredictable. This type of diabetes is caused by the destruction of the cells of the
pancreas that manufacture insulin. An autoimmune type of reaction, in which
the body's immune system turns against itself, is felt to be responsible. Infants
who are breast-fed appear to be at reduced
risk, and some studies have indicated that
cow's milk proteins may play a role in triggering the disease.[1,2]

*Adult-onset diabetes
is almost unheard of in
countries where people
eat high-fiber diets.*

Non-insulin-dependent diabetes mellitus
(NIDDM) is the adult-onset form and is usu-
ally treated by diet alone or in conjunction with pills. It is characterized by a
resistance of the body to the effects of insulin. Some think of it as the milder
of the two types of diabetes, but the same complications affecting life and limb

(literally) occur in both forms of the disease. About 80 percent of people with NIDDM are obese. A high-calorie, high-fat, low-fiber, meat-based diet is the cause. Not surprisingly, the disease is often accompanied by high blood pressure and high blood cholesterol and triglyceride levels, since these problems have the same dietary risk factors as diabetes. This deadly combination greatly increases the risk of heart disease and stroke in the diabetic patient. It is interesting to note that in developing countries where a high-fiber, low-fat diet is still routine, adult-onset diabetes is virtually unheard of. Even in the United States, Seventh Day Adventists, about half of whom are vegetarian, are reported to have only half the death rate from diabetes as the rest of the population.

Complications of Diabetes

The many complications of diabetes are related to the duration of the disease (the longer you've had diabetes, the greater the risk) and to how well blood sugar has been controlled over the years. These complications include heart disease, stroke, kidney disease leading to failure, circulation problems in the limbs, nerve dysfunction in the limbs and elsewhere, increased susceptibility to infection, poorer and slower healing, and various eye problems. Diabetics who have maintained tight control of their blood sugars by complying with dietary and medical measures are at much lower risk than people who have not. A blood test called

Diet is the keystone of treatment.

hemoglobin A_{1c}, which measures linkages between hemoglobin and sugar in red blood cells, indicates how well blood sugar has been controlled in the recent past.

Diet is the keystone of diabetes treatment. The proper choice of foods can keep blood sugar and cholesterol levels down and minimize the complications of the disease. But the benefits of the ideal dietary approach go far beyond this. Appropriate food choices can prevent the vast majority of cases of adult-onset diabetes. Not only that, the disease can actually be reversed in many people who already carry the diagnosis. Clearly, nutrition is of paramount importance in the prevention and control of diabetes.

There is no one diet best for all people who have diabetes. But for most NIDDM patients and many IDDM patients, a high–complex carbohydrate (starch), high-fiber, low-protein, low-fat diet seems to be the ideal for keeping blood sugars under optimal control and reducing the risk of diabetic complications. We're talking about a plant-based diet featuring whole grains that derives 70 to 80 percent of its calories from carbohydrate. The number of calories per day is tailored to the individual patient. This type of diet is similar to that of people in countries with very low rates of adult-onset diabetes. Foods that raise blood sugar the least, such as legumes (beans and peas), pasta, apples, oranges, and sweet potatoes, are emphasized. Smaller, more frequent meals can also improve blood sugar control. Sugar consumption should be kept fairly low, since sugars in the diet can raise blood triglyceride levels. Triglycerides are fats that increase the risk of blood vessel disease, and diabetics often have high levels of these fats. Some researchers have also expressed concern that sugars might participate in an oxidation type of chemical reaction with proteins that may lead to aging changes or diabetic complications.

A number of medical and lifestyle programs have used this high-fiber, high-carbohydrate, low-fat dietary regimen with great success. Many NIDDM patients lose the need for medication altogether. Insulin-requiring diabetic patients can also do quite well, maintaining good blood sugar control and reducing the amount of insulin they must take.[3]

Some doctors have achieved satisfactory results with diets that are fairly high in fat—for example, those including a lot of olive oil. Those doctors usually recommend these diets because they don't feel that a low-fat diet is palatable and acceptable to most people. However, the taste for fat is largely an acquired taste. If given encouragement and cooking suggestions, most people adapt quite well to what seems at first to be a radical change. A low-fat diet also helps with weight loss, which is especially important for most patients with NIDDM.

A good diet has allowed some diabetics to discard their medications.

A warning, though. People who have diabetes, especially people taking insulin, should not change their diets without the advice and consent of their physicians. A dietary change in people on medication could result in a severe bottoming out of the blood sugar, which could have very serious consequences. If diabetic patients improve their diets, their physicians may have to lower their medication dose at the same time to prevent abnormally low blood sugars from occurring. I would also stress once more that there is no one diet ideal for all people who have diabetes. The care of a diabetic patient needs to be tailored to the individual. What improves diabetic control in one individual may worsen it in another. Flexibility is needed.

The Eye: The Body's Showcase for Diabetic Complications

Diabetes can affect the entire eye. The cornea can be involved in various ways. It is normally exquisitely sensitive to touch. In people who have diabetes, however, sensation can become reduced as a result of diabetic neuropathy, the effect of diabetes on the nerves of the body. Also, the cells on the surface of the cornea (epithelial cells) may not stick as tightly to the deeper layers as they should, so scratches or other defects in the cornea are more common, and healing tends to be delayed. The cells that line the back surface of the cornea (endothelial cells) and keep the fluid inside the eye from clouding the cornea are also less healthy in people who have diabetes. As a result, the ophthalmologist sometimes sees tiny wrinkles on the back surface of the cornea.

Occasionally, middle-aged and elderly diabetics suddenly develop double vision, sometimes accompanied by a headache. This is the result of closure of the small blood vessels that nourish any of three major nerves that control eye muscle movement. Fortunately, the double vision usually goes away within three months. Nevertheless, double vision can sometimes be due to other problems, such as aneurysms (weakened, dilated blood vessels) or tumors in the brain, so anyone who develops double vision should have it checked out right away. Some diabetics who have periods of very low blood sugar may transiently complain of light flashes or double vision during these periods, but the visual complaints go away as soon as the blood sugar level is brought up to normal.

Cataract occurs more frequently and at a younger age in diabetics than in nondiabetics. Changes in blood sugar levels result in changes in the amount of sugar inside the lens, and repeated insults of this kind over time may lead to cataract development. A recent study has shown that when the blood sugar is brought down too rapidly in a diabetic who is out of control, some permanent clouding of the lens may occur. Glaucoma may be a little more frequent in people with diabetes as well.

Large swings in blood sugar may cause the vision to blur.

Blurred vision is a frequent complaint in people who have IDDM, especially in people who have large swings in blood sugar and whose diabetes has just been diagnosed. Generally, this occurs because sugar gets into the lens of the eye, drawing fluid into the lens along with it. This imbibing or drawing in of fluid by the lens makes it swell. Since the lens does the focusing for the eye, a change in its shape alters the focus and makes things look blurry. Usually, the person becomes more nearsighted, meaning that distance vision is blurrier. Restoration of the blood sugar to normal eventually results in clearing of the vision, but it can take up to a month after the blood sugar has been stabilized for this to occur. For the same reason, many people who have had high blood sugars for a while, usually without knowing it, experience blurring right after they start taking medication to lower the blood sugar. The reason, of course, is that the shape of the lens is changed now that the blood sugar is lower. Wait until your blood sugar has been stable for at least one month before changing your glasses.

Diabetic Retinopathy: The Greatest Threat to Vision

The greatest concern in diabetic patients has to do with the development of *retinopathy,* a disorder of the retina. Diabetes can damage the tiny blood vessels that nourish the retina. The retina can be compared to the film in a camera: Images of the objects you see are focused on the retina and then transmitted to the brain. The likelihood of developing retinopathy depends on how long the diabetes has been present and, like most diabetic complications, is affected by how well the blood sugars have been kept under control. The majority of people who have had diabetes for over ten years have at least some degree of retinopathy.

After ten years of diabetes, most people have at least some retinopathy.

Damage to the walls of blood vessels causes them to become leaky, and tiny blood vessels sometimes shut down completely. This is called *background retinopathy.* When leakage of this nature occurs, fluid buildup (edema) can occur in the center of the retina (called the *macula*), and this can cause blurring and distortion of vision. The points of leakage, called *microaneurysms,* are sometimes marked by the presence of tiny red dots, which can be seen by the examining physician. Often, however, the microaneurysms can only be detected by performing a photographic type of test called *fluorescein angiography*. In this test, a yellow dye called *fluorescein* is injected into an arm vein, after which numerous photographs of the retina are taken. Areas of leakage can then be easily discerned.

Hemorrhages of various sizes are often present in the retina. They do not affect vision unless they are located in the absolute center of the retina. Another common finding in background retinopathy is the presence of hard exudates. These waxy, yellow spots represent fat-rich leakages emanating from damaged blood vessels, most commonly in the macula. Hard exudates that form very close to the center of the macula are worrisome, because if they reach the very center, the resulting loss of vision can be irreversible.

An even greater threat to vision is the development of *neovascularization*— a condition called *proliferative retinopathy*. This condition is probably triggered by a lack of oxygen in the retina caused by poor circulation. Neovascularization refers to thin, abnormal blood vessels that grow out of the retina and proliferate in front of the retina. They are very fragile and can sometimes bleed. If the bleeding is severe, the eye may become filled with blood, snuffing out vision until the blood absorbs, a process that can take months in severe cases. Eventually, this can result in the formation of scar tissue inside the eye. This scar tissue can apply traction to the retina, pulling it forward and causing what we call a *retinal detachment*. Although surgery can be performed to clean out the hemorrhage and scar tissue and reattach the retina, blindness can sometimes result. To prevent the bleeding in the first place, extensive laser treatments can be performed on the retina.

Laser: It May Save Your Vision, but Don't Get Burned!

The laser treatments performed to make proliferative retinopathy go away are called *panretinal photocoagulation*. These are very extensive treatments in which small burn spots are placed throughout the retina, although not on the abnormal blood vessels themselves. By obliterating some of the retina, the laser treatments may allow more blood to circulate in the remaining retina, carrying oxygen that may promote reversal of the neovascularization. Two or three sessions are usually necessary. Laser is not indicated in everyone with retinopathy but should be done in people who are felt to be at high risk for bleeding. Risk factors for bleeding include very extensive neovascularization,

neovascularization that is present on the optic disk, and the presence of blood in front of the retina, indicating that there has already been bleeding. For the weeks and months after each laser session, the patient is checked at regular intervals to see whether the neovascularization is going away. Since very extensive treatments can affect night vision and peripheral vision, the goal is to do just enough laser treatment to prevent problems but no more than that. The treatments are performed in an office setting and may cause mild discomfort in some people.

Laser treatments have also been advocated as a way of preventing progressive loss of vision from leakage in the macula caused by microaneurysms and hard exudates, the condition we call *background diabetic retinopathy* or *diabetic maculopathy*. The laser is used to obliterate tiny areas of leakage seen on the fluorescein angiogram photos. The Early Treatment Diabetic Retinopathy Study (ETDRS) was performed to determine whether treatment of this kind at an early stage would have long-lasting beneficial effects on vision.[4] The study found that laser treatment of people who had swelling of the macula near its center or hard exudates close to center had only about half the rate of vision loss over a three-year period as people who did not undergo the laser treatment. Soon, "experts" and laser equipment companies were recommending routine laser treatment of all such patients, even those with 20/20 or better vision. To be sure, such treatments have benefited many patients, but there are also a number of drawbacks.

Laser treatments may help prevent leakage, but they do have side effects.

First, the majority of the diabetics in the study, especially those with the best vision at the beginning of the study, did not lose any vision over the three-year period, even when they were not treated with the laser. Thus, because one cannot predict whose vision will worsen and whose won't, many people who undergo the laser treatment do so unnecessarily. This is important, because laser treatments have side effects. Every time the laser applies a burn to the retina, a small piece of the retina is being destroyed. This can create minuscule blind spots that can interfere with the quality of vision. Second, the ETDRS did not really address the question of timing for the laser treatment. It is certainly possible that unnecessary treatments could be avoided by simply following the progress of many patients with diabetic retinopathy closely, performing a laser treatment only if the leakage increased or the vision began to deteriorate.

Certainly if the hard exudate type of leakage is threatening the center of the macula, where it might cause irreversible loss of vision, one would want to perform a laser treatment. But in most cases, there is no such urgency.

Controlling Retinopathy Naturally

There are other approaches to the prevention and treatment of diabetic retinopathy. We have already discussed the importance of good control of the blood sugar in the prevention of diabetic complications. There is no question that diabetics who are conscientious in maintaining tight control have a significantly lower risk of developing diabetic retinopathy. Certain nutritional factors appear to be important as well. One group of researchers looked at differences in dietary patterns between those diabetics who had retinopathy and those who did not.[5] They found that diabetics without retinopathy had higher intakes of carbohydrates (starch) and fiber and lower intakes of protein than those who did have retinopathy.

Consuming less protein may help prevent complications.

The beneficial effect of a lower protein intake may be surprising to some people, but it should not be. Most of us consume much too much protein (up to double the recommended dietary allowance), and excess protein is harmful, especially to diabetics. The American Diabetes Association has recommended for some time that diabetics consume no more than the recommended dietary allowance of protein,[6] because excess protein can accelerate loss of kidney function. Since deterioration of the eyes in diabetics often parallels deterioration in the kidneys, it is interesting to note that too much protein is a risk factor for both problems. The excess protein that people in Western countries consume comes from an animal product–based diet. A plant-based diet, rich in whole grains, vegetables, and fruits, contains a more moderate amount of protein, which is ideal. Fiber, of course, comes only from plant products.

I mentioned earlier that the buildup of hard exudates, the fat-rich leakages in the macula of the eye, is of concern and must be watched closely. The more hard exudates develop in the retina, the greater the likelihood of vision loss. These hard exudates are directly related to cholesterol levels in the blood. People who have higher cholesterol levels tend to have more hard exudates and poorer vision than people with lower cholesterol levels.[7] The question we must ask, then, is whether lowering of cholesterol levels can reduce hard exudates and help stabilize eyesight. If so, we would have an effective nonsurgical alternative to laser treatments. This question has already been answered. More than a half dozen studies published over the past forty years have shown that lowering blood cholesterol levels aggressively, by either dietary or medical means, can make hard exudates go away.

Dr. Walter Kempner, an internal medicine specialist at Duke University in the 1940s, studied the effect of what he called the "rice diet," which consisted of rice, fruit, and fruit juice, on people with uncontrollable high blood pressure. The diet not only helped the blood pressures but also caused large declines in blood cholesterol levels. As an incidental finding, Dr. Kempner noted significant improvement in the retinopathy of two diabetics who participated in his study.

Dr. William Van Eck followed up on these findings in 1959 by placing diabetic patients on a high-carbohydrate, ultralow-fat diet.[8] Not only did all of these patients experience a fall in their blood cholesterol levels, but in eight of ten patients with retinopathy, the hard exudates, some of them quite large, either regressed or disappeared completely. The results strongly suggested that dietary lowering of cholesterol levels can make hard exudates disappear, and Dr. Van Eck suggested that a diet such as this be considered for diabetics who have high cholesterol levels and retinopathy with hard exudates.

Lowering cholesterol levels can clear up leakages and avert the need for laser treatment.

A Swedish study in 1965 employed a similar diet, with fewer than 10 percent of calories derived from fat.[9] In most cases, the hard exudates in these diabetic patients disappeared almost completely. In a number of patients, the number of red dots seen in the retina, indicative of microaneurysms, also diminished. In this, as in all of the other cholesterol-lowering studies, no effect on neovascularization (proliferative retinopathy) was seen. The researchers in this study also noted that improvement in vision may occur as the hard exudates resolve, although this does not happen in most cases.

Not everyone is willing to follow a healthy low-fat diet, so other approaches have been considered. Since substituting vegetable oils like corn oil for fats of animal origin can lower cholesterol levels, another study evaluated diabetics with retinopathy who were placed on a corn oil diet. Here again, not only did cholesterol levels fall somewhat, but there was also a marked reduction in the amount of hard exudate.

Cholesterol-lowering drugs have also been used effectively to improve diabetic retinopathy, proving that it is the cholesterol-lowering effect of the treatments rather than some other dietary factor that is responsible for the beneficial effect on the leakages. Clofibrate and Atromid (a combination of clofibrate and another drug), two of the early medications used to lower blood cholesterol levels, were shown in the late 1960s to bring about a significant reduction in hard exudates just as the dietary approaches had.

Most recently, in 1991, a group of researchers treated six patients suffering from diabetic retinopathy with pravastatin, a potent drug of the "statin" class that lowers cholesterol levels by inhibiting its production by body cells.[10] Another drug, cholestyramine, was added if necessary, the goal being to lower blood cholesterol levels to 150 milligrams per deciliter or less. The average cholesterol level of these patients was 231 before drug therapy and 165 during therapy. All six patients showed an improvement in hard exudates. In four of them, there was an improvement in the number of microaneurysms as well. During the one-year study period, one patient showed an improvement in vision, and five showed no change. Of course, no change is an excellent result, because the whole point of diabetic retinopathy treatment is to prevent loss of vision. Laser treatments do not usually result in any improvement in vision, either.

What is amazing about all of these studies is that although they deal with small numbers of patients, they are absolutely consistent in their results. There is no question that dietary (preferably) or medical treatment to bring

It is an approach that is ignored in most medical practices today.

blood cholesterol levels down can reduce or eliminate hard exudates and, in some cases, microaneurysms. Lowering cholesterol levels, especially by dietary means, obviously confers other health benefits as well. Although neovascularization (proliferative retinopathy) often requires laser treatment on an urgent basis, the treatment of nonproliferative (background) diabetic retinopathy, the type marked by hard exudates and other leakage in the macula, is rarely an emergency. Therefore, the prudent course in most of these cases is to lower blood cholesterol levels, carefully monitoring the retinopathy at regular intervals to make sure no worsening is taking place. If successful, there may be no need for laser treatments, which are expensive and can have adverse side effects. In my own medical practice, I was able to save many people from having to undergo laser treatments in just this way. Sadly, it is an approach that is ignored in most medical practices today.

Magnesium: The Case of the Disappearing Mineral

Most studies of people with diabetes have found that they tend to have lower blood levels of the important trace minerals magnesium and zinc. Diabetics often have excessive losses of these minerals, along with chromium and calcium, in the urine. Low magnesium levels may actually be a risk factor for the development of NIDDM, the usual adult form of the disease, and low chromium levels may reduce sensitivity to the effects of insulin. The consequences of these lower levels are uncertain, but some people have speculated that deficiencies in magnesium or zinc might contribute to diabetic complications. More attention has been focused on magnesium than on zinc, because magnesium deficiency has been linked with high blood pressure, a

Magnesium may help prevent diabetes as well as its complications.

less favorable cholesterol and triglyceride profile, and increased platelet aggregation (the clumping of platelets in the blood leading to clots and hardening of the arteries). All of these effects could increase the risk of diabetic complications.

Some studies have concluded that diabetics with retinopathy have lower levels of magnesium in their blood than diabetics who do not have retinopathy,[11,12] but other studies have found no such relationship. Still, it would be very important to know whether magnesium (and possibly zinc) supplementation might reduce the incidence of diabetic retinopathy and other complications. Unfortunately, no study of this sort has been done.

One of the problems in detecting the extent of magnesium deficiency in diabetics is that the usual laboratory test for magnesium measures the level in the noncellular part of the blood. Most of the magnesium in the body is inside cells, however, so the standard blood test is probably not able to detect a good many cases of true deficiency. Nevertheless, the American Diabetes Association has reached the consensus that diabetics at highest risk of magnesium deficiency should be tested and given magnesium supplements if their blood levels are low.[13] Hopefully, more sophisticated tests for magnesium deficiency will soon be available, and perhaps the question of the effect of supplementation on retinopathy will be answered by a good study. Until then, consuming more magnesium-rich foods, such as green vegetables, whole grains, legumes, nuts, and seeds, should be helpful, and modest supplementation with magnesium, up to the recommended dietary allowance, can be considered as well.

Promising Nutritional Approaches

Some researchers have claimed that improvement in retinal blood circulation might prevent or retard the progression of diabetic retinopathy. It is well known that circulation is a problem in patients with diabetes, as they frequently experience closure of tiny blood vessels that contributes to various complications. The platelets (blood cellular fragments that begin the blood-clotting mechanism) in people with diabetes are "stickier" than they should be. This can trigger the formation of small clumps and clots that can occlude small blood vessels. Magnesium deficiency, as mentioned, may contribute to this problem. The blood in diabetics also tends to have a higher than normal viscosity, and this is at

Vitamin E may prevent blood clots and improve circulation.

least partially due to red blood cells that are less flexible than they should be. These problems can also contribute to poor circulation.

Since *aspirin* is a drug that reduces the ability of the platelets to clump together, some researchers have studied the effect of aspirin on the development or progression of diabetic retinopathy. One study showed that aspirin may help prevent the formation of microaneurysms, the weak spots in blood vessels where leakage can occur. However, another study did not show any beneficial effect of aspirin therapy on the progression of retinopathy. The consensus is that aspirin should not be used for this problem.

Vitamin E therapy may be a more promising approach. Whereas aspirin decreases the ability of platelets to aggregate, vitamin E in doses of 200 international units (IU) a day or higher can significantly reduce the adhesiveness (stickiness) of platelets and is one of the few agents to do so. Interestingly, many diabetics have low levels of vitamin E in their platelets, a condition that increases their tendency to aggregate. This may explain why vitamin E supplementation has more effect on the platelets of diabetics than on those of nondiabetics.

Furthermore, some researchers feel that the antioxidant properties of vitamin E may also have a beneficial effect, since oxidative stress may contribute to the development of diabetic retinopathy. As promising as such therapy seems, no good studies to determine the effect of vitamin E supplementation on diabetic retinopathy have been performed as yet. An added caution is that the effect of vitamin E on platelets may increase one's tendency to bleed, just as aspirin does.

Omega-3 fatty acid supplementation is also a promising type of therapy. These are the polyunsaturated fatty acids associated not only with fish oils but also with flaxseed oil, sea vegetables, fiddlehead ferns, and some range-free eggs. Omega-3 fatty acids decrease platelet aggregation. They also reduce blood viscosity by increasing the flexibility of red blood cells, actions that could certainly benefit diabetics. Because of the potential to reduce the risk of a number of diabetic complications, omega-3 fatty acid supplementation has been evaluated in a number of studies, although not specifically with regard to diabetic retinopathy. The main concern has been that long-term treatment with these fatty acids may worsen blood sugar control in some NIDDM patients, although this is not a problem for IDDM patients. An increased bleeding tendency with this therapy is also a concern. However, some people have speculated that the preponderance of omega-6 fatty acids (from vegetable oils) over omega-3 fatty acids in the average Western diet may increase the risk of diabetic complications. If so, bringing the dietary intake of these two types of fatty acids into balance may be of benefit. Clearly, we must await the results of further studies to see whether omega-3 fatty acid supplementation is beneficial. Because of a lack of evidence at present for the safety and efficacy of omega-3 fatty acids in diabetics, I do not recommend taking such supplements.

Ginkgo biloba extracts, although untested in diabetics, may improve circulation.

Finally, I would mention a promising herbal extract, *ginkgo biloba,* also known as EGb 761. One of the most frequently prescribed medications in France and Germany, this extract, available over the counter as a supplement in the United States, has many interesting components and properties. Some substances in EGb 761 act as potent antioxidants and free radical scavengers. Ginkgolides, compounds that are found only in ginkgo biloba, inhibit the action of platelet-activating factor, a substance in the body that can promote inflammation and clumping of platelets. EGb 761 inhibits the aggregation of platelets, thereby preventing blood vessel blockages. It also reduces blood viscosity, which is usually high in diabetics; increases the flexibility of red blood cells; and stimulates the production of a substance that allows blood vessel walls to relax. All of these properties allow EGb 761 to increase blood flow, especially to areas where circulation is poor.[14,15] Needless to say, this extract may prove to be a most valuable adjunct in the treatment of diabetes and the prevention of diabetic complications, including retinopathy. Be aware, though, that herbal extracts from different companies can sometimes differ quite markedly from each other, and they are not regulated by the U.S. Food and Drug Administration, which investigates them only if possible toxic effects have been reported.

Summary

Nutrition plays a major role in both the prevention and control of diabetes. A healthy diet can help keep blood sugars under optimal control and can reduce risk factors for the circulatory complications of the disease. Diabetic-induced damage to the eye's blood vessels produces retinopathy, a condition that can blur vision and occasionally even lead to blindness. Regular eye examinations are necessary to detect the first signs of retinopathy and follow any retinopathy that may be present. Laser treatments may be indicated to prevent some of the serious complications of retinopathy.

Recommendations

1. Achieve tight blood sugar control with diet and medication if necessary.
2. Consider following a high-fiber, high–complex carbohydrate, low-protein diet, which may reduce the risk of retinopathy, although the optimal diet for a person with diabetes must be determined by the treating physician.
3. Lower blood cholesterol levels to reduce or eliminate the fat-rich leakages called hard exudates that often threaten vision.
4. Consider daily supplementation with modest amounts of calcium (500 to 1,000 milligrams), magnesium (350 milligrams), zinc (10 milligrams), and chromium (150 micrograms). These amounts are present in some multi-vitamin/multimineral supplements. Check with your physician first, especially if you have kidney problems.
5. Consume more vitamin E–rich foods (soy products, whole grains, nuts, dark, leafy green vegetables) or consider supplementation with natural vitamin E, 100 to 200 IU a day, but again, check with your physician first.

CHAPTER TWELVE

Retina and Optic Nerve

Age-Related Macular Degeneration

"Doctor, can't you make the glasses just a little bit stronger?" Mrs. Jones is distressed because it's become difficult to read and drive now. "Well, I'm afraid it's not that easy, Mrs. Jones. You see, the retina of the eye is like the film in a camera. If the film has become exposed or damaged in any way, you won't get good pictures no matter how strong a lens you place on the camera. Your glasses are like that camera lens; all they do is focus the light right on your retina. But if the retina has deteriorated, as is the case in age-related *macular degeneration,* you won't see clearly even with the best possible glasses." This oft repeated dialogue between patient and ophthalmologist reveals the frustration of people suffering from macular degeneration.

It is the most common cause of poor vision among the elderly.

Although many younger people have never heard of age-related macular degeneration, it is the most common cause of poor vision in Americans over the age of sixty. It affects many middle-aged people as well. The disease involves a deterioration of the macula, which is the name given to the central portion of the retina, and it is called "age-related" because its incidence increases with age. Macular degeneration causes blurring, distortion, or, in its most severe form, a large blind spot right in the center of your field of vision. You may look at someone but be unable to see that person's face while you are looking directly at it. The good news is that the disease never causes total blindness, and most people with it are always able to take care of themselves. The bad news is that it can prevent people from driving, reading, and other important everyday functions. To understand the process better and how we might be able to prevent it, let's first take a closer look at the anatomy of the retina.

Parts of the Retina

The *retina* is the delicate inner coat that lines the back wall of the eye (see figure 3.1, page 10). Its photoreceptor layer contains the *rods* and *cones,* specialized cells that receive light impulses from the environment and transmit them, via a network of modulator cells, to the brain. The cones are concentrated in the *macula,* or central retina, and control color vision and fine detail in the center of the field of vision. The rods predominate in the periphery of the retina, and they function mainly when there is little light in the environment. The inner portion of the retina that we have been discussing is called the *neurosensory retina* because of its similarity to sensory nerve tissue elsewhere in the body. The outermost or deepest layer in the retina is called the *pigment epithelium,* so called because its cells contain the pigment melanin, which is also in other pigmented parts of the eye and in the skin. The blood vessel–rich coat of the eye behind the retina is called the *choroid.* Separating the retina from the choroid is *Bruch's membrane.*

The process of macular degeneration begins in the pigment epithelium, although the rods and cones eventually die as well. Throughout life, the pigment epithelial cells ingest and digest debris produced by the rods and cones. If the digestive mechanisms are not working quite right, then abnormal material can build up in the pigment epithelial cells. This material can interfere with the normal workings of the cell, resulting in degeneration. When physicians look into the eyes of patients with macular degeneration, they often see small, yellowish-white spots in the macula. These spots, called *drusen,* are deposits located between the pigment epithelium and Bruch's membrane. Drusen are generally the first visible sign of macular degeneration. In some patients, there is a more diffuse change in the appearance of the retina, with loss of pigment in some areas and a buildup or clumping of pigment in others.

Types of Macular Degeneration

We often differentiate between the "dry" and "wet" forms of macular degeneration. In the dry form there is a slow, inexorable progression of the degenerative process, with more of the drusen and pigmentary changes developing over time. Vision slowly declines, although the rate of loss can vary greatly from one person to another. The wet form of macular degeneration generally begins the same way, but eventually a network of abnormal blood vessels, originating in the choroid layer of the eye, grows beneath the retina. These blood vessels can leak and bleed, wreaking havoc on the retina. When that happens, distortion or loss of the central part of vision can occur almost instantaneously. Permanent damage to the retina results. If these leaking blood vessels are located outside the very center of the retina, they can be obliterated with a laser treatment. Often they are not amenable to such treatment, however. Even if they are, the treatment is not always successful over the long term.

In the wet form, bleeding can occur behind the retina.

Causes of Macular Degeneration

The causes of macular degeneration are not well understood. As with most diseases, there is a hereditary (genetic) component. But I don't like to dwell on this aspect, because it can lead to a fatalistic outlook on life and a lack of desire to make important lifestyle changes. Take skin cancer, for example. People with very fair skin are genetically predisposed to skin cancer. Picture someone with blue eyes and blond hair and a family history of skin cancer who has had a lifetime of sunbathing and other outdoor activities. When that person develops skin cancer at age forty-five, the comment is, "It was inevitable—genetics." Rubbish! If that person had used sunscreen and wide-brimmed hats and avoided excess sun exposure, that person probably would not have cancer. We all have genetic tendencies for different things, but we can modify our risks within those tendencies by conducting our lives appropriately. Since we have no control over who our parents are, we might as well stop blaming genetics for everything and take more personal responsibility for what happens to us.

Don't use genetics as an excuse!

So let us look at some lifestyle factors that may play a role in the development of macular degeneration.

Nutritional Considerations

Zinc: The Crucial Trace Mineral?

The tissues of the eye, especially the retina and choroid layers, have some of the highest concentrations of zinc in the body. The relationship of zinc to retinal health has been studied for many years. People whose zinc intake from food is high have a 40 percent lower risk of developing the early signs of macular degeneration than people whose zinc intake is low. A study published in 1988 examined the effect of supplementing the diet with zinc in 151 patients with macular degeneration.[1] Some of the patients received zinc supplementation, and some received a placebo (sugar pill), but neither the patients themselves nor the doctors examining them knew who was getting the zinc and who wasn't. The dosage of zinc given was 40 milligrams twice a day in the form of zinc sulfate.

People who took zinc lost less vision.

After a one- to two-year follow-up period, people who got the zinc were found to have suffered significantly less visual loss than people who got the placebo. This was only a preliminary study, however. Generally, even a good study should be repeated to make sure that the findings hold up under more intense scrutiny. Certainly, one would want to study larger numbers of patients, people living in different areas and manifesting different lifestyles, before drawing any definite conclusions. One would also want to try different dosages of zinc and look for side effects associated with long-term treatment. Yet not long after the publication of this study, drug companies and ophthalmologists' offices began to push vitamin and mineral supplements containing large amounts of zinc. They were often promoted as a way for physicians to add to their income and get patients to return to their offices.

The evidence for a protective role for zinc is relatively weak.

Recently, researchers in Austria studied ninety-two patients who had developed the exudative (wet) form of macular degeneration in one eye but still had good vision in the other eye.[2] These patients were given either 80 milligrams of zinc once a day or a placebo (no zinc). When zinc is administered in this manner, we would not expect zinc levels in the body to rise quite as much as they would with the 40-milligram twice-a-day dosage employed in the aforementioned study. After two years, evaluation of the status of the better eye showed no significant difference between the two groups (people who got the zinc and people who did not). Therefore, the results of this study do not support the theory that zinc supplementation is protective.

Even if future studies confirm the beneficial effect of zinc in macular degeneration, it would be important to learn what the consequences of high-dose supplementation might be. When used in such large quantities, even minerals like zinc should be considered drugs and not just nutrients. After all, the recommended dietary allowance for zinc is only 11 milligrams a day for men and 8 milligrams a day for women. Could a dose of zinc much larger than that prove harmful? Quite possibly. The more we learn about nutrition, the more we learn that too much as well as too little of a given nutrient can prove harmful.

Consuming excessive amounts of many nutrients can be harmful.

In many areas of nutrition, we have had to learn this lesson the hard way. To give some examples, vitamin D is essential for bodily function and can either be obtained from the diet or manufactured by the skin after sunlight exposure. Too much vitamin D, however, as can occur when milk is fortified with excessive amounts of vitamin D, can be quite toxic to the body. Iron is a mineral needed for blood cell formation and for a healthy immune system, but excess iron may be a major risk factor for heart disease. Perhaps in no area is there greater public misinformation about nutritional requirements than in the area of protein. We do need a certain amount of protein, which comes from vegetables, fruits, grains, as well as animal products. But the average American diet contains one and one-half to two times the recommended dietary allowance. This excess protein is contributing to the epidemic of kidney stones and osteoporosis we are now facing, and it may even be raising our risk for cancer. The lesson we can learn from these and other examples is that although our bodies do require a certain amount of various nutrients for optimal functioning, too much of a given nutrient can be quite harmful as well.

Zinc Supplementation and Copper Deficiency Zinc is no exception to the rule about excess nutrient consumption. Intake of large amounts of zinc can cause copper deficiency. Although we don't hear too much about copper, it is an essential mineral as well. The recommended dietary allowance is 900 micrograms (0.9 milligram) a day. Moderate or severe copper deficiency causes anemia (low red blood cell count) as well as leukopenia (low white blood cell count). Some people have speculated that copper deficiency might also be a risk factor for heart disease. Clearly, copper deficiency would be a most undesirable side effect of any treatment.

Copper deficiency can interfere with the functioning of important enzymes.

To detect copper deficiency, the traditional approach has been to measure the levels of copper and ceruloplasmin (a copper-related protein) in the blood. By this measure, many if not most people taking zinc supplementation for macular degeneration may seem to have no problem. However, we now know that these blood tests are not all that sensitive. One can be mildly copper deficient and still have normal copper and ceruloplasmin blood levels. Newer tests have been devised that do detect the deficiency. One of these measures levels of the enzyme superoxide dismutase in red blood cells. This enzyme depends primarily on copper for its activity, and it has been found to be depressed in people with only mild copper deficiency even when the level of copper in their blood is normal. Superoxide dismutase is an important enzyme, protecting our bodies against oxidant-induced damage. Therefore, a deficiency of it could have serious consequences. Other important enzymes, such as glutathione peroxidase and platelet cytochrome c oxidase, have also been found to be depressed in people with mild copper deficiency.

It doesn't take much zinc to produce a copper deficiency.

What all this means is that we should not take copper deficiency lightly or assume that it does not exist just because the level of copper in the blood is normal. How much supplemental zinc does it take to produce this copper deficiency? Just 25 milligrams twice a day will do it—less than the amount used in the macular degeneration studies.

The question, then, is whether supplementation with copper prevents people who are taking zinc from becoming copper deficient. Most of the supplements that people take for macular degeneration contain 2 milligrams of copper along with 40 milligrams of zinc. Undoubtedly, that helps, but is it really enough copper to prevent deficiency? Further studies are necessary to allow us to know for sure.

Supplementing with copper along with the zinc raises another important question. In the original study on macular degeneration, the patients receiving the 40 milligrams of zinc twice a day did not receive any copper supplementation. Assuming that there was a beneficial effect in the group receiving zinc, how do we know for sure that it was the zinc itself that helped retard the progress of the macular degeneration? A plausible alternative explanation is that a copper deficiency induced by the zinc was responsible for the effect. After all, copper is necessary for new blood vessel formation, which occurs in the "wet" form of macular degeneration. If this explanation were true, then supplementing with copper along with the zinc to eliminate the possibility of copper deficiency might nullify the beneficial effect observed in the original study. More studies are needed to determine whether copper supplementation alters the presumed beneficial effect of zinc on the course of macular degeneration.

Zinc Supplementation and Other Mineral Deficiencies Copper is not the only mineral affected by high doses of zinc, however. One study showed that young women given 25 milligrams of zinc twice a day developed a significant lowering of their serum ferritin levels, a measure of iron stores, as well as a lowering of their hematocrit, which is related to the red blood cell count and hemoglobin level. Thus, it appears that zinc supplementation poses a risk to iron as well as to copper status. Iron deficiency is a serious problem that causes anemia and compromises the immune system.

If zinc supplementation can cause iron as well as copper deficiencies, it is certainly possible that the absorption of other trace minerals could be affected as well. Indeed, there is evidence that zinc supplementation can inhibit the absorption of manganese, an important trace mineral that, among other things, is a cofactor (helper) for one form of the antioxidant enzyme superoxide dismutase. This effect is worsened when copper supplementation is given along with the zinc. Other trace minerals that may be affected by zinc supplementation are cobalt and nickel, since they, along with zinc, copper, iron, and manganese, all belong to the class of elements called *transition metals*.[3]

High doses of zinc could lead to iron, manganese, and other mineral deficiencies as well.

I like to think of the interconnection among minerals as a nutritional ecosystem. When one mineral is consumed in much greater than normal dietary amounts, that is, as a megadose, the delicate ecological balance is upset. Other important minerals may not be absorbed as well as they normally are, leading to possible deficiencies. Therefore, if high doses of a given mineral are found to be effective in the treatment of a given condition, it is important that we assess the impact of that supplementation on the body. We don't want to alleviate one problem but cause another in the process.

Zinc and Cholesterol Levels   Another adverse consequence of consuming large amounts of zinc is its effect on cholesterol levels. Elevated blood cholesterol levels are a major risk factor for heart disease and strokes. We now differentiate, though, between low-density lipoprotein (LDL) cholesterol, the "bad" cholesterol, which increases the risk, and high-density lipoprotein (HDL) cholesterol, the "good" cholesterol, which reduces the risk. Decreasing the HDL cholesterol level can markedly increase the risk of heart disease. And that's exactly what large amounts of zinc can do.

Zinc and Cholesterol in Men   Studies have shown that when men consume 80 milligrams of zinc twice a day, their HDL cholesterol levels fall by approximately 25 percent. LDL cholesterol levels are not affected. Taking even 50 to 75 milligrams of zinc once a day causes a significant lowering of HDL cholesterol levels. This dosage is

Taking too much zinc can lower your "good" cholesterol.

less than that used in the macular degeneration studies. Thus, high doses of zinc might be very harmful through their effect on HDL cholesterol levels.

In contrast, when young and middle-aged men take low dosages of zinc, about 20 milligrams once a day, no significant change in HDL cholesterol levels is observed. Thus, *low*-dose zinc supplementation may not produce the potentially harmful decreases in HDL cholesterol seen with high-dose supplementation, at least not in men in this age group.

Zinc and Cholesterol in Young Women   In a study of young, healthy women who took up to 100 milligrams of zinc once a day, only a transient decrease in the HDL cholesterol levels was observed in the 100-milligrams group. A few caveats should be mentioned, however. First, taking a given amount of a zinc supplement in divided doses, for example, twice a day, as was done in the macular degeneration study, would be expected to result in more zinc absorption than would be seen with once-a-day administration. In this study on the young women, for example, those who consumed 100 milligrams of zinc once a day had zinc levels in their blood only 10 percent higher than in those who consumed 50 milligrams of zinc once a day. Also, the women who volunteered for this study were nutrition students who ate a healthier type of diet than the average American consumes, so the results are not necessarily applicable to the general population.

Zinc and Cholesterol in the Elderly Whereas exercise normally increases HDL cholesterol levels in elderly people, that increase does not occur when they take more than 15 milligrams of supplemental zinc each day. Therefore, it is possible that the older population might be even more sensitive to the effects of zinc supplementation than younger people. People in the over-sixty age group, then, should be cautious about taking large doses of zinc.

Whether copper supplementation can help prevent the fall in HDL cholesterol is uncertain at this point. In the meantime, it seems prudent to perform baseline and follow-up blood tests on people who supplement with large amounts of zinc to make sure that their cholesterol levels are not being adversely affected.

Zinc and the Immune System Zinc is a very important trace mineral in the area of immunity. Our immune systems protect our bodies from infectious diseases and from cancer. Children in developing countries who are zinc deficient because of a poor diet show an increased susceptibility to disease. But what about an excess of zinc? Does supplementation with large amounts of zinc have any effect on the immune system? To assess immune function, researchers often study white blood cells, since they are involved in protecting the body from invaders such as bacteria and viruses.

In one study, eleven healthy men were given 150 milligrams of zinc twice a day for six weeks. This is a huge dosage, over three times that given to the macular degeneration patients discussed earlier. The researchers found that important immune system functions were impaired during the period of zinc supplementation.

Fortunately, other studies on elderly people who consumed lesser amounts of zinc did not demonstrate any loss of immune function. There may even have been a beneficial effect on some aspects of immunity, which is not surprising given the higher incidence of zinc deficiency with increasing age. Nevertheless, a certain amount of caution is in order, as short-term studies such as these do not always reflect long-term effects on the body.

Zinc and Alzheimer's Disease There is now preliminary evidence that zinc may play a role in the development of Alzheimer's disease. This much-feared degeneration of the brain causes progressive memory loss and a decline in mental functioning in general. One interesting finding in Alzheimer's disease patients is that the concentration of zinc in some areas of the brain is altered. In particular, unusually high levels of zinc have been found in the hippocampus, a region of the brain concerned with memory.

Can zinc supplements trigger Alzheimer's disease?

Clumps of proteinlike material called *amyloid* are also found in the brains of people with Alzheimer's disease. Researchers have found that normal body levels of zinc can cause a protein fragment called A beta 1-40 to precipitate into clumps of this amyloid material. This suggests that an alteration in the bodily mechanisms that regulate zinc might play a role in the development of Alzheimer's disease. The findings also give us cause for concern that zinc supplementation in large doses might trigger Alzheimer's disease in susceptible individuals. Hopefully, the question will be clarified by future studies, but until then, we should remain cautious.

Zinc: Summary and Recommendations We conclude that zinc supplementation may help retard the progression of age-related macular degeneration, but the supporting evidence is weak. Zinc supplementation in moderate to high doses carries with it the risks of copper, iron, and possibly other mineral deficiencies; reductions in blood levels of HDL cholesterol, the "good" cholesterol; and possible facilitation of the development of Alzheimer's disease. What, then, should a person with age-related macular degeneration do on the basis of the currently available information?

In any therapeutic intervention, the art of medicine requires a careful assessment of the benefits versus the risks. The Hippocratic dictum, *Primum non nocere* (above all, do no harm), still applies today. Every patient is different, and we must evaluate the risk factors and proclivities of each person to determine which therapy, if any, is appropriate. In the case of macular degeneration, the end result of the disease can be devastating: When you lose your central vision in both eyes, you've lost a good part of your life. Therefore, some risk taking may be worthwhile if sufficient potential benefit exists.

In someone who has already lost the vision in one eye from macular degeneration and is felt to be at high risk in the other eye, my approach has been to treat with moderately high doses of zinc, typically 40 milligrams once a day. There may be some risks, but I want to do everything possible to keep that person from losing the central vision in the remaining eye. I also supplement with copper, even though I do not know for sure whether that alters the effectiveness of the treatment. The blood tests that are most sensitive for the detection of copper deficiency, such as erythrocyte (red blood cell) superoxide dismutase activity, are not readily available in medical laboratories, so one might as well take copper supplements and reduce the risk of developing copper deficiency from the zinc. A multimineral supplement in general is of value, as zinc may interfere with the absorption of other minerals as well. Iron status and cholesterol levels should be checked a few months after the initiation of this therapy.

Modest amounts of zinc should be safe for most people.

For people with mild to moderate signs of macular degeneration but who are not felt to be at high risk for severe loss of vision, I recommend only a multivitamin/multimineral supplement containing 10 to 15 milligrams of zinc. Such a daily supplement is a good idea for anyone over the age of sixty-five, as it has been shown to strengthen the immune system and reduce the incidence of infectious diseases in this age group.

Antioxidants: What They Are and What They Do

Antioxidants are another category of nutrients that some speculate may have protective effects on the retina. The use of antioxidants as supplements has increased dramatically in recent years. Scientists have been concerned that uncontrolled oxidation reactions in our bodies may lead to various diseases. Some have observed that people who consume foods rich in antioxidants seem to have a lower risk of many illnesses. Just in case you're rusty on the subject, let's first look at what we mean by *oxidation* and *antioxidants*.

Oxidative processes occur as part of what we call *oxidation reduction chemical reactions*. A good example would be the formation of rust on a piece of iron. Oxidation has a number of beneficial functions in our bodies. Oxidative reactions are used to generate *adenosine triphosphate* (ATP), a stored form of energy, from the foods we eat. These reactions are also important for proper functioning of the immune system. Therefore, not all oxidation is bad, just excessive or uncontrolled oxidation.

Antioxidants are chemicals that can prevent oxidation reactions from occurring in the body's tissues. They do this by acting as "cannon fodder," becoming oxidized themselves and thereby sparing the DNA, protein, and polyunsaturated fatty acids in the body that might otherwise be attacked. Since polyunsaturated fatty acids form part of the membranes that enclose the cells in our bodies, their oxidation can result in disruption of the architecture of those membranes, impairing important bodily functions.

An antioxidant is similar to a rust inhibitor.

As oxidative chemical reactions occur in the body, molecules can be transformed into free radicals. In the most stable form of any molecules, the electrons are present in pairs. When chemical reactions result in molecules with an unpaired electron, we call those molecules *free radicals*. Free radicals are highly reactive: They can trigger chain reactions in which other molecules are successively "attacked." This can result in damage to cell membranes and other tissues and probably trigger a number of diseases, including cancer.

Antioxidants include vitamins E and C and many of the carotenoids—vitamin A–related compounds such as beta-carotene. Vitamin E itself can be turned into a free radical as it intervenes in chemical reactions, but it can be regenerated to its original form by vitamin C. The minerals selenium, copper, zinc, and manganese are also important in the prevention of the uncontrolled oxidation reactions that can generate the unwanted free radicals.

Antioxidants act as "cannon fodder" to protect our cells from attack.

Can Antioxidants Protect the Retina? There has been much speculation that oxidative damage may play a role in the development of macular degeneration. For example, *peroxidation* (oxidation by a form of oxygen free radical) of the polyunsaturated fatty acids in the rods and cones of the retina could occur. Interestingly, the area just outside the very center of the macula is the area most prone to degeneration, and this particular area has been found to be relatively low in vitamin E and carotenoids, important retinal antioxidants.

The increased risk of macular degeneration in smokers, conclusively shown in a number of studies, may well be related to oxidative processes. Smokers tend to have lower levels of carotenoids and vitamin C, and cigarette smoke contains powerful prooxidants, agents that promote oxidation and free radical formation. Exposure to excess sunlight may also be a risk factor, especially in people with lighter-colored eyes, and again oxidative processes may be involved. This is discussed later in the section on carotenoids in the retina, (see "Carotenoids: The Crucial Antioxidants?" on page 201).

The big question is whether antioxidants, obtained through either food or supplements, can reduce the risk of macular degeneration. The difficulty with food studies is that although they can sometimes discover certain foods or food groups that appear to reduce risk, it is not always clear which substances in those foods are providing the protective effect. Nonetheless, important clues can often be obtained that pave the way for further studies. Another approach is to measure the blood levels of different antioxidants to see whether higher levels of any specific nutrients afford protection.

In one study, the Eye Disease Case-Control Study, the investigators found a greatly reduced risk of neovascular age-related macular degeneration in people with higher blood levels of carotenoids.[4] The neovascular variety is the "wet" form described earlier in which abnormal blood vessels grow behind the retina and cause severe, precipitous loss of central vision. When the researchers combined carotenoid, selenium, vitamin C, and vitamin E measurements, they found that higher levels of these nutrients taken together were also associated with a lower risk of neovascular macular degeneration. However, in other studies on patients with both the dry and wet forms of macular degeneration, the results have been mixed. In one study, increased risk was associated with low blood levels of the carotenoid *lycopene,* a red pigment in tomatoes, pink grapefruit, guava, and watermelon that is twice as potent a quencher of singlet oxygen (an activated form of oxygen although not a free radical) as beta-carotene. Vitamin E from food seems to have a mild protective effect, but, according to at least one study, taking vitamin E supplements may not help.

In summary, there is some indication of a protective effect from certain antioxidants. However, even if we knew exactly which ones were most important, we would still not know whether supplementation is beneficial. The form of antioxidants in the usual supplements is sometimes quite different from the form they assume in nature.

For example, beta-carotene as a supplement is generally synthetic (not natural) and consists primarily of all *trans* beta-carotene, whereas foods contain not only the *trans* form but also several *cis* forms (*cis* and *trans* refer to the three-dimensional configurations of the molecule). There is evidence that the *cis* form may be a more effective antioxidant than the *trans* form. By supplementing with the *trans* form only, you may be "crowding out" the *cis* forms in your body and actually worsening your antioxidant status. Taking large doses of beta-carotene may also reduce the blood levels of the other important carotenoids. These findings may explain recent study results that intimate that beta-carotene supplementation may increase the risk of certain cancers.

> *Antioxidants present in foods may sometimes be more effective than those in supplements.*

As another example, natural vitamin E in foods consists of eight different compounds, four tocopherols and four tocotrienols. The usual vitamin E supplement, however, contains only one tocopherol (alpha-tocopherol). The other tocopherols may be more active in carrying out certain antioxidant functions than alpha-tocopherol is, and by supplementing with alpha-tocopherol only, you may again see a "crowding out" effect in which the levels of the other vitamin E compounds become drastically lowered. If this is true, it may also explain why the small amount of vitamin E derived from food may be more effective than vitamin E in supplement form when it comes to lowering the risk of macular degeneration.

> *Some potent forms of beta-carotene and vitamin E are lacking in most supplements.*

The lesson we must learn is that foods are the preferred source of nutrients. For example, the best way to obtain the full spectrum of vitamin E is by consuming foods such as soy products, whole grains, leafy green vegetables, peanuts, and nuts such as pistachios, pecans, walnuts, and Brazil nuts. Carefully controlled studies may eventually give us more answers, but until then, the value of antioxidant vitamin supplements to prevent macular degeneration remains unproven.

> *Foods are the preferred source of nutrients.*

Carotenoids: The Crucial Antioxidants? We can perhaps infer from the antioxidant studies we've discussed that certain carotenoids may be of value in preventing or retarding the progress of macular degeneration. Carotenoids are chemical compounds related to vitamin A, and they are pigments—colored substances that absorb light. Although most people think of beta-carotene when they think of carotenoids, the fact is that about seven hundred different carotenoids have been found, and humans can absorb at least forty of them. Beta-carotene has been the most studied of any carotenoid, but other carotenoids may be more important in certain circumstances.

In addition to their relationship to vitamin A, carotenoids have important antioxidant functions. Some body tissues tend to accumulate certain carotenoids more than others, and the degree and type of antioxidant protection afforded vary among the different carotenoids. The light absorption properties of carotenoid pigments also provide a means of protecting cells against the harmful effects of light.

In the case of the retina, it has long been known that the macula contains a yellowish pigment. In 1985 it was determined that this pigment consists of the two closely related carotenoids, lutein and zeaxanthin. In infant retinas, lutein is the dominant pigment, but in 90 percent of adults zeaxanthin predominates. Both carotenoids are present throughout the retina, but the concentration of zeaxanthin tends to be higher in the center of the macula, whereas the concentration of lutein tends to be higher in the periphery of the retina. There is evidence that lutein can be converted in the retina to a form of zeaxanthin. This conversion may be important to the retina, since there is more lutein in our blood than there is zeaxanthin.

Lutein may protect the retina from damage caused by light.

The purpose of the carotenoids lutein and zeaxanthin may be to protect the retina from damage caused by excessive sunlight exposure. Light, especially that in the ultraviolet or near-ultraviolet part of the spectrum, may cause the formation of free radicals or other activated forms of oxygen (singlet oxygen) that can be harmful to cells. Blue light may be the most harmful, as it appears that the blue-sensitive cones of the retina are the most vulnerable to light-induced damage. Therefore, a pigment that can absorb light toward the blue end of the spectrum and that can quench singlet oxygen would seem ideal.

Zeaxanthin and lutein both absorb light maximally in this area and are extremely effective quenchers of singlet oxygen, zeaxanthin especially. It is not surprising, then, that lutein and zeaxanthin are the dominant retinal pigments.

Another report from the Eye Disease Case-Control Study Group lends a great deal of support to the theory that consumption of foods rich in carotenoids, especially lutein, can reduce the risk of macular degeneration.[5] These investigators evaluated 356 individuals who had recently been diagnosed with advanced macular degeneration and compared them with a group of control subjects—people with similar personal characteristics who did not have macular degeneration. The participants in the study were asked to fill out a detailed questionnaire to determine how often they consumed any of sixty different food items.

This study found that spinach and collard greens were the two food items most strongly associated with a reduced risk of macular degeneration. The more spinach or collard greens an individual ate, the lower that person's risk of macular degeneration. People who ate five or more servings per week, where a serving was defined as half a cup, either cooked or raw,

People who regularly ate their greens lowered their risk by 86 percent!

had an 86 percent reduced risk of developing severe macular degeneration, as compared with people who consumed less than one serving a month of either of these vegetables. This difference in susceptibility to macular degeneration was highly significant.

The distinguishing characteristic of spinach and collard greens is that they are rich sources of lutein. The analytical techniques used in the past were not able to differentiate between lutein and zeaxanthin, although recent studies show that spinach contains primarily lutein,[6] which is much more abundant in the diet than is zeaxanthin. As mentioned, though, it appears that lutein can be converted to zeaxanthin in the retina. We cannot say for sure that the presence of lutein is the reason for the protective effect of spinach and

Spinach, collard greens, kale, and other leafy green vegetables are rich in lutein.

collard greens, as there are many other chemical compounds in these vegetables as well. I mention this to stress the point once more that foods are the preferred nutritional sources rather than supplements. However, the evidence certainly is suggestive for a protective role for lutein.

Other vegetables are also good sources of lutein. Kale is probably the rich-est, but other good sources include mustard greens, parsley, and turnip greens. These vegetables were not included among the sixty food items on the questionnaire used in this study because most Americans consume them infrequently. Spinach is a staple throughout the United States, and collard greens are in the South. Most of the less commonly consumed dark, leafy green vegetables are nutritional powerhouses, however—rich in minerals like calcium, iron, and magnesium; vitamins; and numerous phytochemicals that may reduce the risk of cancer and other chronic diseases.

The study results did not indicate that consuming only small amounts of foods containing the carotenoid lycopene increases the risk of macular degeneration, despite the recent finding that low blood levels of lycopene are associated with increased risk. Lycopene is the most abundant carotenoid in our bodies, but it has not been found in the macula.

Carotenoids: Summary and Recommendations The evidence strongly suggests that eating more carotenoid-rich foods, especially those rich in lutein, may be the most important step you can take to lower your risk of losing vision from macular degeneration. I recommend trying to eat at least one serving a day of any of the dark, leafy green lutein-rich vegetables. For people with demonstrated macular degeneration who will not eat their vegetables, modest lutein supplementation (about 5 milligrams a day) can be considered, although that route is definitely less desirable than vegetable consumption.

Retinal Hazard of Animal Fats

Many people have wondered over the years whether the risk factors for heart disease are also risk factors for macular degeneration. In fact, many years ago, patients with macular degeneration were often told by their doctors that they had "hardening of the arteries" in the back of their eyes. Not all studies have shown such a connection, however. Recently, some researchers have tried to determine whether cholesterol and saturated fats play any role in macular degeneration.

It is now well established that higher blood cholesterol levels are a major risk factor for heart disease and stroke. Although people have different genetic predispositions for these diseases (as they do for everything), dietary considerations are of the greatest importance. About 20 percent of the cholesterol in our blood comes directly from the cholesterol in the foods we eat. The remaining 80 percent is manufactured by our bodies, primarily from saturated fats. Cholesterol is found almost exclusively in animal products, and saturated fats come primarily from animal products as well. In regions of the world where people consume primarily plant-based diets with relatively little in the way of animal products, blood cholesterol levels are much lower than those of people in Western countries, and the rates of heart disease, stroke, and other chronic degenerative diseases are much lower for people who consume primarily plant-based diets as well.

Cholesterol and saturated fats may increase your risk of macular degeneration.

Studies of blood cholesterol levels have not yielded consistent results. The Eye Disease Case-Control Study Group mentioned before found that high cholesterol levels were a strong risk factor for the development of the "wet" or neovascular form of macular degeneration. Recently, a team of researchers studied over 2,000 Wisconsin residents and tried to determine whether there was any relationship between the type and amount of fat they consumed and their risk of developing macular degeneration of either the wet or the dry variety.[7] The researchers found that high consumption of saturated fat and cholesterol did increase the risk of early macular degeneration. People who consumed large amounts of either saturated fat or cholesterol had an 80 percent or 60 percent higher risk, respectively, of having early macular degeneration than people who consumed small amounts. Thus, the risk appeared to be slightly greater for saturated fat than for cholesterol.

Animal fats accelerate hardening of the arteries in more ways than one.

The one food most strongly linked to macular degeneration was butter. The more butter people ate, the higher their risk. People who consumed a lot of butter had a 50 percent greater risk of early macular degeneration than people who consumed little. Butter is high in both cholesterol and saturated fats, and the type of saturated fat that dairy products contain has a greater tendency to raise blood cholesterol levels than the saturated fats in other food products. People who consumed any lard at all raised their risk by 40 percent. In contrast, people who consumed large amounts of margarine had a reduced risk for early macular degeneration.

This study provides some support for the theory that the consumption of animal products, especially those high in saturated fats, can lead to the development of macular degeneration, just as it can lead to heart disease and blood vessel problems. There are a few reasons why saturated fats may have more harmful effects on the body than cholesterol does. First, eating saturated fat has more of an elevating effect on your blood cholesterol level than cholesterol itself does. As mentioned before, only about 20 percent of the cholesterol in your bloodstream comes directly from cholesterol in the foods you eat. And once your daily intake of cholesterol reaches 300 milligrams, consuming more of it doesn't make much difference. Also, saturated fats affect your tendency to form blood clots. They tend to put you in a hypercoagulable state; that is, your blood forms clots much more easily. This can not only cause blockages of blood vessels but also accelerate the process of *atherosclerosis* (hardening of the arteries) directly. Reducing your saturated fat intake, however, also reduces your cholesterol intake, because the animal products that are high in saturated fats also contain significant amounts of cholesterol.

In summary, there is some evidence that high animal fat intake increases the risk of macular degeneration. We can only speculate as to whether this effect is related to atherosclerosis or some other mechanism. Further studies may give us some answers, but since the development of macular degeneration is such a slow, chronic process, it may take many years to know for sure. But even if some doubt exists as to the exact diet-related risk factors for macular degeneration, you have nothing to lose by adopting the type of diet to which the human body is best adapted. Unlike some new drug or supplement, which may ultimately prove to have unforeseen side effects, a healthy, high-fiber, no-cholesterol, low–saturated fat diet, rich in vitamins and other nutrients unique to the plant kingdom, can only be of benefit to you. There is no reason to delay making the transition. In the words of the great sage Hillel, "If not now, when?"

Dietary factors that may play a role in the development and progression of age-related macular degeneration include zinc; antioxidant vitamins and associated minerals; carotenoids, especially lutein; and fats of animal origin. Supplementation with large amounts of zinc is controversial because of uncertainty regarding its effectiveness and the possibility of long-term adverse consequences. Antioxidant therapy in general has not been proven to be of value, but increased consumption of dark, leafy green vegetables such as spinach or collard greens appears promising from a preventive standpoint. Intake of saturated fats and cholesterol should be reduced or eliminated. The general recommendation, then, is to consume a low-fat, vegetable- and fruit-rich diet with at least one serving a day of spinach, collard greens, kale, or another lutein-rich vegetable. A wide variety of foods assures intake of other important carotenoids, as well as various other antioxidants and phytochemicals. Supplementation with zinc above the recommended dietary allowance can be considered in high-risk cases provided that precautionary steps are taken to assure that copper or iron deficiencies, lowering of HDL cholesterol levels, or other problems do not occur. People over the age of sixty-five should consider taking a general multivitamin/multimineral supplement, and this may contain all the zinc they need.

Resolve to eat a green vegetable you've never eaten before. If not now, when?

A nutritious diet can and should be tasty as well as healthy. There is a widespread misconception that fat makes food taste better. The American preference for fats and animal products is something largely learned, an acquired taste. Once you eliminate the fats and learn to use a wide variety of vegetables, herbs, and spices as the centerpiece of a meal, your tastes will become more sophisticated, and you will enjoy the clean, fresh taste and subtle flavors that food is supposed to have.

I know what you're thinking. Many people have never tasted greens like kale, collards, or mustard. But don't let that scare you off. Consider it an opportunity. Take kale, for instance. It has a pretty, frilly leaf often placed around the margin of salad bars. It doesn't do you much good just to look at it, however. Kale is a cruciferous vegetable, like broccoli or cauliflower. That means that it contains important substances that may help prevent cancer. It is high in fiber, vitamins E and C, and easily absorbed calcium (two cups deliver more calcium to your body than a cup of milk), as well as other important minerals like iron, manganese, magnesium, and copper. It's a good source of beta-carotene and the richest source of lutein, which we've talked so much about. Even better, it's delicious, especially when fresh. Find a good recipe, such as one for colcannon, an Irish dish that can be prepared with kale (or cabbage), mashed potatoes, and onions. Eating more green vegetables is one of the most important steps you can take on the road to good health.

Other Lifestyle Risk Factors

Macular degeneration is another chronic degenerative disease associated with smoking. Several studies have now shown that smoking increases the risk of both the dry and wet forms of age-related macular degeneration. There are certainly a number of known mechanisms that could explain this finding. As discussed before, the components of cigarette smoke have a prooxidant effect on the body, promoting the oxidation reactions that are felt to play an important role in macular degeneration. Smoking causes a decline in certain nutrients in the blood, including antioxidants. Finally, smoking probably has an adverse effect on the circulation to the back of the eye. So if you smoke, you now have one more reason to quit.

Alcohol has also been studied. With regard to wine consumption, the results have been conflicting. In moderation, wine consumption probably does not have much effect one way or the other, but high consumption of alcoholic beverages, including wine, may be slightly detrimental.[8] It is conceivable that a small amount of red wine consumption could even have some protective effects because of the antioxidants present in red grapes. Alcohol by itself has prooxidant properties. Perhaps grape juice may prove to be the best of all for the macula.

High blood pressure has been identified as a risk factor in a number of studies. Presumably, any such effect would have to be attributed to circulatory damage. Most people these days are aware of the importance of keeping their blood pressure under control.

Some people have speculated that exposure to the ultraviolet light from sunlight might be a risk factor, but study results have been inconsistent. The cornea and lens filter out most of the ultraviolet light before it can get to the retina. Still, considering the possible increased risk of other eye problems, such as cataract and pterygium, associated with ultraviolet exposure, it may be wise for people who spend a great deal of time outdoors to reduce their exposure by wearing ultraviolet-absorbing sunglasses or regular glasses.

Staying Dry: Self-Monitoring

The wet form of macular degeneration is much feared because it can wipe out the center of the field of vision in one eye in a matter of days or even less. Although the more common dry form may transform into the wet form in any individual, people who have many large, fluffy-looking, "soft" drusen (the yellowish-white spots in the retina) are at higher risk than people whose retinas show small, waxy, yellow, "hard" drusen. The wet form is caused by the growth of a network of abnormal blood vessels behind the retina, where they can leak and bleed and irreversibly damage the retina. This network of blood vessels can be obliterated by a laser treatment if it is detected before it reaches the center of the macula. Once it reaches the central area, the treatment is stymied by the fact that using the laser in that area would destroy the very part of the macula that we are trying to save. Therefore, the key is to detect the presence of these blood vessels before they have advanced that far.

For people at high risk for the development of wet macular degeneration, regular checks by an ophthalmologist, at least every six months, are mandatory. Sometimes an ophthalmologist can detect signs of leakage and bleeding even before you've noticed any change in your vision. However, monitoring yourself in between visits is also very important. If you are not specifically looking for it, even blurred or distorted vision in one eye can go unnoticed when you're walking around with both eyes open, as most of us do. The way to monitor yourself is to use what we call an *Amsler grid*. This is simply a grid of vertical and horizontal lines in a checkerboard pattern with a prominent black dot in the center. You should be able to obtain these sheets from your ophthalmologist. Once a day, you should check yourself by testing one eye with the other one covered and then reversing the process. Some people tape the sheet in a convenient place, for example, on the refrigerator door or near the mirror in the bathroom. With your reading glasses on, you fixate on the black spot in the center of the grid. As you keep looking at the spot, you determine whether the lines around it look straight and even, as they should, or whether they look at all curved, distorted, or broken. If you suddenly find one day that the lines look abnormal, you should call your ophthalmologist right away and be examined within twenty-four hours, if possible. The abnormal blood vessels behind the retina can grow very quickly, and delaying just one or two days could make the difference between a treatable situation and an untreatable one.

The examination of someone with macular degeneration who reports such new symptoms involves a very careful examination of the macula after pupil dilation. The ophthalmologist looks for signs of swelling of the retina or even hemorrhage. If there is any question at all, the special photographic test called a *fluorescein angiogram* is performed. For this test, a yellow dye called *fluorescein* is injected into a vein in the arm, and a rapid sequence of photographs is then taken through a special camera. The film can be developed right away, and if a network of abnormal blood vessels is found, it can be treated on the spot.

Surgery for Macular Degeneration

No surgery is available for people with the dry form of macular degeneration. There has been some hope that transplantation of cells to the retina could aid people who have already lost a great deal of vision, but research in this area has not really been fruitful to date.

Laser treatment is performed on people with the wet form of macular degeneration when the network of abnormal blood vessels is not under the very center of the retina. The laser obliterates the blood vessels so they cannot leak or bleed. Unfortunately, the procedure is not as successful as we would like. In many cases, the abnormal blood vessels either originate behind the center of the retina or have grown into that area by the time they are first detected. Since the laser treatment destroys the retina as well as the blood vessels in the area begin treated, such treatment is impossible in these situations, since it would wipe out the very vision it is intended to preserve. The other problem is that the condition often returns in an eye even after an apparently successful treatment. Thus, the laser treatment does not save vision as often as we would like.

Photodynamic therapy offers hope for the future.

Another approach under investigation has been to deliver radiation to the retina in the area where the abnormal blood vessels are growing. Radiation is better known as a treatment for cancer, but radiation can also stop noncancerous cells from proliferating. The hope was that this would have a beneficial effect in macular degeneration, but the results so far have not been promising.

A newer approach called *photodynamic therapy* is being studied. With this technique, patients receive an intravenous injection of a substance called *benzoporphyrin derivative,* also known as *verteporfin.* Verteporfin is what we call a *photosensitizer.* When light of the correct wavelength is directed at a tissue containing the photosensitizer, the photosensitizer becomes "excited" and generates activated forms of oxygen, which can damage cell membranes, including those lining the walls of blood vessels. In other words, the process causes oxidation reactions to occur, the very kind of reaction we try to inhibit in the prevention of macular degeneration. This damage can cause blood vessels to shut down. Thus, if successful, it could prove very valuable in the treatment of people in whom the abnormal blood vessels have grown behind the central macula and are thus untreatable by conventional laser therapy. Preliminary results have made us cautiously optimistic, although multiple repeat treatments are often necessary. People whose abnormal blood vessels occur in a very well-defined area are the ones who seem to benefit, at least over the first year or two after treatment. The long-term results are unknown, and many questions remain unanswered.

Age-related macular degeneration, the number one cause of poor eyesight in the elderly, causes irreversible loss of vision. The main hope in dealing with this disease lies in prevention. Following a healthy, low-fat diet, rich in dark, leafy green vegetables and other antioxidant-rich fruits and vegetables; consuming vitamin E–rich soy products, grains, and nuts; supplementing modestly with zinc if necessary; and avoiding smoking should lower the risk dramatically. This approach may not only prevent macular degeneration but also retard its progression in people who have already been diagnosed with the problem.

Retinal Detachment

Detachment of the retina is a serious problem that, until recent times, resulted in blindness. Retinal detachment involves a separation between the neurosensory retina and the pigment epithelium layer. When people think of a detached retina, they are usually thinking of a rhegmatogenous retinal detachment. In this form of the disease, one or more breaks in the retina allow fluid from inside the eye to travel through the break in the retina, dissecting behind the retina and ballooning it forward. The less common form of retinal detachment, tractional retinal detachment, occurs when scar tissue inside the eye, which might be the result of previous bleeding in the eye, tents the retina forward toward the center of the eye.

Risk Factors for Retinal Detachment

Risk factors for rhegmatogenous retinal detachment include aging, myopia, eye injuries, history of cataract surgery, history of previous retinal detachment in either eye, and certain degenerations in the periphery of the retina that cause holes or tears to occur. People with myopia are at higher risk for retinal tears because they tend to develop degenerative changes in the periphery of the retina. Also, because of their longer eyes, the vitreous tends to separate from the retina at a younger age than it normally does, a process that increases the risk of developing a retinal tear. Having had cataract surgery increases the risk of retinal tears and detachment, even years down the road. The risk is even higher if a cloudy posterior capsule, called *secondary cataract,* develops later on (as it does half the time) and a laser procedure has to be done to make an opening in the capsule. Lattice degeneration is a type of change that causes a thinning of the retina toward its periphery, and tears or holes can sometimes form in these thinned areas. About 10 percent of the population have at least a little lattice degeneration in one eye. Retinal detachment is less common in darkly pigmented individuals, probably because there is a stronger bond between the pigment epithelium layer of the retina and the neurosensory retina.

> *Floaters are the little black "cobwebs" or "gnats" that may suddenly appear in your vision.*

Aging increases the risk because of the age-related degeneration of the vitreous. This gel begins to liquefy as we get older, and the portion that remains as a gel begins to shrink. This shrinkage applies traction to the retina in the areas where the vitreous gel is attached. At some point in life, typically when people are in their late fifties or sixties, the traction becomes so great that the vitreous pulls free, at least partially, from where it is attached to the retina. Traction of this nature on the retina often causes a person to see white light flashes. These are often most noticeable in the dark and tend to be toward the side of one's vision. As the vitreous separates from the retina (a process called *posterior vitreous face detachment*), a person may also see little black spots, threads, "spiderwebs," or similar objects. These spots are commonly called "floaters."

What If You See Flashes or Floaters

Anyone who experiences the sudden onset of flashing lights or floaters should see an ophthalmologist within twenty-four hours if possible. The eye needs to be carefully examined through dilated pupils, because about 7 to 8 percent of the time, at least one retinal tear will be found. If the person has reported seeing "thousands" of tiny dots, the chance of finding a tear is much higher. Tears in the retina produce no pain or feelings of discomfort. They are often called *flap tears* or *horseshoe tears,* because one often sees a curved flap

> *A "fresh" tear in the retina has a good chance of leading to a detachment.*

of the torn retina tented up, still attached to the strand of vitreous that caused the tear. The ophthalmologist may even see at this point a tiny amount of fluid that has begun to seep behind the edges of the tear. A fresh tear like this, still being pulled on by some of the separated vitreous, has a significant chance of turning into a full-fledged retinal detachment. Older tears in the retina may occasionally be seen along with evidence that they have scarred down. These older tears are very unlikely to lead to problems. Some tears may be small and difficult to find. One tip-off to the ophthalmologist that a tear is present is the presence of tiny pigment granules in the vitreous. These are liberated when a tear occurs. The ophthalmologist looks extra carefully in such a situation to make sure not to miss a tear.

Treating Retinal Tears

The decision to treat prophylactically with either laser or cryotherapy depends on the risk factors in a given case. For high-risk tears and people who have other risk factors for retinal detachment, treatment designed to seal off the tear and prevent the development of retinal detachment is indicated. This treatment employs either laser or cryotherapy. With laser treatment, the invisible laser beam is directed at the area of the tear and a few rows of small burns are placed in the retina to completely surround the tear. With cryotherapy, a thin probe cooled to far below freezing by liquid nitrogen is applied to the outside of the eye where the tear is located. The freeze produced by the cryotherapy spreads through the wall of the eye so that the retina itself is included in the freeze. These techniques are sometimes compared to welding, but they are really quite different. They do not immediately seal down the retina. They simply create an inflammatory reaction in the area of the tear that, over a period of a few days, causes a scarring reaction. Before that scarring actually takes place, there is still a risk of retinal detachment. These treatments carry only a small risk in themselves, but since there is a small risk, they are generally done only when we feel there is at least a 10 percent chance that a tear will progress to retinal detachment. Risks include creation of new tears and formation of a kind of scar tissue over the center of the retina that causes it to pucker, distorting the vision. (See "Macular Holes and Pucker," page 214). The risks are minimized, however, by avoiding excessive treatment.

How the Retina Detaches

Tears in the retina generally occur in the periphery of the retina because that is where the vitreous is strongly attached to the retina and is also the place where degenerated, thinned areas of retina often develop. Therefore, when a retinal detachment occurs, the detachment is initially located peripherally, not toward the very back of the eye, where the macula is. If the detachment stayed in the periphery, it would not be much of a problem. Unfortunately, most retinal detachments *The sooner a retinal detachment is repaired, the better.*
progress until the entire retina is detached. As a retinal detachment progresses, many people notice a dark shadow that encroaches on their field of vision and becomes progressively larger. This symptom, in addition to floaters and flashing lights, is a warning sign that you may have a detached retina. We like to find retinal detachments before the macula has become detached, because the prognosis for recovering good vision is worse when the macula is involved. Therefore, retinal detachments require surgery on a fairly urgent basis. If we detect the detachment before it has spread to the macula, we want to repair it before it can go any farther. In addition, the retinal cells begin to degenerate immediately in the area of detachment, so it is important to get it reattached as soon as possible to allow maximum recovery of vision.

Surgery for retinal detachment is called a *scleral buckling procedure*. It involves treating the tear or tears, usually by cryotherapy, and by application of a band or "sponge" to the eye to indent it. The indentation of the eye wall brings the detached retina back into contact with the pigment epithelium layer of the retina from which it had separated. Often, a small nick is made in the eye to allow the fluid that has formed behind the retina to drain out. This procedure carries a small risk but facilitates retinal reattachment. The success rate for retinal detachment surgery depends on different factors, but, on average, is about 90 percent. If unsuccessful, the surgery can usually be repeated. An interesting alternative to scleral buckling is pneumatic retinopexy. In this procedure, after treatment of the tear as above, air or sometimes a gas called *sulfur hexafluoride* is injected into the eye to push the retina back against the back wall of the eye. This procedure may be useful in cases where the retinal tear is so far back on the eye that performing a scleral buckling procedure would be impractical or too likely to cause problems.

The tractional type of retinal detachment, as opposed to the rhegmatoge-nous type, is not associated with retinal tears. It is often seen in people with dia-betes who have had repeated hemorrhages into the vitreous. The eye is able to clear some of the blood, but a certain amount of scar tissue inevitably occurs, and this scar tissue can pull the retina forward, detaching it. This problem requires a major operation called a *vitrectomy*, in which special instruments are inserted into the eye to cut and remove the scar tissue, thereby relieving the traction. If the macula is involved in the tractional detachment, the surgery should be done soon if there is to be any chance for restoration of vision.

Macular Holes and Pucker

The *macula* is the very center of the retina and therefore its most important part. A problem with the macula in an eye causes a blur, blind spot, or distor-tion in whatever we are looking at with that eye. Unfortunately, many retinal problems affect primarily the macula.

Macular Holes

A *macular hole* is a hole in the center of the retina that in most cases probably occurs because of traction from the vitreous onto that area. The *vitreous* is the gel that fills the inside of the eye, and it shrinks with age. At the interface between the vitreous and the retina, a scar tissue–like film called an *epiretinal membrane* may form. This membrane may then contract and pull on the retina, resulting in the formation of a macular hole.

In some cases, people complaining of a change in vision have been found to have traction on the macula but no definite hole. Studies have been done to determine whether performing a major operation called a *vitrectomy* may prevent the development of a hole. In this operation, tiny instruments are inserted into the eye, and some vitreous is removed in such a way as to relieve the traction. Although some of the results have been promising, it is impor-tant to remember that vitrectomies carry a small risk of complications such as cataract and retinal detachment. However, if the eye is being closely fol-lowed and the situation is rapidly deteriorating, it may well be a reasonable thing to attempt. Complicated surgical procedures have also been proposed for eyes that already have full-fledged macular holes. Again, the potential benefits have to be weighed against the risks. It is safe to say that the jury is still out on this issue.

Macular Pucker

Formation of epiretinal membranes over the center of the macula, as described above, usually does not result in macular hole formation. However, this condition, also known as *macular pucker* or *cellophane maculopathy* (because the membrane has a crinkly, shiny look similar to cellophane), is a common cause of vision problems in the elderly population. The membrane causes the center of the macula to become wrinkled. This can have anywhere from a mild to a severe distorting effect on vision. In some cases, objects may appear smaller than normal. Macular pucker does not always get worse with time, however. Frequently, it just stays the same, and in perhaps 10 percent of cases, it actually improves as the membrane separates itself from the retina. As with macular holes, surgery (vitrectomy) can be done to try to remove the membrane. The surgery is fairly successful in bringing about an improvement in vision, but because of the potential for cataract development and retinal complications, it should be reserved for people who have fairly severe loss of vision.

High Blood Pressure and the Eye

High blood pressure, or hypertension, affects blood vessels throughout the body. It is a major risk factor for heart attacks as well as for strokes. Before major attacks such as these occur, the blood vessels undergo changes in response to the blood pressure. Special X-ray techniques are required to see the blood vessels in the heart or brain, but the eye is the one place where they can be seen directly! Observing the branches of the arteries and veins as they course over the retina provides a wealth of information, although they can also be seen on the conjunctiva, the clear membrane over the white of the eye.

Effects of High Blood Pressure on the Eye

As part of the routine eye examination, we dilate the pupils and closely examine the back of the eye. The arteries, with their oxygen-rich blood, are lighter in color than the veins, which appear dark red. We look at the width of the arteries. These blood vessels are narrower in people who have high blood pressure. With time, indentations occur in the walls of the veins at the points where the arteries cross over them. If the blood pressure is very high, other signs of what we call *hypertensive retinopathy* also develop. Small hemorrhages of various types appear in the retina. Some are flame shaped, indicating that they are located around the inner surface of the retina, where the nerve fibers are. Others, located deeper in the retina, look like little red dots and blots.

> *Uncontrolled high blood pressure can damage the retina and optic nerve.*

Sometimes a tiny blood vessel shuts down, resulting in the death of a tiny segment of retina. This is signaled by what is commonly known as a *cotton wool spot*—a little, fluffy, feathery, whitish spot near the surface of the retina signifying the death of nerve cells at that location. Hard exudates, yellowish fat-rich leakages from the damaged blood vessels, can sometimes be seen near the center of the retina or in other areas toward the back of the eye. Edema in the macula can result in some blurring of vision. In very severe high blood pressure, the optic nerve may even become swollen and undergo permanent damage. The higher the blood pressure, the greater the degree of hypertensive retinopathy.

Vein Occlusions

High blood pressure is also a major risk factor for the development of retinal vein occlusions. Sometimes just a branch of a vein becomes blocked off. In the worst case, the *central retinal vein,* the main vein that drains blood away from the retina, can become blocked. A vein occlusion such as this produces extensive hemorrhaging and leakage and usually causes significant blurring of vision. It also predisposes to other serious problems, including *rubeosis of the iris,* an abnormal growth of blood vessels on the iris that can block off the drainage channels of the eye and lead to a severe, very difficult to treat form of glaucoma. Neovascularization of the retina can occur, a growth of abnormal, fragile blood vessels that can bleed and fill the eye with blood. (See "Retinal Blood Vessel Occlusions," page 217.)

Role of the Ophthalmologist in Diagnosing Hypertension

Because so many people are screened these days for high blood pressure, and because so many effective blood pressure–lowering drugs are now available, we see hypertensive retinopathy much less frequently than we used to. However, the ophthalmologist is sometimes the first one to suspect high blood pressure in a given individual. If typical hypertensive retinopathy is present, the ophthalmologist checks the blood pressure right away and refers the patient to a primary care physician for treatment if it is elevated. The eyes can truly be a window to the rest of the body.

Retinal Blood Vessel Occlusions

Robbing any bodily tissue of its circulation is a major threat to its existence. The retina depends on the bloodstream for its sustenance. If the blood supply to the retina were completely shut off for forty-five minutes, the retina would die. Occlusions or blockages can occur either on the arterial side, which brings blood to the retina, or on the venous side, which drains the blood away.

Arterial Occlusions

A central retinal artery occlusion occurs when the main artery that brings blood to the retina becomes blocked off. Branches of this artery may become blocked as well. There are many different causes for these blockages. Commonly, a piece of cholesterol breaks off, either from the ophthalmic artery behind the eye or from the carotid arteries, which carry blood from the heart up the neck and give rise to the ophthalmic arteries. Occasionally, we can even see the cholesterol deposit, especially if it breaks into tiny pieces that then travel downstream and lodge in the smaller blood vessels of the retina. They appear yellowish, and we may sometimes see one during the course of a routine eye examination in a person who has had no symptoms whatever. If we do, that person may need to undergo testing to evaluate the major arteries.

Change in lifestyle can help prevent blood vessel occlusions in the eye, as elsewhere.

A blockage can also be caused by a tiny piece of calcium that comes from an area where there is hardening of the arteries or possibly from a heart valve. People with irregular heartbeats, such as atrial fibrillation, can sometimes release tiny blood clots from their heart that can travel to the eye, causing occlusions. A very important cause of central retinal artery occlusion in elderly people is *temporal arteritis,* also known as *giant cell arteritis.* This is an autoimmune type of inflammation in the arteries that can lead to blood vessel occlusions, including strokes. It is clear, though, that the main risk factor in most arterial occlusions of the eye is atherosclerosis, or hardening of the arteries. The same kinds of lifestyle change that can help prevent heart attacks and stroke—healthy diet, exercise, and so on—can also prevent blood vessel occlusions in the eye.

Symptoms of Arterial Occlusions

A central retinal artery occlusion causes a complete blacking out of vision in the involved eye. If the blacking out of vision does not resolve within the hour, the eye may go blind from permanent retinal damage. In some cases, the blacking out may be transient. It may occur gradually, similar to a shade being pulled down over the eye, but much more commonly it is a diffuse graying or browning out of the vision. The vision may then return in

Transient loss of vision may be the warning sign of an impending stroke.

ten to thirty minutes. We call such an episode a *transient ischemic attack,* or TIA. It indicates that a temporary blockage has occurred, and it is an important warning sign of an impending stroke.

Special testing should be performed to evaluate the blood vessels. It is not something that should be ignored. Younger people without hardening of the arteries may rarely experience temporary loss of vision in one eye, but it may often be just a form of blood vessel spasm, similar to what one occasionally sees in people with migraine.

To test for the possibility of temporal arteritis in an elderly person, we generally ask about symptoms associated with this disorder. For example, does the person have pain in the temples or extreme tenderness to touch in these areas or on the scalp? Does the jaw become painful with chewing? If there is any suspicion at all, a blood test called a *sedimentation rate* is performed, which is usually abnormal in people with temporal arteritis. The definitive test is a biopsy of one of the arteries lying under the skin in the area of the temples. The biopsy can show whether the characteristic inflammation is present in the walls of those arteries.

A central retinal artery occlusion is one of the few true emergencies in ophthalmology. If the vision in one eye blacks out completely, you need to be checked immediately. If one ophthalmologist cannot see you right away, find another. When we examine the eye, we usually find that there is no light perception. In other words, the person cannot even tell light from darkness in the eye. The arterial blood vessels are narrow and thread-like. The whole retina has a pale appearance because of a lack of circulation. Once the diagnosis is made, treatment is begun. Even if several hours have elapsed after the loss of vision, it is worth treating, because probably at least a tiny bit of blood has been getting through to the retina, barely keeping it alive.

Sudden loss of vision should always be checked out immediately.

Treating Central Retinal Artery Occlusions

Many techniques have been tried, but good studies on these techniques have been lacking. An injection of lidocaine, an anesthetic that can also cause blood vessel dilation, can be given behind the eye. Massage of the eye by alternately pressing on the eye and then releasing the pressure can be a very useful way to try to dislodge whatever is blocking the artery. In the process, the massage gradually lowers the fluid pressure in the eye, which may make it easier for blood to get through the arteries. Some ophthalmologists insert a tiny needle and withdraw a small amount of fluid from the anterior chamber of the eye. The purpose is to lower the pressure in the eye suddenly and promote blood flow. Pressure-lowering eye medications can also be used. Patients can also be admitted to the hospital so that they can be placed on oxygen for twenty-four hours, hopefully increasing the amount of oxygen delivered to the retina. There is much hope that the so-called clot-busting drugs used to treat strokes and heart attacks may also prove useful in central retinal artery occlusion. The risks of such therapy (from bleeding) must be carefully weighed against the possible benefits.

When only a branch of an artery is obstructed in the eye, this type of aggressive therapy is usually not done, because much less visual loss is involved and because people sometimes don't even notice the change in vision in the one eye right away. A branch arterial occlusion such as this does require some testing to determine the source of the occlusion, however.

If temporal arteritis is diagnosed by blood testing and by biopsy, high doses of cortisone medication are administered and must often be continued long term. Because of the possible side effects associated with this medication, careful monitoring by a physician is necessary.

Vein Occlusions

When the central retinal vein, the main vein that drains blood away from the retina, becomes occluded, the vision usually becomes blurred but does not black out completely. The vein occlusion affects the circulation to the retina, although many people who have central retinal vein occlusions may already have somewhat compromised circulation because of hardening of the arteries in the neck or closer to the eye. The typical appearance of the retina in this situation has been called one of "blood and thunder." Severe hemorrhaging and leakage from the blood vessels are seen throughout the retina, and the veins appear dark and swollen. In contrast to this picture is a less severe type of central retinal vein occlusion called *venous stasis retinopathy*. In this form, there is much less hemorrhaging, the vision may remain fairly good, the circulation to the retina is fairly good, and the prognosis over all is much better. Occlusions of branches of the central retinal vein also occur. Sometimes the indentation of the veins by the arteries that cross over them may play a role.

Risk Factors for Vein Occlusions

High blood pressure and a high intraocular pressure (IOP)are two major risk factors for vein occlusions. High blood pressure needs to be adequately controlled by lifestyle change (weight loss, low-salt vegetarian diet, and exercise) and drugs; and high intraocular pressure, the main risk factor for glaucoma, can be controlled with pressure-lowering eyedrops if

People without obvious risk factors may need to undergo special testing.

necessary. In some cases, special testing can be done in people with vein occlusions to determine whether any unusual blood abnormalities are present that may have contributed to the occlusion. Such abnormalities may include a strong tendency for blood clot formation or an increased blood viscosity.

Treating Vein Occlusions

Many treatments have been tried for vein occlusions, and almost all have been abandoned. For example, warfarin (Coumadin), which reduces the ability of the blood to form clots, does not appear to have any value. More promising are agents that reduce the blood viscosity, a property that might also prove useful with arterial occlusions. In one study, troxerutin, a derivative of a flavonoid, seemed to cause significant improvement in people with vein occlusions. Troxerutin reduces the clumping of red blood cells and the blood viscosity. Standardized ginkgo biloba extract, a common herbal supplement, and omega-3 fatty acids, such as flaxseed oil and fish oils, also effectively reduce blood viscosity.

Complications After Vein Occlusions

The concern in the more severe type of vein occlusion in which the blood flow to the retina has been compromised is that neovascularization will develop. *Neovascularization* refers to the abnormal blood vessels that grow in response to a lack of oxygen stemming from poor circulation. Neovascularization on the optic nerve and retina can lead to severe hemor-

Abnormal blood vessel growth may cause bleeding or glaucoma.

rhages into the eye. These hemorrhages can then form scar tissue and detach the retinas. Neovascularization of the iris can also occur, a condition known as *rubeosis iridis*. These blood vessels then grow into the area where the trabecular meshwork, the drainage channels of the eye, is located. The result is a very difficult to control form of glaucoma called *neovascular glaucoma*. Neovascularization of both the retina and the iris can lead to loss of the eye.

In people who are felt to be at risk for the development of neovascularization of the retina or iris, or who have already devel-

Laser treatments may sometimes be helpful.

oped the problem, laser treatment of the retina can be effective. This is called *panretinal photocoagulation*, the same type of treatment that is performed in diabetics who have neovascularization as a result of their disease. These extensive laser treatments, in which hundreds of burns are applied through-out the retina, not only can prevent neovascularization but also can make it regress after it has already appeared. Laser treatments are also sometimes indicated in people who have branch vein occlusions. The treatments may help improve vision by reducing leakage of fluid from the blood vessels, but normally this should not be done until at least six months have elapsed, because the leakage from branch vein occlusions often improves on its own with time. In selected cases, laser treatments can also be done in people with branch vein occlusions who have developed neovascularization. Obviously, anyone who has a central or branch vein occlusion must be followed closely by an ophthalmologist at regular intervals to make sure that complications such as neovascularization are not occurring.

Presumed Ocular Histoplasmosis Syndrome

This problem of the retina and choroid, known as either *ocular histo* or *presumed ocular histoplasmosis syndrome* (POHS), is seen primarily in people who have lived in the area of the Mississippi River and its tributaries. Many people from Missouri, Illinois, Indiana, and Kentucky are afflicted with this disease. In other parts of the country, it may be seen in people who lived in the Mississippi River Valley area in the past but left many years ago.

It usually occurs in people who have lived in the Mississippi River Valley area.

Histoplasmosis is an infection caused by *Histoplasma capsulatum,* a fungus that lives in the soil. Ocular histo does not represent an active infection of any kind. Although it is unproven, we think that it is the result of an inapparent infection by *Histoplasma* at some time in the past. If the infection did cause any symptoms when it occurred, it may have seemed like nothing more than a cold.

When we examine the retina in someone with ocular histo, we see whitish chorioretinal scars—scars in the deepest layers of the retina and in the blood vessel–rich choroid layer next to it. These scars are commonly known as *histo spots.* Also common is scarring adjacent to the optic disk, the oval-shaped por-tion of the optic nerve where it enters the back of the eye. All these areas of scarring are felt to be the result of the previous unrecognized infection.

How Ocular Histo Harms the Eye

The real problem with ocular histo is that the damage caused to the deepest layers of the retina allows a process called *subretinal neovascularization* to develop. Subretinal neovascularization also occurs in people with other conditions that cause scarring or degeneration in the retina, for example, age-related macular degeneration; injuries that cause breaks in Bruch's membrane, the layer between the retina and the choroid; and high myopia (extreme near-sightedness). *Subretinal neovascularization* means that blood vessels from the choroid layer travel through the breaks in Bruch's membrane and grow in a network behind the retina, where they can bleed and damage the retina. Since the process most commonly occurs in the macula, the damage can wipe out the most important part of our vision, leaving a large blind spot. Obviously, if this occurs in both eyes of an individual, that person is legally blind.

On examination of the eye, subretinal neovascularization is suspected whenever retinal hemorrhage is seen in a person with the other findings of ocular histo. Sometimes

A special test can detect the bleeding blood vessels.

the network of abnormal blood vessels appear as a fuzzy, dirty gray color. The presence and extent of subretinal neovascularization can be determined by a test called a *fluorescein angiogram*. This is a photographic test in which rapid sequence photos are taken through dilated pupils immediately after giving the patient an injection of fluorescein, a yellow dye, in an arm vein. The camera uses a special filter to detect the dye, which causes blood vessels to light up as the dye moves through the bloodstream.

Treating Subretinal Neovascularization

If subretinal neovascularization is present but is not under the very center of the retina, then laser treatment can be employed. The laser obliterates the blood vessels that have formed behind the retina so that they cannot grow and bleed any more. The laser treatment itself can have complications and cause some loss of vision, but the odds are still in your favor. Of course, the same problem could recur in the future. To detect any future problems, affected individuals can monitor their own vision with an *Amsler grid,* a sheet with a checkerboard pattern of horizontal and vertical lines. This sheet, which can be obtained from an ophthalmologist, can be used daily. If you notice any change, for example, if the straight lines become wavy or crooked in any area, notify your ophthalmologist immediately. Note that although we think that this disease originated from a fungus infection, it does no good to treat with antifungal antibiotics, because there is no longer any active infection by the time these other problems have surfaced.

Toxoplasmosis

Toxoplasmosis is a parasitic infection caused by a one-celled organism called *Toxoplasma gondii*. It can affect many tissues of the body, including the eyes and the heart. The most severe manifestations of the infection are seen when it is transmitted by pregnant women to their offspring before birth. In the eye, it causes a *retinochoroiditis* (infection of the retina with a secondary inflammation of the choroid layer that is in contact with the retina). The inflammation can sometimes fill the eye with cellular debris, reducing the doctor's ability to see the retina when examining the eye. Darkly pigmented scars in the retina are the signs of previous infection, which can recur many times. A blood test can also tell us whether a person has been infected by *Toxoplasma* in the past. Toxoplasmosis is actually a *zoonosis*—a disease of nonhuman animals that can be transmitted to humans. People can acquire it after contact with the litter of an infected cat, who may become infected after coming into contact with infected rodents. Keeping cats inside is one way to prevent this problem. But the most common way of acquiring this infection is eating undercooked meat, such as beef, lamb, or pork. Even just handling uncooked beef can transmit the infection. In one study, Seventh Day Adventists, whose religion encourages a vegetarian diet, had only about one-fifth the rate of infection from toxoplasmosis as a control group of people that resembled the general population. Suppression of the immune system, as seen in patients with AIDS, can also allow toxoplasmosis to recur.

The infection is commonly acquired by eating undercooked meat.

Although an active toxoplasmosis flare-up can sometimes burn itself out on its own, the infection also has the potential to destroy the macula. Therefore, when the eye is threatened by the inflammation, intensive treatment is necessary.

Treating Toxoplasmosis

Normally, treatment entails use of three different drugs concurrently. A corticosteroid (cortisone type of drug) is used in high doses to reduce the dangerous inflammation and is then tapered as quickly as the inflammation allows. A sulfa drug, such as sulfadiazine or triple sulfa, is combined with pyrimethamine (Daraprim).

Treatment generally requires three different drugs.

Both drugs affect the ability of *Toxoplasma* to utilize folate, one of the B vitamins. Since the two drugs interfere with different chemical reactions involving folate, they are said to be *synergistic*. This means that their combined effect is more than what you would expect just by adding one to the other. Of course, some people are allergic to sulfa drugs. In that case, another effective drug called *clindamycin* is substituted. The tetracycline class of antibiotics, which includes minocycline, has also been shown to be effective against *Toxoplasma* and can be used if needed. Finally, an antibiotic called *spiromycin*, which is available in Europe for treatment of toxoplasmosis, can be obtained in the United States, but only by filing a special application.

Side Effects of Treatment

These drugs can have serious side effects. For example, pyrimethamine can cause aplastic anemia, a life-threatening shutdown of the bone marrow, which stops producing blood cells. Because of this possibility, a few precautions are taken whenever pyrimethamine is prescribed. First, we do a baseline blood test to measure the blood count, including the platelets. These tests are repeated weekly as long as the pyrimethamine is being taken. If the blood count falls, we can discontinue the drug before things have gone too far. Second,

Corticosteroids reduce the inflammation but weaken the immune system.

we treat at the same time with folinic acid, a different form of folate that our bodies can use but *Toxoplasma* cannot. This reduces, although does not completely eliminate, the possibility of aplastic anemia.

Corticosteroids, of course, have many potential side effects, including impairment of healing and of the immune system. It's true that it sounds paradoxical to treat an infection with a drug that impairs immunity and increases the risk of infections. And, in fact, corticosteroid medication is never used to treat *Toxoplasma* infections elsewhere in the body, for just that reason. But the inflammation in the eye can be quite harmful to the delicate eye structures. Therefore, we compromise. We use corticosteroids to combat the inflammation but resolve to taper their use as quickly as we can.

Clindamycin, the other drug sometimes used to treat toxoplasmosis, can infrequently cause a very serious side effect called *pseudomembranous colitis*. This represents an infection of the large intestine by a bacterium called *Clostridium difficile*. This bacterium is an opportunist that takes over after many of the "good" bacteria in the large intestine have been killed off by the clindamycin. This colitis, which occurs in no more than a few percent of people who take clindamycin, causes diarrhea, although diarrhea can also occur with clindamycin therapy even if pseudomembranous colitis is not present. If someone is found to have pseudomembranous colitis, another antibiotic must be given to eradicate the *Clostridium difficile* infection. From this discussion of the possible side effects of pyrimethamine, corticosteroids, and clindamycin, it should be clear why we treat toxoplasmosis only when a very significant threat to vision exists.

Optic Nerve Problems

The *optic nerve* is the connection between the eye and the brain. You might even think of the optic nerve as an extension of the brain. Problems involving the optic nerve may interfere with the transmission of the image seen by the eye to the brain, where our higher consciousness recognizes the image. Many types of insults can occur to the optic nerve, and we discuss the main types here. Glaucoma, a disease of the optic nerve, is discussed in chapter 10.

Symptoms of Optic Nerve Disorders

People who are having optic nerve problems often complain of problems with their eyesight and poor color vision. The eyesight problem may present as a large blind spot in the center of the field of vision along with a greatly reduced visual acuity. If color vision is affected, a red object may have a very washed out appearance or simply appear darker to the involved eye than to the good eye. In some cases, the loss of vision may be so subtle that the person does not even recognize it. Any time someone is found to have reduced vision in an eye for which there is no obvious explanation, we do a visual field test to look for clues that might suggest the presence of an optic nerve problem.

Detecting Optic Nerve Problems

Besides measuring the visual acuity and performing color vision and visual field tests, we check the pupils carefully. The pupils of both eyes constrict when light is shone in either one. After checking each pupil individually, we shine the light back and forth between the two eyes, a procedure known as the *swinging flashlight test*. As we go back and forth, the pupils should remain constricted in both eyes. However, if the pupil in one eye appears to dilate a little when the light comes over to that eye (instead of remaining constricted), we call that a *Gunn pupil* or a *relative afferent pupillary defect*. This is an abnormality that strongly suggests optic nerve malfunctioning, although very severe macular degeneration or a retinal detachment involving the macula could also cause it.

Tests that are part of a routine eye examination detect most optic nerve problems.

Careful examination of the optic nerve often yields important clues. If the problem was of fairly sudden onset, the optic disk, which is the optic nerve where it enters the back wall of the eye, may look normal or, in some conditions, swollen. It also swells if there is increased pressure in the fluid around the brain. If the condition has been long-standing, the optic disk may appear pale because of a loss of nerve fibers. We can also examine the nerve fiber layer of the retina in the area around the optic disk. Changes in this layer can be seen if nerve fibers have been lost. Glaucoma, of course, is a long-standing, progressive degeneration of the optic nerve, but the changes in the appearance of the optic nerve are usually fairly distinctive for glaucoma.

Sudden changes in vision from an optic nerve problem suggest a blood vessel shutdown or perhaps an inflammation. Slow, insidious, progressive changes make us worry about the possibility of a tumor or an aneurysm (weakened, dilated artery) pressing on the optic nerve somewhere. Visual field testing can sometimes yield important clues as to the location and cause of the optic nerve disorder. In addition to the examination conducted in the office, other testing procedures, such as brain scans, are sometimes indicated.

Optic Neuritis

Optic neuritis is an inflammation of the optic nerve. It may involve the optic nerve where it enters the back of the eye, or it may involve the portion of the optic nerve in the orbit (socket) behind the eye. Vision is often severely affected because of blind spot formation in the center of the field of vision, and there may be significant loss of peripheral vision as well. Since the straplike muscles that control eye movement are in the vicinity of the optic nerve behind the eye, optic neuritis involving the optic nerve as it travels through the orbit often causes pain when the eye moves.

Poor color vision is a common finding.

When we examine an eye with optic neuritis, we often find not only poor visual acuity but also a loss of color vision, a common finding with other optic nerve problems as well. The optic disk may appear swollen, but it may also look perfectly normal if only the portion of the nerve behind the eye is involved in the inflammation. Visual field testing may show that a large central blind spot may connect with the eye's normal blind spot off to the side.

Causes of Optic Neuritis Although optic neuritis may be caused by virus infections and rarely by bacterial infections, most cases are felt to be a form of autoimmune disease, in which the immune system of the body begins to attack itself. This type of optic neuritis is usually seen in young adults, more commonly in females than in males. When it is not linked to any other disease, we call it *idiopathic* (cause unknown). However, there is an important link between optic neuritis and another important nerve disease of young adults, multiple sclerosis. Multiple sclerosis causes lesions in many parts of the central nervous system (that portion that includes the brain). Optic neuritis can be a sign of multiple sclerosis, and it may, in fact, be the very first sign of the disease to appear. If you have optic neuritis, then what are the chances that you will ultimately be diagnosed with multiple sclerosis? If you are female, and you look about fifteen years into the future, there is at least a 75 percent chance that you will eventually have multiple sclerosis. If you are male, the chances are only about one in three. Although these are worrisome statistics, remember

Optic neuritis may sometimes be the first sign of multiple sclerosis.

that multiple sclerosis is not always the severe, progressive, crippling disease that first comes to mind. Many people may only have a mild form of multiple sclerosis that stops progressing after a certain point.

Besides the vision testing and eye examination performed in the office, people diagnosed with optic neuritis often undergo a brain scan by magnetic resonance imaging (MRI). This type of scan uses a powerful magnet rather than X rays to produce a three-dimensional picture of the brain. The involved optic nerve probably appears thickened on such a scan, but what we are really looking for are lesions in the brain that tell us whether someone is likely to develop multiple sclerosis in the future.

Prognosis for Optic Neuritis Most people with optic neuritis show spontaneous improvement in vision over a period of weeks or months. Usually, most of the lost vision returns, but not quite to its previous level. The question, then, is whether any treatment is beneficial. Treatment with large doses of oral corticosteroids (cortisone), potent anti-inflammatory medication, does not alter the ultimate outcome. Treatment with extremely large doses of intravenous corticosteroids may prolong the time before multiple sclerosis is diagnosed, if it is going to develop at all, but does not improve the outcome of the optic neuritis. Since taking large doses of corticosteroids involves a little risk, there is no point in taking them if they are not going to help. It's a little hard to be afflicted with a disease and do nothing about it but wait and see how it will turn out, but sometimes that is the best approach. We call that "tincture of time."

"Treatment" of optic neuritis does not improve the outcome.

Some, but not all, studies have suggested that people with multiple sclerosis who consume diets that are low in fat, especially saturated fat, the type that predominates in meat, may do better than people on higher-fat diets. Whether such a diet would be beneficial to people suffering from an attack of optic neuritis has never been studied. However, a healthy diet can't hurt.

Ischemic Optic Neuropathy

The term *optic neuropathy* simply means that there is something wrong with the optic nerve. *Ischemic* means that there is inadequate blood flow. Therefore, *ischemic optic neuropathy* refers to optic nerve damage caused by interruption of the circulation. There are two main categories of ischemic optic neuropathy. One is associated with temporal arteritis, and the other is not.

Temporal Arteritis

Temporal arteritis is also known as *giant cell arteritis*. This is an autoimmune kind of inflammation, meaning that the body's immune system mistakenly attacks some of the body's own tissues. Temporal arteritis is a disease of older people, usually over age seventy. Sometimes they may have been feeling poorly for a while, with headaches, muscle aches, and occasionally even weight loss and fever. They may have tenderness over their temples or discomfort when they run a comb through their hair. Their jaw may become tired and achy after chewing a short while. In other people, however, the symptoms may be minimal or absent. Symptoms are caused by an inflammation in arterial walls, which can cut back on the circulation to some areas of the body.

In the eye, temporal arteritis can cause an occlusion of the central retinal artery. (See "Retinal Blood Vessel Occlusions," page 217.) It can also bring about closure of the small blood vessels that bring blood to the optic nerve. This produces what amounts to a stroke of the optic nerve. The severe loss of vision that it typically produces occurs fairly suddenly, sometimes over a period of hours or in a stuttering manner over a few days. This loss of vision is not accompanied by pain in the eye or other symptoms.

Diagnosing Temporal Arteritis When we examine the eye in someone with the temporal arteritis form of ischemic optic neuropathy, we may see swelling of the optic disk. The visual acuity is often extremely poor, accompanied by loss of much of the field of vision. Unfortunately, this loss of vision is frequently irreversible. However, the diagnosis of temporal arteritis must be made with great urgency because of the risk that the optic nerve in the other eye may also become affected, not to mention the possibility of a stroke in the brain.

A blood test called an *erythrocyte sedimentation rate* is performed. This test can be performed immediately by the laboratory and the result obtained. Temporal arteritis usually causes a large elevation of this sedimentation rate, although many other diseases as well as aging itself can affect the sedimentation rate. If temporal arteritis is still suspected as a strong possibility, then a temporal artery biopsy can be performed. In this minor surgical procedure, an incision is made in the skin over one of the arteries in the temple area or on the side of the face near the ear. Interestingly, if temporal arteritis is present, the skin often does not bleed because of the poor circulation from the inflamed arteries. When the artery is located, a segment of it is removed and sent to the pathology department for microscopic examination. The

Biopsy of an artery is necessary to diagnose temporal arteritis.

pathologist makes many tiny slices of the arterial segment and examines them to see whether the typical inflammation caused by temporal arteritis is present in their walls. However, it takes a few days for the pathologist to complete this work. The question, then, is what to do in the interim.

Treating Temporal Arteritis If we suspect that temporal arteritis is present, we immediately begin treating with high doses of oral corticosteroids (cortisone) to combat the inflammation and hopefully prevent involvement of the other eye. In fact, if the temporal artery biopsy has to be delayed for a day or two, the corticosteroids can still be started, because they do not affect the results of the biopsy after such a short time. Why do the biopsy at all, then? Because treatment of temporal arteritis with corticosteroids often continues for a fairly long time, until the disease burns itself out, and we would not want to subject someone to the risks associated with long-term corticosteroid therapy unless we were sure it was truly needed. We usually have the person's internist or other primary care physician monitor the situation to make sure that no complications are arising from the use of these drugs.

Ischemic Optic Neuropathy Without Temporal Arteritis

Ischemic optic neuropathy can also occur in people without temporal arteritis. These are typically middle-aged to elderly people who commonly have small blood vessel disease throughout their bodies. They often have high blood pressure or diabetes, diseases that affect the circulation. When some of the small blood vessels that nourish the optic nerve shut down, vision is lost, although the loss is often not as severe as that seen with temporal arteritis. Swelling may be seen in the optic disk, but it often affects only part of the disk.

If a diagnosis of nonarteritic (nontemporal arteritis-associated) ischemic optic neuropathy is made, there is no specific treatment known to affect the end result. Could an agent like ginkgo biloba extract, which lowers the blood viscosity and thereby promotes better circulation, be of benefit? We don't know at present. What we can do, however, is to treat any of the factors that caused the blood vessel problems to begin with. For example, we can make sure that the blood pressure and diabetes (if present) are under good control, and we can try to modify the lifestyle factors, such as diet and exercise, that contribute to blood vessel problems as well.

Other Optic Nerve Disorders

Many other problems can cause optic neuropathy, damage to the optic nerve. Such damage may be suspected when the vision has declined, when color vision has become poorer in an eye, or when testing the pupils reveals that one pupil does not react as much to incoming light as the other pupil does.

Injuries can damage the optic nerve. Head injuries may cause fractures in the bones of the head and thereby traumatize the optic nerve passing by them. In some cases, a bone fracture is not even necessary. A hard hit to the temple, for example, may cause a tear in an optic nerve. Rarely, the optic nerve may be injured by a needle being used to inject an anesthetic behind the eye. An operation in the orbit (socket) behind the eye to remove a tumor could cause inadvertent nerve damage,

Optic nerve damage has occurred during cosmetic surgery to remove excess eyelid skin.

as could a decompression procedure, in which one or more fractures are purposely created in the walls of the orbit. Surgery such as this may be done in people with severe thyroid gland–related eye problems. Rarely, blindness because of optic nerve damage has been attributed to blepharoplasty surgery, which removes excess eyelid skin and fat. The damage in this case may occur when the surgeon pulls on the fat pads around the eye to remove them, in the process putting traction indirectly on the blood vessels behind the eye and tearing them.

Severe blood loss, as might occur in an accident, can damage the optic nerves by reducing the amount of circulation to them. Blood vessels nourishing the optic nerve can also become blocked, for example, by a piece of calcium that breaks free from a diseased heart valve.

Nutritional factors may play a role in some cases. *Tobacco alcohol amblyopia* refers to optic nerve problems in smokers and alcoholics, but it is not clear how much of a role the tobacco and alcohol play as compared with the B vitamin nutritional deficiencies commonly seen in these people.

Vitamin B_{12} deficiency can cause optic neuropathy along with nerve damage elsewhere. About one in eight adults in the United States over the age of sixty-five is vitamin B_{12} deficient as a result of aging changes in the stomach and small intestine. Although this deficiency is a well-known cause of anemia, nerve damage can occur before the anemia develops. Therefore, vitamin B_{12} deficiency should always be considered as a possible cause of optic neuropathy, and elderly people should probably be screened for vitamin B_{12} deficiency about every two years to prevent the possibility of irreversible nerve damage. Deficiency of other B vitamins, such as folate and thiamin, can also cause optic neuropathy.

One out of eight people over age sixty-five has vitamin B_{12} deficiency.

We have discussed the optic neuritis associated with multiple sclerosis, but other autoimmune diseases like lupus can also affect the optic nerve, probably because the vasculitis (blood vessel inflammation) seen in these conditions can shut down small blood vessels.

People who have an elevated pressure in the fluid around the brain eventually suffer optic nerve damage. Such an elevated pressure may be caused by tumors and other problems, or no other problem may be found, in which case the condition is referred to as *benign intracranial hypertension* or *pseudotumor cerebri*. Many tumors can cause progressive optic nerve damage by pressing directly on the nerves. Such tumors include *meningiomas* (benign tumors of the lining around the brain and optic nerves), optic nerve gliomas, pituitary gland tumors, and tumors that have spread to the brain. Tumors in the orbit can also press on the optic nerve and cause it to degenerate in a slow, progressive manner. Aneurysms of the brain may press on the optic nerve as they enlarge, or they may bleed, with the resultant blood clot putting pressure on the optic nerve and causing its nerve fibers to die off. Aneurysms usually require urgent surgical treatment.

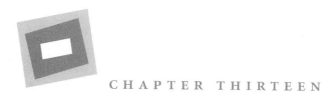

CHAPTER THIRTEEN

Special Topics

Uveitis

Uveitis (or *iritis*) refers to an inflammation of the part of the eye that we call the uvea. The *uvea*, which comes from the Greek word for grape, consists of the heavily pigmented structures: the *iris* (the brown or blue ring around the pupil); the *ciliary body*, which contains a focusing muscle and secretes fluid into the eye; and the *choroid*, the middle coat of the back wall of the eye, sandwiched between the retina and the sclera (see figure 3.1, page 10). If the inflammation involves only the front part of the eye, the area around the iris, we call it *iritis*. If we see inflammation in the *vitreous*, the gel that fills the large, back chamber of the eye between the retina and the lens, we call it *vitritis*. If the most forward part of the vitreous is involved, the inflammation is termed *cyclitis* (or *anterior vitritis*), whereas if the part near the retina is involved, it is called *posterior vitritis*. If both iritis and cyclitis are present, the term is *iridocyclitis*.

Uveitis often falls into the category of autoimmune disease. This means that the immune system of the body, which normally defends the body against foreign invaders like bacteria and viruses, has turned against certain body tissues, attacking them as though it does not recognize them as being part of the body. Some other diseases that are felt to be autoimmune diseases include rheumatoid arthritis, lupus, type I (juvenile) diabetes, and some types of thyroid gland disorders. We often don't know exactly why this autoimmune reaction occurs. In some people, there is a genetic tendency for some kinds of autoimmune disease. We think that, at least in some cases, an infection in the body by a virus or bacterium may somehow begin the process.

Uveitis may be caused by other diseases, but in most cases, no specific cause is found. Some of the diseases that can be associated with uveitis include ankylosing spondylitis (a kind of arthritis affecting the spine), psoriasis, syphilis, tuberculosis, sarcoidosis, toxoplasmosis, cytomegalovirus infection, ulcerative colitis (and less commonly Crohn's disease), multiple sclerosis, and many more. In general, if someone has an episode of iritis for the first time, and it involves one eye only, we generally do not test for these diseases. However, in more complicated situations we do.

Symptoms of Uveitis

Symptoms vary widely depending on the type of inflammation that is present and its location in the eye. The most common presentation for iritis, in which the inflammation is toward the front of the eye, is extreme light sensitivity with some redness (dilated blood vessels) of the affected eye. Other eye problems, such as a scratched cornea, can also cause light sensitivity. However, in iritis, the eye hurts just as much when light is shined into the other eye!

Pain, light sensitivity, and redness are the main symptoms.

That's because even when light enters one eye only, the pupils in both eyes constrict. The muscles of the iris in an eye with iritis are in spasm, and anything that makes the pupil constrict causes pain. Thus, when light is shone in the opposite eye and the pupils of both eyes constrict, the eye with iritis feels the pain.

Another distinguishing feature of the eye with iritis is the type of redness. Often the redness is more marked in the area around the cornea than elsewhere. In addition, it is a "deeper" kind of redness. The redness is caused more by the deeper blood vessels near the sclera than by the blood vessels located toward the surface of the conjunctiva. This is something more easily discernible by the ophthalmologist than by you.

Some cases of iritis have very few symptoms. These cases are the ones more likely to be related to an underlying medical problem. They tend to have an insidious onset rather than the explosive presentation described earlier. The iritis may be present for some time before the diagnosis is made.

When the uveitis presents in the form of vitritis rather than iritis, there is often little or no pain or light sensitivity. In some cases, the vision becomes blurred, and small spots are seen in the field of vision. These spots are caused by clumps of debris that form as a result of the inflammation.

Diagnosing Uveitis

The visual acuity may be normal or reduced, depending on the degree of inflammation inside the eye. If the eye is extremely light sensitive, then it may be extremely difficult at this point to examine the eye. The tip-off that iritis is the cause of the light sensitivity is the fact that pain is evoked by shining a light in the other eye, as mentioned earlier. However, if we can get close to the eye, we often find that the pupil in the eye with iritis is a little smaller than the pupil in the other eye. Spasm in the iris muscle around the pupil causes this difference. By obtaining some magnification with the slit lamp, we can see tiny cells floating in the aqueous humor. These cells are white blood cells that are released when inflammation is present. We can also see what we call *flare* in the aqueous humor. Flare means that we can actually see the beam of light from the slit lamp traveling through the aqueous humor. This is similar to being able to see the beam of light coming from a movie projector in a dusty room. Normally, one

Scarring in the eye may cause glaucoma.

cannot see the light as it travels through the fluid of the eye. However, when inflammation causes protein to be released into that fluid, the light traveling through it becomes visible. Flare and cells are important findings in the diagnosis of iritis.

If we look closely, we can also see small clumps of cells that form on the inner surface of the cornea. These clumps of cells are called *keratic precipitates*. In acute iritis, the type that usually causes pain, these keratic precipitates are tiny and discrete. In the chronic, painless form of iritis, the clumps become fairly large and greasy looking. Rarely, clumps of cells can also be seen on the iris.

The longer iritis has been present, the more likely we are to see adhesions (scarring) between the iris near the pupil and the lens behind it. The changes in the aqueous humor create a "sticky" kind of situation that promotes these adhesions, which we call *synechiae*. The formation of synechiae is undesirable because they not only distort the pupil but also can form in a continuous band around the entire pupil. This prevents the aqueous humor from being able to travel through the pupil into the anterior chamber of the eye, where it can drain out in the normal manner. If this happens, a severe pressure rise, a form of glaucoma, occurs. Synechiae can also form in the front of the eye in the angle where the iris meets the cornea. This is where the drainage channels of the eye are, so synechiae in this region can also cause glaucoma.

We check the lens for the presence of cataract. Both the uveitis itself, if left unchecked, as well as the treatment for it—corticosteroid medication—can cause cataracts.

We also examine the vitreous to detect the presence of cells. If we see cells, then we know that vitritis is present. Sometimes vitritis can coexist along with iritis, and sometimes it may be present by itself.

The pressure in the eye with iritis is frequently lower than in the normal eye. This occurs because inflammation suppresses the formation of aqueous humor. However, the cellular inflammatory debris created by the iritis can sometimes clog up the eye's drainage channels. If this occurs to a significant degree, then the pressure may actually be higher in the involved eye.

We then examine the retina closely. Some forms of infection, such as toxoplasmosis or cytomegalovirus, may cause retinitis, which is usually easy to discern. The blood vessels coursing over the retina are also examined for signs of vasculitis. Finally, we examine the macula for the buildup of fluid that can be seen with moderate to severe uveitis.

Determining the Causes of Uveitis

In someone who (1) has iritis in both eyes, or (2) has iritis that has recurred in one eye, or (3) has vitritis along with iritis, or (4) has the chronic, insidious form of uveitis, we generally do special testing to look for the cause, guided by the patient's past medical history.

Does the person have any symptoms of arthritis in the spine, such as stiffness on getting up in the morning? An X ray of the spine may yield subtle clues about the presence of arthritis. Genetic testing can also determine whether the person has a tendency for this form of arthritis, as well as for iritis. Does the person have any symptoms suggesting urinary tract inflammation? *Reiter's syndrome* is a disease of uncertain cause marked by iritis, occasional conjunctivitis, arthritis, and urethritis (inflammation of the urethra). Is there any chance the person could have acquired a venereal disease? Syphilis is easy to test for and easy to treat should it be present. Is there a history of tuberculosis? A skin test for TB and a chest X ray may provide important information. Does the person have a form of colitis, such as ulcerative colitis? Are there any skin lesions suggestive of psoriasis, another cause of iritis? Could sarcoidosis be present? This is a poorly understood inflammatory disease that can affect many parts of the body. A blood test and X rays can help in the diagnosis. Does the person have an immune system problem, either from a disease like AIDS or as a result of chemotherapy or organ transplant medication? Cytomegalovirus is a cause of infection of the retina and uveitis in patients with immune system disorders. Are there scars on the retina characteristic of old toxoplasmosis infection? (*Toxoplasma* is a one-celled parasitic organism acquired prenatally from one's mother, from infected cat litter, from eating meat, and so on.) It is important to diagnose any underlying medical problem causing the uveitis, because eradication of the uveitis may depend on appropriate treatment of the causative medical condition.

Treating Uveitis

Two types of treatment exist: nonspecific treatment to quell the inflammation, and specific treatment of any underlying medical problem.

Nonspecific treatment invariably involves dilation of the pupil with eyedrops. These drops are called *cycloplegic eyedrops*. They temporarily paralyze the sphincter muscle of the iris, thereby allowing the pupil to dilate. *Dilating eyedrops and corticosteroids put the eye at rest and quell the inflammation.*

They also temporarily paralyze the ciliary body, which contains the muscle the eye uses for near focusing. These actions accomplish two things: (1) They put the eye at rest, reducing the pain and light sensitivity caused by muscle spasm; and (2) they can break synechiae (adhesions) that have formed between the iris and the lens and can hopefully keep new synechiae from forming. Cycloplegic eyedrops vary in strength and duration of action, but their bottles always have red caps for easy identification. Cycloplegics commonly used include atropine, scopolamine, homatropine, cyclopentolate, and tropicamide.

239

Nonspecific treatment also includes corticosteroid (cortisone) medication. Corticosteroids inhibit the inflammation by a number of mechanisms. They are available in both eye drop and ointment form, and they come in different strengths. Prednisolone acetate 1 percent is one of the most potent, while predisolone acetate ⅛ percent is a weaker preparation. Ointment tends to be used only at bedtime to avoid blurring of vision during the day. Initially, the drops may be prescribed anywhere from three times a day to hourly. After the inflammation has responded, the drops must be slowly tapered rather than stopped suddenly to avoid rebound inflammation. Eyedrops or ointment such as this is used when iritis is present. If the uveitis consists of vitritis only, these medications are generally not effective because they don't penetrate into the back areas of the eye.

When vitritis is present, the corticosteroid medication is delivered by other means. One way of accomplishing this is to give an injection right next to the eye. We call this a *subconjunctival injection,* because the medication is injected under the conjunctiva. The corticosteroid medication is gradually released from this location and reaches all parts of the eye. Some studies indicate that this is the most effective way of getting corticosteroid drugs into the vitreous. A subconjunctival injection causes just mild discomfort at the time it is given, but the eye usually feels quite sore over the next twenty-four hours. People sometimes say it feels as if they had been kicked in the eye by a mule (or at least what they imagine that would be like).

The alternative to a subconjunctival injection is to take the corticosteroid medication by mouth, something occasionally done if the uveitis involves both eyes or if the patient refuses to have an injection. This approach not only delivers the medication to the eye but also subjects the entire body to significant amounts. Corticosteroid medication can cause numerous side effects. In the eye, it can raise the intraocular pressure, causing secondary glaucoma that can damage the optic nerve, and it can cause cataracts after months of use. All forms of corticosteroids, whether given as eyedrops or delivered into the body as a whole, can cause these eye problems. However, systemic corticosteroids (given by mouth or by intramuscular or intravenous injection) impair the immune system, increasing the risk of serious infection, especially after prolonged use. An inactive tuberculosis infection in the lungs can suddenly become active. Corticosteroids delay and interfere with healing. Psychological

Corticosteroid (cortisone) treatment can have many side effects.

effects, including depression, may occur. People sometimes eat ravenously and gain weight. Fluid retention can develop. The blood sugar may become elevated in susceptible people, blood pressure may rise, and peptic ulcers may recur. In rare cases, the hip joints or the kidneys may be severely damaged.

Because of this multitude of possible side effects, we never prescribe large doses of corticosteroids without carefully evaluating the benefit/risk ratio. However, in many cases, corticosteroids are definitely indicated, especially when losing an eye is a possible consequence of not using them. If you are taking corticosteroids, report promptly any symptoms you think you may be having to your doctor.

In some people, the uveitis does not resolve completely with treatment, or it recurs as soon as the medication is tapered down. These individuals may need to continue corticosteroid treatment at the lowest possible dosage indefinitely. Obviously, it would be nice if we had a safer long-term alternative to corticosteroids. The nonsteroidal anti-inflammatory drugs (NSAIDs), commonly used for arthritis, have been tried, but without much success.

One patient of mine suffered from a chronic uveitis (primarily vitritis) in one eye that was presumably caused by her sarcoidosis, an inflammatory disease that can also cause lung problems, among other things. She required corticosteroids by mouth, and whenever I tapered her below a certain level, the uveitis surfaced again—very frustrating. Finally, I suggested she take some ginkgo biloba extract at 80 milligrams three times a day—double the usual dose, in addition to her corticosteroid. This extract has a mild inhibiting action on platelet-activating factor, a substance involved in inflammation. I slowly tapered her off her corticosteroid, except that this time, her uveitis did not flare up again! One day, she returned to the office complaining of symptoms in her eye along with a flare-up of her lung problems from the sarcoidosis. The uveitis had *returned*. On questioning her, I found that she had absentmindedly stopped taking the ginkgo biloba on her own, and the recurrence of both of her problems followed soon thereafter. I put her back on the same regimen, and once more I was able to taper her off the corticosteroids by maintaining her on the ginkgo biloba.

Obviously, the previous anecdote is simply that—an anecdote. We can't say for sure that the ginkgo biloba had a beneficial effect. But it might have, and it certainly deserves further study. Ginkgo biloba certainly does not have the anti-inflammatory strength of corticosteroids and should not be used in place of them. But simply to try the ginkgo biloba as a supplement seemed warranted, considering the potential hazards associated with long-term corticosteroid use.

Get plenty of rest, avoid stress, and eat a healthy diet.

While we're talking about "natural" treatment modalities, we should talk about general supportive measures for the patient with uveitis. Avoidance of any stress, physical or emotional, is important. A major physical stressor is lack of adequate rest. Make sure you get enough sleep every night. Eat a balanced diet with plenty of fruits and vegetables. I have seen many patients with immune-mediated inflammatory disorders who suffered a major setback when their bodies became stressed for one reason or another.

Treating Specific Causes of Uveitis

When someone is found to have a previously undetected medical problem that is now causing uveitis, the internist or family physician must often share in the care with the ophthalmologist.

Treating the uveitis may not always necessitate treatment of the underlying problem. *Ankylosing spondylitis,* a form of arthritis in the spine, affects 1 out of every 500 to 1,000 people and is more common in men than in women. The iridocyclitis (both iritis and cyclitis) is treated nonspecifically with cycloplegic and corticosteroid eyedrops. *Psoriasis* affects primarily the skin but can also cause arthritis and uveitis. Again, nonspecific treatment of the uveitis is all that is necessary. The same applies to *Reiter's syndrome* (arthritis, urethritis, conjunctivitis, and iridocyclitis) and inflammatory bowel disease (*ulcerative colitis* and *Crohn's disease*).

Syphilis is a venereal disease that has always been much less common than others, such as gonorrhea or chlamydia infections. But the bacterium responsible for syphilis causes a chronic infection in the body that can affect many organ systems, including the brain, spinal cord, eyes, and heart. Congenital syphilis causes a number of deformities in the newborn infant, but syphilis acquired during life is quite serious as well. A syphilis infection can go through several stages, termed *primary, secondary,* and *tertiary syphilis.* Primary syphilis can cause a sore on the genitals that eventually resolves. Secondary syphilis includes other manifestations that occur as the bacterium spreads throughout the body. Tertiary syphilis involves the late, most serious complications. Uveitis is a common manifestation of secondary syphilis, and a blood test for syphilis is almost always part of the medical testing done for uveitis. If the blood test is positive, then additional confirmatory tests, sometimes including a spinal tap, are done. Penicillin or another antibiotic is then administered in high doses.

Although we generally do not see uveitis associated with rheumatoid arthritis in adults, it is a common feature of *juvenile rheumatoid arthritis*. Interestingly, those children who only have a few joints involved have a much higher risk of developing iridocyclitis than do those whose arthritis involves many joints. Often, the iridocyclitis occurs in what seems to be a quiet eye, causing no symptoms at all, and a significant amount of damage can occur to the eye by the time the iridocyclitis is diagnosed. Therefore, children who are felt to be at high risk should undergo routine screening eye examinations.

Sarcoidosis is a chronic inflammatory disease that affects the lungs, bones, eyes, and other tissues. It can cause a chronic uveitis, often primarily involving the vitreous of the eye, and may occasionally affect the optic nerve or retina. Chest X rays sometimes show large, calcified lymph nodes between the lungs. A blood test may show a high level of angiotensin-converting enzyme. Other blood test abnormalities are occasionally found as well. If the eye appears to be involved, the inside lining of the lower eyelid can be biopsied, especially if any small nodules appear to be present there. The biopsy result may support a diagnosis of sarcoidosis. Treatment of any uveitis is nonspecific, however, as corticosteroids represent the only form of treatment for sarcoidosis.

Toxoplasmosis, a parasitic infection caused by *Toxoplasma gondii,* is a cause of retinochoroiditis, an infection primarily of the retina and secondarily of the choroid layer of the eye. (See "Toxoplasmosis," page 224.) Pregnant women can transmit it to their offspring, and it is most commonly acquired by eating undercooked meat or by coming into contact with the litter of infected cats. In some cases, a marked uveitis can accompany the retinochoroiditis, sometimes severe enough to obscure the view of the retina. The uveitis and retinal inflammation are treated by high doses of oral corticosteroids, while the infection of the retina is treated with combinations of antitoxoplasmosis drugs, which include sulfa drugs, pyrimethamine, clindamycin, and the tetracyclines. The corticosteroids impair the immune system, of course, but their use is essential if the sight and the eye itself are to be saved.

Headaches

Eye problems cause headaches less frequently than most people think. In most people, the mild blurring of vision that necessitates a change in glasses does not cause headaches. Eye muscle problems may occasionally cause headaches. The most common of these would be a *convergence insufficiency,* a weakness of the muscles that turn the eyes inward. (See page 107.) Many headaches feel as though the pain is located in or behind the eyes, but that does not necessarily mean that there is an eye problem. Also, rest assured that a feeling of pressure in the eyes is not a sign of glaucoma (unless the eye pressure is extremely high, which is rare).

Headaches may result from a number of causes, including migraine, allergy, elevated fluid pressure around the brain, circulation problems to the brain, and head injuries. But the most common cause of headache, by far, is muscle tension.

Muscle Tension Headaches

Muscle tension headaches often result from stress. Some people handle stress better than others do. For people who have no outlet for their stress, the stress may become localized in the muscles of the head, including those that surround the eye. Muscle tension headaches are not associated with any particular activity, such as reading (unless the reading material is very stressful!). In fact, people often wake up with the headache. So much for restful sleep.

> *Muscle spasm on the back of the head can cause what feels like eye pain.*

Sometimes a stressful event causes a headache, but even after the stressful event is gone, the headache remains. This type of chronic headache may persist until the vicious cycle is broken.

One form of muscle-related headache is called *greater occipital neuralgia.* This is a kind of headache pain that follows the distribution of certain nerves on the head. People who have greater occipital neuralgia typically complain of pain in or behind the eye, but on examination, they have an area of tenderness on the back of the head right at the base of the skull. Why should muscle tension in the back of the head cause eye pain? It has to do with a phenomenon called *referred pain.* This means that when people experience a problem along one branch of a nerve, they often experience and localize the pain as though it were coming from a location in the territory of one of the other branches of that nerve. In the case of greater occipital neuralgia, the same nerve that sends a branch to the muscles at the back of the skull also sends a branch to the muscles near the eye. When the muscle in back goes into spasm and pinches the nerve, the person feels it in the eye. Greater occipital neuralgia can be caused by stress-related muscle tension, although it may sometimes be associated with arthritic problems in the neck.

Eliminating muscle tension headaches may not be easy, but you can try a number of approaches. Obviously, if there is a source of stress in your life, such as job-related stress, you can take steps to eliminate it. You can also work at reframing things in your mind so that they don't bother you as much. For example, if you are stressed out by having to wait in lines or in rush hour traffic, try to look at it positively. Think of it as an opportunity to improve yourself by developing the attribute of patience. Or consider it an opportunity to think through in your mind some dilemma you've been facing. Things are stressful only if you allow them to be stressful to you.

Muscle relaxation techniques are safe and effective.

Muscle relaxation techniques are very useful. Many of us walk around with tensed muscles without even being aware of it. The remedy for this is to get in touch with your body and become aware of how it is behaving. Try this. Lie down in bed on your back with your legs uncrossed, or just sit back in your chair, and breathe slowly and deeply, in and out. Try to relax completely. Begin with your toes and your feet. Are they completely limp? If not, allow them to relax. Then mentally move up to your ankles, legs, and thighs. Allow them to loosen up and become completely relaxed. Then concentrate on your abdomen. Allow it to follow the pattern of your breathing. Allow the outward movement of your abdomen to draw in your every breath. Then relax your fingers, hands, arms, and shoulders. If they are tense, become aware of that tension and learn to recognize when those muscles are tense and when they are not. Then concentrate on your neck and head. Let them completely relax. Is your forehead drawn into furrows? If so, relax your forehead muscles and note the difference. This type of muscle relaxation exercise should be done not only whenever you are showing signs of tension, but also routinely, to keep yourself from tensing up.

Massage, biofeedback, even acupuncture—many other techniques may be worth trying. Should you take pain medication? You should when necessary, as it may also help break the cycle of pain and muscle spasm. Avoid addictive prescription medications, however. Learning to become aware of tight muscles and to relax them is more effective in the long run and certainly a healthier alternative.

Migraine

Migraine is a common disorder, affecting one out of six women and about one in twenty men. Migraine headaches are sometimes called *vascular headaches,* referring to the fact that they involve both constriction and dilation of blood vessels of the brain during the headache's various phases. Many forms of migraine exist. In *classical migraine,* the person experiences visual changes, called an *aura,* followed by a headache. Some people can get the headache without experiencing the aura, while others may have the aura but not get a headache. Migraine without a headache? Exactly. We call this *acephalgic migraine.* (*Cephalgia* is the medical term for headache.) Some people have the aura followed by headache when they are younger, but then have the aura without a headache when they become middle-aged or older.

When I see people who I suspect may be suffering from migraine, I always ask them two questions. First, do you have car sickness now, or did you as a child? For some reason, a history of motion sickness is somewhat more common in migraine sufferers. Second, do you get a headache when you eat something that is very cold? Experiencing pain, usually on the forehead between the eyes, after eating something cold is strongly correlated with migraine. They are often termed *ice-cream headaches.* What I have found to be very interesting is that most people who answer yes are puzzled about why I asked. They assume that everyone who eats ice cream gets a pain in the head! Apparently, it is not a common topic for discussion. In my experience, it is unusual to find someone with migraine who does not give a history of ice-cream headaches.

Ice-cream headaches go hand in hand with migraine.

Symptoms of Migraine The aura of migraine may be difficult to understand for people who have never experienced it. Visual changes are the most common manifestation of the migraine aura because the arteries that supply the part of the brain that controls vision are the ones most likely to constrict. However, other parts of the brain can occasionally be affected, producing transient paralysis of one side of the body or perhaps involving one of the nerves that controls eye movement, causing double vision. In any case, the aura usually lasts less than an hour.

Visual auras usually involve blind spots in either the left or right half of the field of vision of each eye. The auras often include what we call *scintillations,* jagged lines or abstract figures of varying configurations that may not be too noticeable at first but then become more prominent while enlarging and flickering wildly. People who experience the aura often have to stop what they are doing and just close their eyes. The blind spots can be quite frightening, especially the first time they are experienced. Although the vision generally returns to normal at the conclusion of the aura, rarely one may find permanent damage as one would see in someone who has suffered a stroke. For example, one might occasionally see a Horner's syndrome in someone who has suffered repeated attacks of migraine. Horner's syndrome refers to nerve damage that causes a mild drooping of the upper eyelid and a slightly smaller pupil in the eye on that side. Rarely, people may also complain of small, permanent blind spots.

I had a patient, a smoker, who suffered from migraine. During the aura of one attack, the vision completely blacked out on the left side of his vision in each eye. Unfortunately, it never returned. He was left with this disabling loss of vision, possibly because the blood vessel spasm associated with smoking prolonged the constriction of his arteries and resulted in a stroke in the vision part of his brain. A word to the wise is sufficient.

Some physicians are puzzled when they see the occasional patient who has the migraine aura but no headache thereafter. Although this phenomenon, acephalgic migraine, is well known to ophthalmologists and neurologists, the average physician may not be aware of its frequency or the fact that it even exists. But what about the middle-aged or elderly patient who

Migraine without the headache is a common phenomenon.

develops what sounds like a migraine-related aura, even though that person has never experienced a migraine in the past? Migraine usually begins in children or young adults. To occur for the first time in older people is unusual.

Visual changes that may be very similar to the auras of migraine may be seen in adults experiencing circulation problems to the brain because of hardening of the arteries. In other words, they may represent a warning sign that the individual is at risk for a stroke. In someone like this, appropriate testing of the circulation to the brain must be performed so that preventive measures aimed at reducing the chance of a stroke can be carried out.

The headache caused by migraine often involves only one side of the head. Generally, the same side of the head is not involved with every attack. Migraine often causes a severe, throbbing headache. It may strike suddenly, or it may come on more gradually. The headache is often accompanied by nausea and heightened sensitivity to light and sound. It is easy to understand why migraine is sometimes called a "sick headache." The migraine sufferer must often just go to bed and wait out the attack.

In an older person, vision changes similar to those of migraine may be the warning sign of a stroke.

Treating Migraine Pain medication may be all that is needed if the headache is not severe. *Fiorinal*, a combination of aspirin, caffeine, and butalbital (a barbiturate sedative), can be effective, and it is also available with added codeine for more severe headaches. Aspirin can also be combined with acetaminophen and caffeine for use in mild cases. Besides aspirin, other drugs of the nonsteroidal anti-inflammatory class, such as naproxen, are effective and can also be taken routinely to prevent migraine attacks. To avoid the risk of addiction, strong narcotics should be used only occasionally.

Other drugs used to treat migraine include *ergotamine* and *dihydroergotamine,* members of the drug class called *ergot alkaloids.* They are available in many forms and can be taken by mouth, sprayed in the nose, or injected. Ergotamine is sometimes taken orally along with caffeine after the aura of migraine appears to prevent or diminish the headache. It can cause nausea, however, adding to the nausea that is part of a migraine attack. Because ergot alkaloids constrict blood vessels, there is also some concern that they may prolong the period of reduced circulation to parts of the brain and increase the risk of permanent brain damage.

Treating the muscle tension component can be helpful.

A newer class of drugs, commonly known as the *triptans,* can also be given by mouth, by injection, or sprayed into the nose. They are effective in lessening or shortening the headache in migraine, but the headache can return after the medication wears off. As newer drugs, they are fairly expensive.

Finally, it is important to note that although migraines are "vascular" headaches associated with dilation of arteries in the brain, there is often a muscle tension component to migraine headaches as well. Therefore, treatment of the muscle tension component, as discussed earlier, can also be effective in reducing the amount of pain.

Preventing Migraine Many drugs have been tried and found to be somewhat effective in preventing migraine attacks. Beta blocker drugs, such as propranolol and timolol, when taken regularly, can reduce the frequency of migraine. These drugs can have side effects, however. They can cause asthma attacks in predisposed people, worsen the blood cholesterol profile, and cause feelings of tiredness and depression. Calcium channel blockers such as verapamil, frequently used to treat high blood pressure, can also prevent migraine. Antidepressant medication of the tricyclic class and an antiepilepsy drug called *valproate* have also been used with some success. And, as mentioned before, nonsteroidal anti-inflammatory drugs, commonly used to treat arthritis and for pain relief, also appear to have preventive properties.

In the herbal area, feverfew *(Tanacetum parthenium)* seems to help prevent and treat migraine headaches, although it is probably not as effective as the beta blockers. It also has anti-inflammatory properties. Feverfew herbal extracts are often standardized according to their content of parthenolide, which may be the main active component. Feverfew can be irritating to the inside of the mouth and is very bitter, so it is often taken in the form of capsules or tablets.

Extracts of the herb feverfew may reduce the frequency of attacks.

Like aspirin and the other nonsteroidal anti-inflammatory drugs, feverfew can inhibit the function of the platelets in the blood, which are involved in the first step of blood clot formation. Therefore, caution should be observed in people who have a bleeding tendency. The long-term consequences of taking feverfew continuously are not known, but it appears to be fairly safe. There may be some rebound effects in terms of migraine attacks, anxiety, and inflammation in the body after discontinuing it. If you decide to take feverfew, do so with your physician's knowledge and choose a brand from a well-established company that labels its product with the parthenolide content. Do not ask a health food store clerk for medical advice.

Hormonal factors can play in important role in migraine. For example, birth control pills may have an effect, in one direction or the other, on the incidence of migraine headaches. Therefore, the presence of migraine may influence the choice of birth control bills or hormone replacement therapy.

Many foods have been suspected of triggering migraine in sensitive individuals. Cheese, chocolate, and red wines are some of the more commonly mentioned foods, but it varies widely from one person to another. The best thing for you to do is to try to determine whether eating some food product is often followed by a migraine headache. If you suspect a given food, try eliminating it from your diet and see whether you develop fewer headaches. Newer research suggests that high-fat diets, especially those rich in animal fats, promote migraine. A diet high in complex carbohydrates (starch) and low in fat may be very helpful as a preventive.

Dairy products or other foods may trigger migraine in some people.

Other Headache-Related Eye Problems

Many major brain problems can cause both headaches and eye problems. For example, brain tumors may not only cause headaches but also cause double vision by pressing on some of the nerves that control eye movement. They may damage the optic nerve, either by pressing directly on the optic nerve fibers as they pass through the brain or by raising the fluid pressure inside the head, which in turn applies pressure to the optic nerves. An aneurysm, by bleeding suddenly, may cause similar problems. Nerve palsies caused by the shutdown of small blood vessels, as often seen in diabetics, are sometimes accompanied by pain around the involved eye. Some eye medications, such as pilocarpine, a drug used to treat glaucoma, may cause a headache, although in the case of pilocarpine, it is often termed a brow ache.

Fortunately, most headaches are not caused by serious problems such as brain tumors or aneurysms. But any new headache, especially one that persists or is different in quality from a person's "usual" headaches, deserves medical evaluation.

Thyroid Disorders

Thyroid gland problems are about nine times more common in women than in men. The thyroid gland produces two important thyroid hormones known as *T4* and *T3*. Both overactive (hyperthyroid) and underactive (hypothyroid) conditions can develop, upsetting the body's metabolism.

Hypothyroidism

People who are *hypothyroid* may feel tired and sluggish, gain weight, and even have some memory loss. They frequently develop swelling, which can include the area around the eyes. The hairs on the outer portion of their eyebrows may be lost as well. Dry eye syndrome is also more common than in the average person and may require the use of artificial tear drops. Hypothyroidism may occur on its own or be present after treatment for hyperthyroidism. A less common cause is iodine insufficiency, seen in people who do not consume iodized salt, fish, or sea vegetables and live in an area where the soil in which foods are grown is low in iodine. People who eat a lot of raw cruciferous vegetables, such as cauliflower and broccoli, may also become hypothyroid. Those vegetables contain substances that are said to be *goitrogenic*—they interfere with the formation of thyroid hormones. People with these latter forms of hypothyroidism sometimes develop a *goiter*—an enlarged thyroid gland that can be felt on examination.

Tiredness, weight gain, and memory loss are some of the symptoms.

Hyperthyroidism

An overactive thyroid gland may be associated with nodules, little bumps on the thyroid gland, that produce excess thyroid hormones, or more commonly may be caused by *Grave's disease,* an inflammatory autoimmune condition in which the entire gland becomes overactive. Autoimmune diseases are those in which the body's immune system turns against itself, producing different kinds of inflammatory problems.

Hyperthyroidism can produce weight loss, hair loss, nervousness, palpitations, and many other symptoms. It produces a multitude of problems associated with the eyes that we call *thyroid ophthalmopathy.* People who smoke are at increased risk for these eye problems. If you smoke, this should certainly make you want to quit if nothing else does. Interestingly, the eye problems seem to be a separate phenomenon from the symptoms that arise elsewhere in the body. In fact, some people don't even develop the eye problems until their hyperthyroidism is treated (by surgery, treatment with radioactive iodine, or drugs that suppress

Smoking increases the risk of thyroid-related eye problems.

the thyroid gland). Radioiodine treatment in older people seems to carry with it a higher risk of ophthalmopathy as compared with surgery or drugs. In some people, any thyroid-related eye problems already present can become worse after the thyroid hormone levels have become normalized. Just as perplexing, some people develop the eye problems even though they do not have and have never had elevated thyroid hormone levels. We say that such people have *euthyroid* (neither hyper- nor hypo-) *ophthalmopathy*. Obviously, there is still a lot about the thyroid gland that we do not understand.

Symptoms of Thyroid Ophthalmopathy

People with thyroid ophthalmopathy have very uncomfortable eyes, and it is extremely difficult to make them comfortable. They complain of burning, grittiness, feeling of something in the eye, tearing, and light sensitivity. A number of the changes that occur around the eye can explain this. Eyelid retraction often occurs. This means that the eyes are open wider, and the white of the eye is often visible on top as well as below, something that does not normally occur. When they look down, the upper eyelid may lag somewhat rather than following the eye downward as it should. People also tend to develop *exophthalmos*, a forward protrusion of the eyes that results from inflammation in the fat and muscle tissue in the socket behind the eyes. Hyperthyroidism is the most common cause of exophthalmos, whether in both eyes or just one. The wider opening of the eyes from the eyelid retraction and the protrusion of the eyes from the exophthalmos make the surface of the eye dry

The eye muscles may become thickened, and double vision may occur.

out quickly, and this undoubtedly contributes to the symptoms. In fact, if the exposure of the cornea becomes severe enough, it can become ulcerated, clouded, and may eventually perforate, resulting in loss of the eye.

In many people with thyroid ophthalmopathy, the eye muscles are affected by the inflammation. They become thickened and scarred. This thickening can easily be seen with a computed tomography (CT) scan, a three-dimensional type of X ray. Involvement of the muscles in this way causes them to become dysfunctional. For example, when the inferior rectus muscle, the muscle below the eye that turns the eye downward, becomes scarred, it loses its flexibility and tethers the eye down, preventing it from moving upward. As different muscles become affected to differing degrees in the two eyes, double vision can result. The tethering effect can also make the pressure in the eye go up when the eye looks in certain directions. Finally, because of the swelling in the orbit tissues, the optic nerve can become squeezed and badly damaged. Frequent examinations, including visual field testing, may be necessary in high-risk patients to make sure that the optic nerve is not being compromised. Eventually, after a period of two to three years, the inflammation of the various tissues caused by thyroid ophthalmopathy tends to burn itself out. The eye situation is then stable.

Treating Thyroid Ophthalmopathy

Treatment depends on the nature and degree of the problems. Irritative symptoms can be treated with frequent instillation of preservative-free artificial tear drops, which are sold over the counter. Such drops come in different brands, and you should try the different varieties to see which one makes your eyes feel the best. Sunglasses can help with light sensitivity and retard the evaporation of tears from the eye. The retraction of the eyelids may get better when the thyroid hormones are brought down to normal levels. If it doesn't, a simple operation can be performed on *Mueller's muscle,* one of the muscles of the upper eyelid, to lower it to a more acceptable level. Obviously, this does not have to be done if the cornea is not drying out, but some people desire it for cosmetic reasons.

Reducing the exophthalmos is a more difficult task. In some cases, treatment with corticosteroids can be used to reduce the inflammation behind the eye. If that does not work, we might consider performing a decompression procedure in which the bones of the orbit are fractured, thereby allowing some of the fat tissue behind the eye to exit the orbit and allowing the eyeball to sink back somewhat. There is some risk to this type of surgery, including risk to the optic nerve and a small risk that an eye muscle might become entrapped in the area of fractured bone. Decompression is performed when pressure-related damage is occurring to the optic nerve or the cornea is in danger from exposure. In a small percentage of cases, it is done for cosmetic reasons. If you are considering having surgery for cosmetic reasons, be sure you are informed of the surgical risks.

When inflammation in the eye muscles causes double vision, a mild form of radiation therapy to the orbit can sometimes improve but not cure the problem. To lessen or eliminate double vision, prisms can be incorporated into eyeglass lenses, and this is often a good temporary fix. If the muscles change with time, the prisms can be changed as well. Ultimately, however, surgery on the muscles may be contemplated if there is more than just a mild double vision problem. Such surgery generally involves removing a scarred muscle where it is attached to the eyeball and sewing it back on with an adjustable suture. The suture is adjusted the day after the surgery so that the muscle ends up in the right position. It is done this way because the results would be very unpredictable otherwise.

Although eye muscle surgery such as this can be successful, it should only be done if the eye positions and movement have been stable for a minimum of six months, that is, the inflammation from the thyroid disease has burned itself out. There is no point in performing surgery if the eye muscles are going to continue to change afterward.

Another approach that has been tried is to inject botulinum toxin into a muscle. This is the toxin that causes the dreaded form of food poisoning called *botulism,* but in this case the toxin is used in a positive way, causing a temporary mild paralysis of a muscle to favorably affect muscle balance.

In summary, hyperthyroidism, or Grave's disease, can have a profound effect on the eyes. The problems it produces can be very complex, and every case is different. The proper outlook is to work to make the best of the situation. Although things will probably never be perfect, they can at least be made tolerable. The real challenge facing researchers will be to learn how to prevent thyroid ophthalmopathy from occurring.

Parkinson's Disease

Stiffness and tremor are the hallmarks of Parkinson's disease, but eye problems associated with the disease can interfere with functioning as well. People with Parkinson's usually develop a stare because they don't blink as frequently as they used to. Involuntary eyelid closing is also frequent. Eye movement disorders are apparent on examination, although they do not always cause problems from a functional standpoint. For example, the eyes may not move much in an upward direction, something that occurs to a lesser degree in many people as they age. The eyes may have difficulty fixating on objects and following them as they move. These problems are all caused by the degeneration in the brainstem seen in people with Parkinson's disease. This degeneration results in low levels of dopamine, an important chemical messenger in the brain.

Low dopamine levels may cause other vision problems. Special tests measuring electrical activity in the eye and brain, such as the visual evoked potential (VEP) and the electroretinogram (ERG), have shown abnormalities in people with Parkinson's. Symptoms caused by these abnormalities include poorer vision, reduced color vision, and difficulty determining the correct location of an object. It is not clear whether all of these vision problems are the result of the degeneration in the brain or whether some may be due to lowered dopamine levels in certain cells of the retina.

The lack of blinking can make reading difficult.

The lack of blinking often causes problems, especially with reading. Blinking is necessary to keep the front surface of the eye moist and preserve the quality of the tear film that coats the cornea. With inadequate blinking, dry spots form on the cornea, causing discomfort and interfering with vision. Furthermore, without the windshield wiper–like motions of the eyelids, the quality of the tear film suffers greatly. Oily debris builds up in the tear film, making it "dirty." This destabilizes the tear film and allows dry spots to appear on the eye much sooner than they would otherwise. As a result of these problems, along with the dryness of the eyes that often accompanies aging, people with Parkinson's disease may have difficulty reading and seeing clearly in general.

The ultimate solution to the eye problems seen in Parkinson's disease will be better treatment or even prevention of the underlying disease. Better drugs are being developed, and surgical treatments are being investigated. Dietary treatment can be valuable as well. Many patients with Parkinson's disease develop an on-off syndrome, in which the symptoms of Parkinson's come and go. Higher-protein diets seem to contribute to the problem, inhibiting the absorption of L-dopa-containing medication such as Sinemet and interfering with its ability to enter the brain. A healthy fruit- and vegetable-based diet, lower in protein than the average American diet, can help alleviate this problem.

Preservative-free artificial tear drops, sold over the counter, can be used as a way of lubricating the eye and temporarily improving the quality of the tear film. However, because of the involuntary spasmodic closing of the eyelids that is often present, instilling the drops may not always be too easy, and the drops' effect may last for no more than fifteen minutes. Use of an eye-wash to flush out the debris and wet the eye may also be helpful. Above all, it is important that the cause of the visual problems be recognized so that unnecessary surgical procedures, such as cataract surgery, are not performed.

A lower-protein diet can enhance the medication's effect.

Herpes Infections

Herpes is a virus that at times causes active infection and at other times remains in an inactive, latent state. There are two main forms that infect the eyes, *herpes simplex* and *herpes zoster*, the latter better known as *shingles*. Herpes viruses can involve many parts of the body, and their effects on the eye can sometimes be sight threatening. Since the effects of each type of herpes virus are quite different, we will approach them separately.

Herpes Simplex

There are two strains of herpes simplex: *herpes simplex type I* and *herpes simplex type II*. We generally think of herpes simplex type I as the strain that causes cold sores and fever blisters and occasionally infects the eye. Herpes simplex type II is most closely associated with genital herpes infections. However, either strain can affect either part of the body. Sophisticated testing can differentiate between the two strains, but in practice this is not done because it makes no difference with regard to treatment or prognosis.

Conjunctivitis from herpes simplex may look identical to any other viral infection.

When herpes simplex infects the eye, there is usually a history of previous cold sore or fever blister formation. Ninety-nine percent of the time, only one of the eyes is affected, even in people in whom the disease recurs many times. A common first episode of herpes around the eye is an infection of the eyelid near its margin. Tiny blisters may be seen on the eyelid, especially toward the margin.

These resolve without treatment, just as fever blisters and cold sores go away on their own. Herpes simplex can also cause *conjunctivitis,* commonly known as *pinkeye.* The red, watery eye can be indistinguishable in appearance from the conjunctivitis caused by the usual upper respiratory cold viruses. Therefore, a person can have conjunctivitis caused by herpes and not even know that is what it is.

A much more serious situation develops when herpes infects the cornea, a condition called *keratitis.* Involvement of the cornea

Herpes infections produce a characteristic lesion on the cornea.

may produce minimal symptoms at first, perhaps slight light sensitivity and a scratchy feeling in the eye. On examination, the earliest signs may be just some dotlike areas on the surface of the cornea where a few of the cells have sloughed off. Even an ordinary virus infection can look this way. If the infection does not go away on its own at this point but instead progresses, it forms a characteristic lesion on the surface of the cornea called a *dendrite.* A dendrite represents a defect in the surface layer of cells in the cornea, and this defect has a branching shape, with limbs coming off of other limbs. This branching pattern represents the pathway of the virus as it grows through the corneal cells. Generally, the dendritic keratitis (infection) caused by the herpes virus is so characteristic in appearance that a herpes infection is diagnosed by this alone. Virus cultures, which may take weeks to yield results, or any other testing procedures are not necessary. Another finding with a herpes infection of the cornea is that the cornea loses some of its sensation. If the uninfected eye is touched with a little wisp of cotton, you certainly feel it. When the infected cornea is touched, you may feel nothing at all.

Untreated corneal herpes infections may become even more advanced. Large layers of corneal surface cells slough off, and the infection is then called *geographic* or *amoeboid keratitis.* The area where the cells have been lost has a large, irregular shape, like the appearance of a country on a map or an amoeba under a microscope. Geographic keratitis has a worse prognosis than the earlier dendritic keratitis. It may be harder to eradicate and is more likely to lead to other complications. Herpes keratitis that cannot be controlled can lead to scarring of the cornea and extensive loss of vision.

Treating Herpes Simplex Infections Herpes infections on the cornea may resolve spontaneously without treatment, but usually they persist and become worse. Several antiviral drugs are effective at eradicating the active infection. It is important to use them exactly as prescribed because of the sight-threatening nature of herpes infections. Trifluridine (Viroptic) is an eyedrop usually instilled every two hours except during sleep, for a total of about nine times a day. After the infection starts to respond to the treatment, the frequency of eyedrop use can be reduced. Treatment is continued until all signs of active infection are gone, which usually takes one to two weeks. Along with the antiviral medication, a dilating (cycloplegic) eyedrop is usually prescribed, especially if there are any signs of inflammation inside the eye that is putting the eye muscles into spasm.

An alternative antiviral medication is vidarabine (Vira-A). It comes in the form of an ointment that you instill every four hours while you are awake, or a total of five times a day. It is less expensive than Viroptic and may be easier for people who cannot keep up with the more frequent eyedrop use. As with any ointment, Vira-A may blur the vision somewhat.

One other antiviral medication is available in both eyedrop and ointment forms. It is called idoxuridine and is less expensive than the other two medications. However, it is more likely to cause toxic effects to the eye with extended use. Such side effects may include loss of cells from the surface of the cornea and scarring in the tear drainage passageways, both of which are problems that the herpes virus itself can cause.

One other note: It is very important not to use corticosteroid (cortisone) eyedrop medication when an active infection of the cornea with herpes simplex is present, because doing so makes the prognosis much worse. As I have already pointed out, a herpes conjunctivitis may look just like any other eye infection. That is exactly why corticosteroid eyedrops should never be used in the treatment of what looks like a routine eye infection.

Do Herpes Infections Return? Although treating a corneal herpes infection usually makes the active infection go away, the virus never disappears entirely. It hides in nerves behind the eye in a latent, inactive form. It always has the potential to come back. We know that within two years after the first episode of herpes keratitis, there is a 25 percent chance that the active infection *Mild iron deficiency may increase the risk of recurrence.* will come back. If it does come back, the chances of further recurrences in the future are even greater.

What makes a herpes infection come back? A number of factors have been proposed. Anything that impairs the immune system, such as physical or emotional stress, may provide the trigger. One study indicated that even very mild iron deficiency may increase the risk of recurrence,[1] which is consistent with our knowledge of iron's role in immunity. Good nutrition in general, with consumption of a good variety of fruits and vegetables, is also known to enhance immunity. Extensive sunlight exposure may be a trigger in some people. Hormonal factors may be important—some women may suffer recurrences around the time of their menstrual periods. Fever may also stimulate reactivation, so fevers should be lowered with appropriate medication. A recent study, however, showed no correlation between any potential trigger, including psychological stress, and recurrences of the disease, so the role of any factor in causing recurrences remains controversial.

Herpes Simplex and Other Eye Complications As if the problems already discussed aren't enough, the herpes virus has a lot more mischief in its bag of tricks. At times, a cloudy inflammatory swelling, called *disciform keratitis,* may appear in one part of the cornea. This type of keratitis does not represent an active herpes infection but rather is a type of immune response to inactive virus protein that has remained in the cornea. Although there may be no active infection here, disciform keratitis needs to be treated because it can scar the cornea, thereby causing blindness. This presents a tricky problem, because corticosteroid medication is used to treat this kind of inflammation. As mentioned earlier, we avoid use of this type of medication in active herpes infections because it promotes virus growth. In the situation where there is no active virus infection, corticosteroids can actually make the virus become active again.

So how do we deal with disciform keratitis? Very cautiously. We use just enough corticosteroid medication to bring the inflammation under control while at the same time treating with antiviral medication to help keep the virus from becoming active again. The metaphor about being between a rock and a hard place would definitely be applicable here. A dilating eyedrop is also normally used to control any secondary inflammation inside the eye.

Uncommonly, the herpes simplex virus may infect the retina. This manifestation of the disease generally indicates a compromised immune system, as you would find in people who have AIDS or are receiving powerful chemotherapy for cancer or to prevent rejection of a transplanted organ. Antiviral drugs are given intravenously when people have a serious infection such as this.

Herpes Zoster (Shingles)

The *herpes zoster* virus, which causes shingles, is exactly the same virus that causes chicken pox in children, although in that situation the virus is usually known as *varicella zoster*. Shingles usually represents a reactivation of the virus that has remained in the body ever since the childhood chicken pox infection. Shingles may also sometimes occur after an adult is exposed to someone with chicken pox. You may be surprised to learn that it was an ophthalmologist who first noted the connection between chicken pox and shingles, an observation that ultimately led to the discovery that both diseases were caused by the same virus! Although shingles itself represents an active infection, it is not as highly contagious as chicken pox is, but caution should still be observed.

Shingles is more likely to occur in people with weakened immune systems.

Shingles may occur in people of any age, but it is more common in older people because of the weakening of the immune system associated with aging. It may occur in people with an undiagnosed cancer such as lymphoma, which affects immunity. It also is commonly seen in people with AIDS and other immune system disorders. It may even be the very first problem associated with the human immunodeficiency virus (HIV) infection, which causes AIDS.

Herpes zoster, or shingles, has a well-earned reputation as one of the most painful diseases. The explanation is that the virus grows along nerves and can damage them. Shingles usually affects only the left or the right half of the body. The trunk is frequently involved, and so is the area around the eye. Shingles can occasionally become systemic and infect the whole body, a problem seen most often in people with severely damaged immune systems.

As the tip of the nose goes, so goes the eye.

Herpes zoster ophthalmicus is the name we give to shingles infections around the eye. In some cases, pain may be present even before the characteristic skin rash appears. The blistery skin rash occurs on one side of the forehead, on the upper eyelid, and on the eye itself, and it may even affect one side of the nose right down to the tip. The eye is often but not always involved. Because of the way the nerves are set up, it has long been known that when the tip of the nose is affected, the eye almost always becomes affected by the virus.

When someone develops the classic appearance of shingles on the forehead and near the eye, the eye should be closely examined over the next four to seven days to detect the onset of eye infection. (This means you should see an ophthalmologist even if the shingles was diagnosed by another physician.) The eye may become red, a form of infection of the conjunctiva. The cornea may develop tiny areas where some of the outer layer of cells sloughs off. It may develop a form of dendrite (branching lesion) somewhat different in appearance from the dendrite caused by herpes simplex infections. Later, cloudy patches may also develop, and these represent a form of immune reaction of the body to virus protein that remains in the cornea. Herpes zoster often causes a marked iritis, an inflammation inside the eye that can badly damage it. Inflammation toward the back of the eye, specifically in the retina, can also occur, especially in a person with immune system problems. Rarely, the optic nerve itself may be damaged. Occasionally the nerves from the brain controlling the eye muscles become involved with the infection, causing the muscles to become palsied.

One of the dreaded complications of shingles anywhere on the body is called *postherpetic neuralgia*. This is the severe, persistent pain that occurs after the active infection is over. The pain, which can be difficult to treat, is caused by damage to the nerves along which the virus had been growing. Learning how to prevent this neuralgia would be a major medical advance and has been a focus of medical research for some time.

Treating Herpes Zoster Treatment is directed at ending the active infection and preventing complications, even though the virus always remains in the body. Several antiviral drugs exist, but they must be begun as soon as possible after the first signs of infection appear. People who begin the treatment within three days of the onset of the rash do much better than people in whom the initiation of treatment is delayed.

Treatment of shingles must begin as soon as possible.

In my own experience, the severity of corneal problems and iritis, as well as pain, is greatly reduced with the treatment. Unfortunately, postherpetic neuralgia can occur whether the drugs are used or not, although they may reduce the risk of developing this problem.

The drugs currently used are *acyclovir* (Zovirax), *famcyclovir* (Famvir), and *valacyclovir* (Valtrex). The initial studies on herpes zoster were done with acyclovir, which was shown to enter the eye in adequate concentrations to be effective. Acyclovir is taken five times a day, whereas the other drugs are taken three times a day, and a week to ten days is the usual course of treatment. The cost varies widely depending on the drug chosen and whether a generic equivalent is available.

Before the advent of these antiviral drugs, treatment with corticosteroids was often employed because of some indication that it might reduce the incidence of postherpetic neuralgia in people over the age of sixty. However, corticosteroids suppress the immune system somewhat, and in the case of herpes zoster infections in people whose immune systems are already compromised, corticosteroids might increase the risk of having the infection spread throughout the whole body. These days, use of corticosteroids is generally reserved for elderly patients who are having severe symptoms.

There is a very significant risk of developing a secondary bacterial infection in the skin in the area of the rash; antibiotic ointments are generally used to reduce this risk. I usually recommend that a thin film of bacitracin/polymixin double antibiotic ointment be applied to the area of the rash twice a day. The ointment also soothes the skin. Even if no bacterial infection sets in, scarring may occur in the area of the rash, especially when the blistering has been severe.

If significant eye problems develop, then eyedrops are prescribed as well. If there is inflammation, dilating drops help put the eye at rest. Corticosteroid eyedrops are usually used if a significant amount of iritis is present. If some of the outer layer of corneal cells has sloughed off, sulfa or antibiotic eyedrops may also be used to prevent a secondary bacterial infection. The antiviral eyedrops used to treat herpes simplex infections have no role in the treatment of herpes zoster.

Sometimes patches of corneal clouding and inflammation can occur after the active infection has subsided. These problems are caused by the immune system, which is reacting to the presence of protein from the virus that remains in the cornea. Anti-inflammatory eyedrops may be necessary to control this type of problem, which, in rare cases, can even persist for years.

Many drugs have been studied for the treatment of the severe pain associated with postherpetic neuralgia, but the results have not been promising in most instances. Cimetidine, a drug used to decrease acid secretion in the stomach and treat ulcers, may be of some value, especially if begun soon after the rash appears. Capsaicin (Zostrix), a substance derived from chili peppers, can reduce pain when applied to the skin, but it should not be used until the skin has completely healed from the rash. It is a treatment certainly worth trying, and you should give it at least a few weeks to see whether it is helpful. Many other treatments, including biofeedback, acupuncture, and nerve blocks, have been tried with varying degrees of success.

AIDS

The *acquired immunodeficiency syndrome* (AIDS) is caused by the *human immunodeficiency virus* (HIV). The virus, which is usually spread either sexually or through the blood, destroys the white blood cells that fight off infection. People who have AIDS, therefore, are subject to many serious infections that are extremely rare in the general population. In the eye, a number of sight-threatening infections occur, especially in the retina. The weakened immune system may also allow certain cancers to appear. Almost all AIDS patients show some retinal blood vessel abnormalities, which may look on examination very similar to the blood vessel problems in diabetics.

Cytomegalovirus Retinitis

The most common AIDS-related infection in the eye is *retinitis* (infection of the retina) caused by *cytomegalovirus* (CMV), a virus that can be acquired as a venereal disease or through the blood, just like HIV. However, it usually does not cause any symptoms and is kept under control by the immune system. Before the advent of AIDS, active cytomegalovirus infections in the eye and elsewhere in the body were fairly rare. They were seen primarily in people whose immune systems had been suppressed by drugs, such as the antirejection drugs used in organ transplant patients and the chemotherapy drugs used in cancer patients. The rise in

One-third of people with AIDS ultimately develop retinal cytomegalovirus infections.

cytomegalovirus retinitis cases brought on by AIDS has led to an intensive search for better ways to control this infection.

Cytomegalovirus retinitis affects about one-third of AIDS patients during the course of their illness. People with CMV may have visual disturbances such as blurring and loss of areas of their field of vision. They may also see spots or light flashes. Examination of the retina by the ophthalmologist reveals whitened areas accompanied by extensive hemorrhaging. The rest of the eye generally looks fairly normal. Mild *iridocyclitis,* inflammation in the fluid inside the eye, may be present in people with a history of CMV retinitis but does not necessarily mean that the infection is currently active.

The CMV infection causes the retinal cells to die in the area of whitening. Even if the virus is successfully treated, it always remains in the body and has the potential to recur (and frequently does). The retinal destruction also puts the eye at high risk for retinal detachment, a problem that threatens the sight in the eye and requires surgery. Both the CMV infection itself and retinal detachment can cause blindness.

Regular eye exams by a conscientious physician are crucial to the AIDS patient.

Several potent drugs have been shown to be effective in the treatment of CMV. *Gancyclovir* and *foscarnet* are the two most frequently used, and gancyclovir is sometimes even administered in the form of an implant inside the eye that slowly releases the drug over time.

Cidofovir is a newer drug that is also effective. All of these drugs have possible severe side effects and should be administered by a physician experienced in their use. It also appears that treatment of the underlying HIV infection itself and the improved immunity that results may aid in the control and resolution of CMV retinitis.

Regular eye examinations by a competent and conscientious ophthalmologist are of great importance to the AIDS patient. "A stitch in time saves nine" certainly applies here; early detection and close follow-up can make the difference between success and failure in treatment. The following anecdote should illustrate this point.

D. was a forty-four-year-old man with AIDS who had been a patient of mine for almost eight years. Almost two years after he had been diagnosed with the HIV infection, he came in for a routine eye exam and had no complaints about his eyes at that time. His visual acuity was excellent at 20/15 in both eyes, although he seemed a little uncertain with the right eye. A careful examination of his eyes showed that he had just a trace of cells floating in the aqueous humor of his right eye, along with a few in the vitreous. When I examined the retinas, they looked fine except for one area in the far periphery in the right eye, where whitening and hemorrhages were seen. All of these findings could have easily been missed with a cursory examination. He was then seen in consultation by a retinal specialist, who confirmed the diagnosis of CMV retinitis. D.'s internist began him on gancyclovir treatment, which put the retinitis into remission, and he was then followed monthly by the retinal specialist. But the story does not end here.

Over the next year, D. observed that his peripheral vision was gradually declining in the right eye, especially at night. However, no change had been found in his retina to indicate that the CMV infection had become active again. When he finally returned to me, his visual acuity had fallen only slightly to 20/20. Although I did not see any whitening of the retina, I was concerned that the CMV was active, so I had his internist switch him from gancyclovir to foscarnet. A careful visual field examination showed that he had very extensive loss of his field of vision in the right eye. He saw another retinal specialist on his own and said that he was told that the AIDS was causing blood vessel closure that was destroying his vision, but that the CMV was not active.

At this time, none of the protease inhibitors were available; these drugs are now an important part of AIDS therapy. But I had just read a newspaper article stating that a lottery would be held to determine which patients would be allowed to try Crixivan, one of the first protease inhibitors, on an investigational basis. I gave the information to D., and he entered the lottery. He won, beating ten-to-one odds, but his internist did not want to deal with the paperwork. So he found another physician who would administer the Crixivan to him. Soon thereafter, I recommended that D. see Dr. Gary Holland, a renowned expert on the effects of AIDS on the eye. He confirmed my impression that the CMV infection was still active and causing retinal destruction, even though the retina did not appear to be actively infected. He recommended a small increase in the dose of foscarnet. Follow-up visual field tests were then performed regularly and showed that the visual field loss was not progressing.

It is important to find doctors who will go the extra mile for you when necessary.

The tribulations experienced by the patient in this story illustrate the importance of performing meticulous examinations, listening to a patient's complaints, and going the extra mile when necessary. This is especially important when you have a life- and eye-threatening illness like AIDS. Obviously, in today's health care environment, it is not easy to find physicians who will spend the time required to deliver optimal care, but it is worth trying.

Other Forms of Retinitis in AIDS

Both of the herpes viruses, herpes zoster and herpes simplex, occasionally cause retinitis. The herpes zoster virus lies dormant in the body following childhood chicken pox infection, while the herpes simplex virus can be acquired in a number of ways, sometimes via the sexual route. These viruses may also cause *keratitis*, infection of the cornea (see "Herpes Infections," page 256) and mild iridocyclitis, an inflammation inside and toward the front of the eye. Both of these infections require intensive antiviral drug treatment. In some cases, people with AIDS take one of these drugs, acyclovir, prophylactically to prevent future herpes outbreaks.

Mycobacterium avium intracellulare is a bacterium that is a cousin to the bacterium that causes tuberculosis. However, it does not spread the way tuberculosis does, and it tends to cause disease only in people whose immune systems are not working properly. It can cause infection throughout the body, including the lungs and digestive system. In the eye, it is an unusual cause of retinitis. Drugs that are used to treat tuberculosis are also used to treat this disease, but, as with the other causes of retinitis, the best we can hope for is to suppress the infection, not completely eradicate it.

Toxoplasmosis, a chronic infection by the one-celled parasite *Toxoplasma gondii*, can also become active when the immune system is suppressed. In the eye, it causes a retinitis that can destroy vision. Toxoplasmosis is acquired by eating meat that is not well cooked and by coming into close contact with the litter of infected cats. People who have the HIV infection should avoid these risky acts. Toxoplasmosis in the eye is treated with several drugs that are potentially toxic to the body. (See "Toxoplasmosis," page 224.)

Toxoplasmosis is often acquired by eating undercooked meat.

Syphilis, the well-known venereal disease, can also sometimes lurk in the body in an inactive form and then resurface when HIV impairs the immune system. Syphilis is a cause of uveitis, but it may also cause retinitis. A blood test can usually confirm the diagnosis. Treatment consists of high doses of penicillin given intravenously. Other bacteria only rarely cause retinitis or other infection inside the eye.

Other Retinal Problems

Some causes of retinitis can cause the retina to detach. In the usual form of retinal detachment, one or more tears occur in the retina, allowing fluid in the eye to seep through the tears and dissect behind the retina, ballooning it forward. This is an all-too-common effect of cytomegalovirus infections. Surgical repair of the retinal detachment is necessary to avoid blindness. (See "Retinal Detachment," page 210.)

The HIV infection causes blood vessel problems in the retina in most people with AIDS. The small hemorrhages, leakages, and evidence of small blood vessel shutdown look very similar to background diabetic retinopathy, which is caused by diabetic-induced damage to the walls of blood vessels. As in diabetics, changes in the blood vessels of the conjunctiva can also be seen. If enough fluid leakage from the damaged blood vessels occurs, some blurring and distortion of vision may be present. Small blood vessel closure may also cause damage to the optic nerve. Exactly how AIDS causes these blood vessel problems is not known, but it does not appear to be the result of infection (other than the underlying HIV infection).

Eyelid Problems

The herpes simplex and herpes zoster viruses discussed earlier can affect the facial skin, including the eyelids. Tiny blisters are seen in the area of the rash, and as these blisters break, bacterial infections can set in. Herpes zoster, which grows along nerves, has a tendency to affect the nerve whose distribution includes one side of the forehead up to the midline, the eye on that side, and the nose on that side. *Molluscum contagiosum,* a virus infection that produces tiny nodules in the eyelid, often around the eyelashes, occasionally

Kaposi's sarcoma may look like a broken blood vessel on the eye.

flares up in people with AIDS. It sometimes becomes noticed when it causes the eye to become red.

Kaposi's sarcoma is a skin cancer seen in many AIDS patients. It may affect the eyelids as well as the conjunctiva, which lines the inside of the eyelids as well as the outer surface of the eye. When it affects the conjunctiva, its reddish appearance may make it look almost identical to a subconjunctival hemorrhage. Kaposi's sarcoma may be difficult to treat, and chemotherapy may be necessary.

Summary and Recommendations

Many serious eye infections and other problems are common in people with HIV infection. These problems may cause no symptoms at first, so regular examinations by a competent, conscientious ophthalmologist are essential. Effective treatment for many of these conditions is available, but it is most effective when the conditions are discovered early in their course. Any new visual symptoms should be checked out as soon as possible.

Antiviral treatment aimed at HIV itself can often keep the immune system strong enough to prevent the onset of many of these eye problems. General supportive care, including adequate rest and a healthy diet rich in vegetables and fruits, is important as well. A diet deficient in calories can suppress the immune system, so try to eat enough even if your appetite is not good.

Optimizing Infant Vision

The miracle of vision begins before birth, as the visual system, from the eyes to the brain, develops along with the rest of the body. This developmental process continues after birth until the visual system is mature. Just as in adults, the condition of the retina is often the limiting factor in determining how well the young eye will see. Recent research shows that nutrition is of major importance in determining how well the retina functions and how quickly good vision develops in the growing child. Of course, just because vision develops rapidly does not necessarily mean that it will be better in the long run. But it is a sign that nutritional needs are being adequately met.

The perfect food for infants is mother's milk, not cow's milk.

The perfect food for infants is milk. No, not cow's milk. Cow's milk has been found to cause intestinal bleeding in some infants and to promote anemia, prompting the Committee on Nutrition of the American Academy of Pediatrics to recommend that cow's milk not be given to infants under one year of age.[2] Cow's milk, which is intended for baby cows, is very different from human milk, being lower in iron, vitamin E, and essential fatty acids and too high in sodium, potassium, and protein. So it is mother's milk that is the perfect food. Infants who are breast-fed appear to have numerous advantages over their formula-fed counterparts. Among other things, they develop better vision[3,4] and have higher IQs.[5] Formula is a poor second choice. The better vision and brain development appears to be related to the essential fatty acids that mother's milk contains. Fatty acids are the building blocks of fats, and essential fatty acids, also known as *polyunsaturated fatty acids,* are those that we must obtain from our food in small amounts.

The retina contains specialized cells called *rods* and *cones*. When we look at an object, light coming from that object is received by the rods and cones, which then transmit impulses to the brain so that our higher consciousness can recognize what we are seeing. The membranes of these rods and cones, like those of the brain, are rich in certain polyunsaturated fatty acids. These fatty acids, the same ones present in mother's milk, appear to play an important role in both eye and brain development.

Polyunsaturated Fatty Acids

You need a bit of a chemistry lesson to understand polyunsaturated fatty acids. Fatty acid molecules are classified according to their length (the number of carbon atoms they contain) and their structure (the number and location of double bonds, which are double linkages between carbon atoms). Polyunsaturated fatty acids contain two or more double bonds. You may have heard of omega-3 and omega-6 fatty acids. These are the two main classes of polyunsaturated fatty acids. An omega-3 polyunsaturated fatty acid is one in which the first double bond occurs between the third and fourth carbon atom in the chain. In an omega-6 polyunsaturated fatty acid, the first double bond occurs between carbon atoms 6 and 7. This seemingly small difference makes

The retina and brain are rich in the omega-3 fatty acid DHA.

a big difference in their properties. The shortest omega-3 fatty acid is called alpha-linolenic acid, and it is present in dark, leafy green vegetables, walnuts, soy products, and other foods. The longer omega-3 fatty acids are called *eicosapentaenoic acid* (EPA) and *docosahexaenoic acid* (DHA). Both EPA and DHA can be obtained directly from certain foods or manufactured to some extent by our bodies, using enzymes that lengthen alpha-linolenic acid.

The retina and the brain are rich in DHA, one of the long-chain omega-3 fatty acids. We think that these fatty acids allow the membranes of the retina and brain to be more fluid (less stiff), facilitating their ability to transmit signals. If an infant is deficient in DHA, other polyunsaturated fatty acids may substitute for it, but the retina and brain may not function as well.

DHA: Food for Thought (and Vision)

Infants acquire DHA in one of several ways. First, they are born with a certain amount of DHA that they obtain through the bloodstream of their mothers. This prenatally acquired DHA, which depends on the mother's diet during pregnancy, declines after birth. To replace it, the infant's diet must then supply either DHA (ideally) or its precursor, the shorter alpha-linolenic acid. Human milk, as opposed to cow's milk, is an excellent source of DHA (as well as EPA), and its concentration in the milk is related to the mother's blood levels and her dietary intake. Currently available infant formulas do not contain DHA and EPA; the only omega-3 fatty acid they contain is alpha-linolenic acid, which the infant must then convert to long-chain fatty acids such as DHA. However, this conversion is not very efficient, and formula-fed babies end up with lower levels of DHA in their blood, eyes, and brains. Preterm infants may show even more of a difference, as they are usually born with lower blood levels of DHA than full-term infants. Therefore, it is clear that infants fed human milk maintain a much better DHA status than infants fed formula.

Significance of the DHA Level in Infant Brains and Retinas The evidence is that the DHA level in infant brains and retinas is important, especially in premature infants. Some studies have shown that supplementing formula with DHA may lead to improved mental functioning at twelve months of age and beyond as compared with infants who drink formula without DHA.[6] Special

techniques have also been used to study vision in infants. In one such study of premature infants, those who were fed either human milk or formula supplemented with DHA showed significantly better vision and retinal function at both thirty-six and fifty-seven weeks of age than did infants fed regular formula.[2] Although human milk may contain other substances

Breast-fed babies may develop better minds and vision.

besides DHA that may hasten vision development, it does appear that DHA itself plays an important role in the process.

In summary, we now have a great deal of data that implies that breast-fed infants develop visual and mental functioning skills more rapidly than their formula-fed peers. The difference is apparently explained by the DHA content of human milk, which leads to higher levels of DHA in the growing infant. Since formulas in the United States do not currently contain DHA, the message is clear. Breast-feeding of newborn infants should be done for as long as possible. Even if the U.S. Food and Drug Administration approves the addition of DHA to formula, as it probably will in the near future, human milk, with its complex blend of nutrients, will remain the infant food of choice.

Drug Side Effects

All medications have side effects. Even vitamins can have side effects, especially when taken in large amounts. Recognition of early problems stemming from the use of medication is important if permanent damage is to be avoided. We discuss here some of the major drugs and supplements that are known to have ocular side effects.

Anti-inflammatory (Arthritis) Drugs

Corticosteroids are drugs related to the hormone cortisone. They suppress inflammation and are therefore used to treat diseases like rheumatoid arthritis, lupus, asthma, and many others. The main side effects on the eye have to do with cataracts and glaucoma. Although we are most concerned when the drugs are given orally or in eyedrop form, inhalation of these drugs can also cause the same problems with the eyes. Long-term use of moderately high doses of corticosteroids can cause a posterior subcapsular type of cataract. The cloudy area interferes with light traveling through the center of the pupil. It is a particularly disabling form of cataract because it makes you prone to "light blindness"—sharply reduced vision when you're out in the sunlight or when lights such as headlamps from other cars are directed toward you. The cataract can progress fairly rapidly if you continue to take the corticosteroid medication. The risk of cataract development varies from person to person, but on the average, it takes about six months of prednisone (the most commonly prescribed corticosteroid) at a dosage of 20 milligrams a day to produce the earliest sign of cataract.

The other major ocular side effect, an elevated intraocular pressure that we call *secondary glaucoma,* takes only a few weeks to develop. Some people have a genetic predisposition to secondary glaucoma. If it is not detected, the high pressure can cause irreversible optic nerve damage. Therefore, people who must take corticosteroids on a long-term basis should have their eyes checked by an ophthalmologist at least every six months. The prescribing physician should try to keep the dosage at the lowest possible level. Of course, corticosteroid eyedrops and ointments can also cause these problems. They should be prescribed only when necessary and only by an ophthalmologist.

Hydroxychloroquine (Plaquenil) is a drug derived from chloroquine, and both of them were originally used to treat malaria. Now they are used to treat autoimmune diseases like lupus and rheumatoid arthritis, with hydroxychloroquine being the one usually prescribed. These drugs can become deposited in the eye tissues, mainly the retina and the cornea. The risk depends both on the daily dose and on the length of time the medication has been taken. This toxicity is generally seen only with daily doses of 300 milligrams or more. Most people at this dosage eventually show a very fine dusting of the corneal surface, although it does not affect vision unless it becomes more severe. Fortunately, the buildup in the cornea is generally reversible after the drug is stopped. In the retina, however, irreversible damage may occur, so problems there are more serious than those in the cornea. The drug tends to accumulate in the macula. Therefore, it is important to detect any such changes in the macula as early as possible, so that the hydroxychloroquine can be discontinued before any measurable effect on the vision occurs.

People taking hydroxychloroquine should have their eyes checked by an ophthalmologist every six months for as long as they take the drug. The first visit should include a baseline examination, before the drug is started, so that results of tests in the future can be compared to the first one. The visual acuity should be carefully checked each time. The retina is closely examined. We look for any changes in the pigmentation of the center of the macula. In particular, we look for the tiny light reflex that shines back at us from the center of the macula. A change in this light reflex or the loss of this light reflex could be the first indication of hydroxychloroquine toxicity to the retina. A visual field test is performed to make sure there are no blind spots or a more subtle loss of sensitivity in the central portion of vision. We pay special attention to the central ten degrees of vision, and it is often helpful to use a red light as the target rather than the usual white light, since defects to the red light may appear earlier on. Another useful test is a color vision test, such as the Farnsworth-Munsell 100 hue test. In this test, round, colored tiles are placed in order as the hues become darker or lighter. A change in color vision could also signal hydroxychloroquine toxicity.

Most people become worried about their eyes when they start taking this drug. The good news is that there's no real cause for concern. Retinal toxicity from hydroxychloroquine is quite rare, much rarer than the toxicity seen when chloroquine was used. It was because of the experience with chloroquine that we were worried about what hydroxychloroquine could do. Only once have I seen a case of marked toxicity from hydroxychloroquine. This occurred in a young woman who was taking 600 milligrams a day for almost ten years and never had her eyes checked during this time. Her vision was moderately reduced in both eyes, and there was a severe buildup of hydroxychloroquine in her corneas. In fact, her corneas were so cloudy that we could not even determine the condition of her retinas. She stopped taking the hydroxychloroquine, and by six months later, about half of the cloudiness in her corneas had resolved, accompanied by improvement in her vision. But this was simply a case in which the eyes had been neglected. So don't be overly concerned about taking hydroxychloroquine. Just make sure you have your eyes checked as you are supposed to, and be sure you go to a conscientious ophthalmologist who takes the time to check all of the important items.

Tranquilizers and Antidepressants

A number of the medications in this category carry warnings that people who have glaucoma should not use them. In fact, in people who have chronic open angle glaucoma, the usual variety, the effect on the intraocular pressure is so small as to be insignificant. The problem is actually in people whose eyes have what we call *anatomically narrow angles*. These individuals have a very narrow entranceway to the location of the eye's drainage channels, and they may be prone to angle-closure glaucoma. Some of these drugs, by dilating the pupil slightly, can cause the angle inside the eye to close down, precipitating a large rise in eye pressure. But people who have chronic angle-closure glaucoma or are felt to be at high risk for attacks of angle-closure glaucoma should not be walking around with this condition. They need to have a small laser procedure called an *iridotomy*, which creates a small hole in the iris and virtually eliminates the possibility of angle closure. Therefore, the only people at true risk from these drugs are people who have narrow angles but don't know it and people who know they have narrow angles but haven't done anything about it. So if you have glaucoma, check with your ophthalmologist, but in general, using this type of drug poses no problem.

Some major tranquilizers can cause other eye problems. Drugs in the *phenothiazine* class, which includes chlorpromazine (Thorazine), thioridazine (Mellaril), fluphenazine (Prolixin), trifluoperazine (Stelazine), and others, are generally used to treat psychotic conditions. Such drugs are fairly safe for the eye, but they can cause pigmentary deposits on the surface of the lens and on the back surface of the cornea. Thioridazine in particular can cause pigmentary changes and damage to the retina, although usually only at higher dosages and when the drug has been used for a long time.

Anticancer Drugs

Tamoxifen (Nolvadex) is a drug that opposes the action of estrogen, and it is widely used as a treatment for breast cancer. This drug, especially when used at the upper end of the dosage range, can occasionally deposit itself in the eye, in both the cornea and the retina. In the cornea, the superficial deposits may look similar to what one sees with the antimalarial and antiarthritis drugs hydroxychloroquine and chloroquine, that is, a fine dusting on the surface of the cornea. What we look for in the retina are glinting deposits just outside the retina's center. Since this can affect vision, the dosage is usually lowered (or the drug discontinued) if such a problem is found. Therefore, regular eye examinations by an ophthalmologist are indicated for women taking tamoxifen long term.

Many drugs used in chemotherapy can irritate the eyes, but the irritation usually goes away on its own with no permanent damage. The irritative effects may include blepharitis, redness of the eyes, and tearing. Of course, in cases where the hair is lost, hair loss may also occur from the eyebrows and eyelashes. *Vincristine,* a drug that can affect the nervous system, can affect the nerves around the eye as elsewhere, and droopy eyelids or double vision may result, albeit transiently in most cases. Oncologists (cancer specialists), who prescribe the drugs used in chemotherapy, are generally well informed about the possible side effects and can handle most of these problems, although they can request a referral to an ophthalmologist if necessary.

Cholesterol-Lowering Drugs

Niacin, also known as *nicotinic acid* or *vitamin B₃,* is used in high doses to lower cholesterol levels. People who take these megadoses need to be under the supervision of a physician in case toxicity develops. In the eye, very large doses may rarely cause a fluid buildup in the center of the retina, which we call *macular edema.* This edema can blur and distort the vision. Fortunately, the problem generally resolves after the niacin is discontinued.

The most frequently used drugs today to lower cholesterol levels are commonly known as the *statins.* Six statins are now available in the United States, and they are extremely effective, with cholesterol reductions in the range of 20 to 60 percent usually reported. They inhibit an enzyme and thereby prevent the cells of the body from manufacturing cholesterol. When the first of these drugs, *lovostatin,* was introduced, there was concern that it might cause cataract, because preliminary studies showed that dogs who were given enormous doses of the drug developed cataract. (No other animal species did.) Of course, there is often not much correlation between what happens in one species of animal and what happens in another, and extremely large doses also do not reflect what occurs with the proper therapeutic dosage. In any case, people who took lovostatin had their eyes carefully monitored for cataract development, which did not occur. The evidence indicates that there is no reason to have routine screening examinations of your eyes just because you are taking a statin.

Other cholesterol-lowering agents are also considered safe for the eyes. Of course, garlic and oat bran are probably the safest of all!

Drugs for Tuberculosis

Tuberculosis (TB), once a major cause of death, has tapered off along with other infectious diseases that were major public health problems in the past. However, TB has had a slight resurgence lately for several reasons. First, many people have a dormant, inapparent TB infection. However, AIDS, which suppresses the immune system, can make the TB become active again. The emergence of AIDS has thus led to some increase in active tuberculosis. Second, to a much lesser degree, some U.S. immigrants have brought TB with them. Third, strains of the tubercle bacillus resistant to many of the usual drugs used to treat TB have evolved and often defy treatment. So tuberculosis remains a disease to be reckoned with.

Two drugs commonly used to treat TB, *ethambutol* primarily and *isoniazid* (INH) to a lesser degree, can cause toxicity to the optic nerve. Optic nerve problems can reduce vision greatly and may cause blind spots and color vision problems. Therefore, anyone starting to take either or both of these drugs should undergo a screening eye examination to establish a baseline and regular follow-up examinations, with the time interval dependent on the drug dosage. Visual acuity testing, careful visual field testing, color vision testing, and examination of the optic nerve are usually employed. Changes in medications or dosages may be necessary if there is any evidence of optic nerve compromise.

Sildenafil (Viagra)

Sildenafil (Viagra), a drug used to treat impotence, has a transient effect on the retina. A small percentage of men using this drug may complain of light sensitivity, blurring, or a blue-green tinge to their vision. Recently, a case[7] was reported in which a diabetic man developed proliferative diabetic retinopathy within six months after beginning treatment with sildenafil. There are some theoretical reasons why sildenafil might have this effect. Since impotence is a common problem in long-standing diabetics, and since many may be prescribed sildenafil, doctors are monitoring them to see whether sildenafil may, in fact, promote progression of retinopathy, which can cause serious bleeding into the eye.

CHAPTER FOURTEEN

A Primer on Nutrition

N UTRITION IS THE MOST IMPORTANT DETERMINANT OF HEALTH and the backbone of preventive medicine. Many people are aware of the role good nutrition can play in preventing heart disease and cancer, but most chronic eye diseases are also related to the foods we eat. In fact, the nutritional and other lifestyle factors that benefit our eyes are often precisely the same factors that benefit all of our organs. Medicine has made many major advances in recent

Good nutrition is a feast for the eyes.

years. But if we can avoid smoking and eat the amount and type of food for which our bodies are adapted, we will have a greater impact on our health than have all the drugs, surgeries, and other technological advances of medicine.

Nutrition as a science has changed dramatically over the past hundred years. At one time, we were concerned about the malnutrition caused by nutritional deficiencies. Today, we are still plagued by malnutrition, but not a malnutrition of deficiencies, at least not a deficiency of vitamins, minerals, and protein. Today's malnutrition is often a malnutrition of excesses—excesses in fats, sugars, protein (yes, protein!), and overly refined products. The deficiencies are now in fiber and phytochemicals, the "nonessential" nutrients found in products of the plant kingdom: vegetables, fruits, whole grains, and nuts and seeds. This new type of malnutrition does not cause our immediate demise, but it is responsible for the epidemic of chronic, degenerative diseases that afflict our affluent society.

Sight-threatening manifestations of vitamin deficiency diseases, of course, are still a major problem in the world's developing nations. These manifestations are caused by a lack of food and by other factors, such as intestinal parasites. But the Western nations have the lion's share of chronic degenerative diseases like diabetes, a major cause of blindness and a direct consequence of our dietary lifestyle.

The ideal diet is one that maximizes the consumption of fresh vegetables, fruits, and whole grains and minimizes the use of animal products. Plant foods, with their fiber, antioxidant vitamins, minerals, and phytochemicals, are felt to play a significant role in the prevention of chronic diseases. It has been estimated that if people simply increased their consumption of fruits and vegetables to five to eight servings a day, the death rate from cancer would be cut in half.

The ideal diet maximizes consumption of vegetables, fruits, and grains.

Animal products, in contrast, are closely linked with the development of most of our serious chronic diseases. The types of fat and protein in these products are felt to be the main culprit. Consider some of the evidence. The Lifestyle Heart Trial showed that coronary artery disease can actually be reversed by lifestyle changes, including a low-fat vegetarian diet (free of fish, poultry, and beef), exercise, and meditation (stress reduction).[1] The implication is that the vast majority of heart attacks are preventable and that heart disease is not inevitable but rather the result of patterns of food consumption for which our bodies were not intended. Studies now show that other diseases can be prevented as well, including some of our eye diseases.

Can this be? Haven't animal products always been an important part of a healthy, normal diet? A World Health Organization study group published a report in the form of a book entitled *Diet, Nutrition, and the Prevention of Chronic Diseases.*[2] They observed that *Homo sapiens*, the human species, "has subsisted for

Today's malnutrition is mainly one of excesses.

most of its history on low-fat high-fiber diets, rich in vitamin C and many other micronutrients, to which it presumably adapted biologically to achieve optimum function." They pointed out, however, that the industrial revolution brought about "radical changes in methods of food production, processing, storage, and distribution."

Eventually, this led to decreased consumption of complex carbohydrates and increased consumption of fats and sugars. The result has been "the emergence of a range of chronic noninfectious diseases." In other words, our affluence and gluttony have created malnutrition in the form of nutritional excesses. Feeding into this mind-set has been the influence of certain food industry groups, such as the meat and dairy industries, which have convinced most of us that their products are not only desirable but necessary.

We have seen what happens to people who move from developing countries to our "civilized" Western societies. As their dietary habits change, so does their health. They assume the risk for chronic diseases of the country to which they have moved. We see similar changes when people who remain in their own countries assume Western habits. So much for genetics as an excuse! With that in mind, we will now look at basic nutritional principles.

Energy Sources

Carbohydrate, protein, and fat are the three main sources of calories in our diet. Even when we are not exercising, our bodies need a certain amount of fuel and basic building blocks to keep all systems going. If energy requirements are not met, weight loss occurs, and the immune system and other important bodily functions are impaired. The findings from nutritional research have led to the recommendations that we increase the proportion of complex carbohydrate and decrease the proportions of protein and fat in the diet. Let us now take a closer look at these three classes of nutrients.

Carbohydrate

To chemists, *carbohydrates* are compounds that contain the elements carbon, hydrogen, and oxygen. The basic carbohydrate unit is the *sugar,* of which there are many types. We sometimes refer to sugars as *simple carbohydrates.* Long chains of chemically linked sugars are called *complex carbohydrates,* better known as *starch.* Complex carbohydrates that are not digestible represent a form of fiber. Carbohydrates are the body's principal energy source.

Sugars are derived primarily from fruits and vegetables. Many people who claim they eat no sugar would be surprised to learn how much is naturally present in the foods they eat. Added sugars in the diet come from white sugar (sucrose), brown sugar, molasses, honey, refined fructose, high-fructose corn syrup, rice syrup, maple syrup, fruit juice concentrates, barley malt syrup, and others.

Excess sugar consumption is one of the characteristics of the modern diet. But exactly what are the health consequences of consuming too much sugar? You will hear many different answers. On the one extreme, some mainstream nutritionists say that there are only two problems: "empty" calories from sugar that are taking the place of more nutritious foods and an increased incidence of dental caries (cavities). On the other, there is the common health food store myth that "sugar" is akin to a dangerous addictive drug, making people hyperactive, and sick to their stomach and causing every disease from A to Z. In reality, the truth lies somewhere between the two.

Eating too much sugar can make you lose important minerals.

Heavy consumption of sugar-rich, refined "junk foods" such as soda, candy, cakes, and cookies that take the place of whole foods certainly can lead to nutritional deficiencies, dental problems, and obesity. But the problems go beyond that. High sugar intake can cause loss of calcium in the urine, potentially increasing the risk of osteoporosis and kidney stones. Loss of other important minerals, such as magnesium, zinc, and chromium, may occur as well. Some immune functions may be weakened. Sugar, especially fructose, may contribute to elevated blood levels of triglycerides, fats that increase the risk of heart disease and stroke. A recent study indicated that sugar added to drinks and desserts may be a risk factor for cancers of the gallbladder and bile ducts.

The other type of carbohydrate, *starch,* should be the major source of calories in the ideal diet. Don't be confused by the archaic designation of potatoes and rice as "starches." Complex carbohydrate, or starch, is widely distributed among plant foods, especially grains, vegetables, nuts, and seeds. Animal products are lacking in starch.

Protein

It is not *protein* per se but *amino acids,* the building blocks of protein, that our bodies must obtain from the diet. That is because our digestive enzymes and by our intestinal cells break down almost all the protein we consume into amino acids before they are absorbed into the bloodstream. We obtain twenty amino acids from our food. Nine of these amino acids are called *essential amino acids,* meaning that they must be derived directly from food because our bodies cannot manufacture them from other amino acids.

Proteins serve a number of important functions in our body. There are structural proteins that provide the structure for the skin, nails, cornea, lens, and other tissues. We also have *enzymes,* specialized proteins that act as the catalysts that speed up chemical reactions in our body. *Immunoglobulins* are proteins better known as *antibodies,* part of the immune system. Some amino acids are used to synthesize other substances, such as hormones or chemical transmitters in the brain.

All vegetables, fruits, and grains contain protein.

One of the most frequently asked questions about healthy, plant-based diets is "Where will I get my protein?" Apparently, most people have been brainwashed into thinking that only certain foods contain proteins. Have you ever heard the expression *protein foods?* I suspect this term was devised by certain food industry groups that wanted to persuade people that their food products were the only sources of protein. Obviously, they were successful, proving the old adage that when people keep hearing the same thing again and again, they start to believe it.

Think for a minute about a cow—and all the protein in its meat and milk. Where did the protein come from? Cows don't normally eat meat (except perhaps in this day of mad cow disease); they're herbivores (vegetarians), consuming large quantities of grains and grasses and the like. Obviously, all their protein comes from plants. The fact is that all whole foods—grains, vegetables, nuts, and fruits—contain protein. So long as you consume enough of them to maintain your weight, you should obtain an adequate amount of protein.

Another commonly heard misconception is that plant products do not contain "complete" protein, meaning that they lack one or more of the essential amino acids. Perpetuators (or should I say perpetrators?) of this myth go on to say that one must "complement" proteins, combining one food with another, for the body to be able to use the protein. This myth began many years ago when it was found that rats grew best when fed proteins from different foods combined in this way. However, rats are not human beings and have very different dietary requirements. Humans do not require amino acids in the same proportions as rats do, nor do they need to combine them in any way.

The reality is that the protein from each plant individually does contain all of the essential amino acids. The only protein I know of that does not is gelatin, which comes from the skin, bones, and hooves of cows. It is true that some plants contain protein with an amino acid composition that does not exactly match the profile of the amounts of each of the amino acids recommended for humans. But no one ever said they have to match. All that is required is that you con-sume at least the recommended amount of each essential amino acid over the course of a day. The proteins of certain plants may be slightly low in certain amino acids, but that does not mean that they don't have any, as implied by the ridiculous term *incomplete protein*.

> *The protein in each and every plant contains all of the essential amino acids, the required building blocks of protein.*

For example, corn is often cited as a vegetable relatively low in the amino acid tryptophan, but it still has some. In fact, if an adult male ate nothing but eight cups of corn a day, he would still be consuming the recommended amounts of all nine essential amino acids. If you ate enough of any one veg-etable's protein to meet your daily protein requirement, you would also be meeting your requirement for each of the essential amino acids. Thus, the con-cepts of complete protein and protein complementation are fallacious. Only in rare circumstances—for example, in dealing with a patient in kidney failure who must consume the least protein possible—is it necessary to arrange food choices in such a way that the amino acids consumed are in exactly the same proportions as they are listed in the recommended daily amounts.

If that is so, you might ask why people in the poorer, developing countries who subsist primarily on grains, corn, and the like have such a high incidence of protein deficiency. The reason is that these people are not eating the quan-tities of corn or any other food we've been discussing. They are consuming a low-calorie as well as a low-protein diet because they can't get enough food to eat. In addition, many suffer from parasitic infections, which also compromise their nutritional status.

The recommended dietary allowance (RDA) for protein is 63 grams for men and 50 grams for women. Most people in the United States and other Western countries consume one and one-half to two times that amount. The dictum "if a little bit is good, then more must be better" seems to apply. However, it doesn't work that way. We are learning the hard way that protein is one of those nutrients, like fat, that we should limit. We need to consume some protein, which is not difficult, but too much may be harmful. Excess protein in the diet, especially animal protein, which is more acidic, causes calcium to be lost from bones and concentrated in the urine, leading to osteoporosis and kidney stones. Furthermore, on a typical high-protein diet, we cannot even digest all the protein we eat. About 12 grams of protein a day may travel down to our large intestines undigested and be transformed there into potentially cancer-causing chemicals.[3] Dietary moderation and modification could avoid these problems.

Fat

Fats, also known as *lipids,* have developed a bad reputation, but they do have a number of important roles to play. They are components of the membranes that surround our cells, and their properties help to regulate many of the functions of those cells. Certain fats make up the sheath called *myelin* that surrounds our nerve cells. Cholesterol is needed to produce the various steroid hormones, such as cortisone and the sex hormones, as well as the bile acids, which aid in fat digestion. Lipoproteins (molecules with both fat and protein components) containing cholesterol and other fats in the bloodstream act as carriers for fat-soluble vitamins and other substances. Last but not least, fats serve as a way to store energy. Unfortunately for many of us, the body lacks its own liposuction device, so fats do have a way of building up on us when we consume too much of them.

Fats have a way of building up on us when we consume too much of them.

The negative side of fats is well known. Excess body fat, especially around the abdomen, is a major risk factor for many diseases, including heart disease, high blood pressure, and diabetes. Elevated blood cholesterol levels have been the bane of our society and have greatly increased our rates of heart disease and stroke. Excess fat can also suppress our immune systems, increasing our risk of developing certain cancers.

There are different types of *fatty acids,* the building blocks of fats. They include *saturated, monounsaturated,* and *polyunsaturated fatty acids.* Let us examine the differences among them.

Fatty acids are organic molecules (molecules are individual units), which means that they consist of chains of carbon atoms. These carbon atoms are bonded to each other. In some cases, this may be a single bond, whereas in other cases, it may be a double bond, a much stronger linkage.

You may have heard of saturated fats, the type most often of animal origin and that our bodies use to make cholesterol. When we say that a fatty acid is saturated, we mean that there are no double bonds, only single bonds, between the many carbon atoms in the chain. If one double bond is present in a given fatty acid molecule, then we have a monounsaturated type of fatty acid. Oleic acid, the predominant fatty acid in olive oil, is of this type. If two or more double bonds are present, then we are dealing with a polyunsaturated fatty acid, the type most common in vegetable oils.

It gets just a little more complicated. Polyunsaturated fatty acids may be of the omega-3 or omega-6 variety. An *omega-3 polyunsaturated fatty acid* is one in which the first double bond occurs between the third and fourth carbon atoms in the chain. In an *omega-6 polyunsaturated fatty acid,* the first double bond occurs between carbon atoms 6 and 7. Both omega-3 and omega-6 fatty acids are sometimes called *essential fatty acids,* because we require a small amount of them in our diets.

There is no such thing as a no-fat diet.

As with protein, many people have misconceptions as to which foods contain fats. We often hear people say, "I'm on a no-fat diet." On further questioning, however, we find that they are eating fish, chicken, and most other things. There is no such thing as a no-fat diet. It would be incompatible with survival. All whole foods—grains, vegetables, fruits, and of course animal products—contain fat. So-called nonfat or skim milk derives 5 percent of its calories from fat. Most other products advertised as fat free contain some fat as well. Fat is a natural part of everything that grows. Whole wheat is about 5 percent fat. Certain refined products like sugar and alcohol do not contain fat, but everything else that we eat does. That is why it is difficult to develop a fatty acid deficiency. If someone who avoided animal products also avoided whole grains, subsisting on white bread and other products containing white flour only; avoiding all added fats; and consuming many processed foods in which the naturally occurring fat has been removed, it is possible that person would develop an essential fatty acid deficiency. The problem can be avoided, therefore, by consuming whole grains and by not eating too many so-called fat-free processed foods.

It should be clear that it is not necessary to use any added fats, such as oils or margarine, in cooking or other food preparation. The foods we eat contain all the fats we need. You can cook in vegetable broth or water instead of oil. Oil-free salad dressings can be prepared. Bread or toast can be eaten alone (the best way with fresh bread!) or with a low-fat spread. Although this may seem harsh at first, people who decide to eat a very low-fat diet find that their taste for fat goes away after a few months. Fatty foods then seem rich and distasteful, while low-fat foods seem clean and fresh. Many subtle flavors that had not been appreciated before come to the fore.

Fiber

Fiber comes only from plant products. It consists mainly of indigestible carbohydrates, many of which are derived from the cell walls of plants. Many years ago it was called *roughage,* and its usefulness was felt to be limited to the avoidance of constipation. Some medical "experts" even derided people who advocated high-fiber diets as a general preventive health measure. Now we know differently. Diets

Fiber comes only from plant products.

high in fiber are associated with lower risks of developing heart disease, cancer, diabetes, high blood pressure, elevated blood cholesterol levels, and obesity. It is often difficult to distinguish, though, between the protective effects of the fiber itself and the protective effects of other components of fruits and vegetables, since they all occur together in the same foods.

We often differentiate between *soluble* and *insoluble fiber*. The terms simply indicate whether a given type of fiber dissolves in water. However, the designations are useful because the two types of fiber have different properties. Insoluble fiber, such as that in wheat bran, helps ensure a rapid transit time of food through the bowel, helping prevent constipation and associated problems such as hemorrhoids and diverticulosis. Soluble fiber, found in oat bran, legumes (beans, peas, and lentils), fruits, and other foods, can lower cholesterol levels and help keep sugars from being absorbed into the bloodstream too quickly.

In most cases, it is not necessary or desirable to add fiber in the form of bran to foods. Excess fiber could interfere with mineral absorption. Simply eating a variety of whole grains, fruits, and vegetables supplies all the fiber you need. Occasionally, as in the case of a high blood cholesterol level, addition of fiber to foods could be tried, but for most people, the fiber naturally present in foods is sufficient, provided the fiber has not been removed from those foods, as in white bread.

Vitamins

Vitamins are chemicals necessary for normal body functioning. The minimum amount that should be obtained from the diet is not necessarily the amount that allows optimal functioning. To help us determine how much we should be consuming, the Food and Nutrition Board established the recommended dietary allowances (RDAs) and the newer dietary reference intakes (DRIs). There is nothing magical about

Excesses of any nutrient may cause problems.

vitamins, however, and we should not assume that consuming amounts far in excess of the RDA is beneficial or free of adverse effects. The more we learn about nutrients, be they vitamins, minerals, or protein, the more we come to realize that excesses may cause problems, either by way of direct toxic effects or by creating imbalances with respect to their relationships with other nutrients.

Some people express concern that in switching to a healthy, plant-based diet, they may develop vitamin deficiencies. There is no cause for worry. A diet rich in fruits and vegetables not only helps protect against many of our chronic degenerative diseases but can also easily meet all nutritional needs. We will next look at the major vitamins and show just why this is so.

Vitamin A

Vitamin A is a group of related substances that are important for maintaining a strong immune system, proper *cellular differentiation* (specialization of cells in their functions), a healthy retina, and good quality tears that keep the eye moist. A deficiency can cause a form of dry eye syndrome as well as night blindness. Vitamin A has been

Vitamin A has been used to treat retinitis pigmentosa.

used in the treatment of *retinitis pigmentosa,* a hereditary degeneration of the retina. One study showed that supplementation with 15,000 IU of vitamin A palmitate each day can help slow the progression of the disease.

Vitamin A itself is found in animal products, but the body can convert a number of plant chemicals called *carotenoids,* such as beta-carotene, alpha-carotene, gamma-carotene, and beta-cryptoxanthin, to vitamin A. These carotenoids come from vegetables and fruits. Although vitamin A in large doses can be toxic, beta-carotene is generally well tolerated because the body converts only as much as it needs to vitamin A. Beta-carotene and the other carotenoids have important antioxidant activity as well, which may help protect against chronic diseases.

Whereas synthetic beta-carotene supplements contain primarily one form of beta-carotene, all-*trans*-beta-carotene, natural sources contain a mixture of all-*trans* and several *cis* forms of beta-carotene. The *trans* and *cis* designations refer to the shape or configuration of

Beta-carotene from foods may be a stronger antioxidant than the beta-carotene in most supplements.

the beta-carotene molecule. Recent evidence suggests that the *cis* forms of beta-carotene may be much more effective antioxidants in the body than the all-*trans* form. Foods rich in beta-carotene include carrots, sweet potatoes, spinach, kale, apricots, pumpkins, cantaloupe, collard greens, and Swiss chard.

Thiamin (Vitamin B₁)

Thiamin (vitamin B_1) acts as a coenzyme for certain chemical reactions in the body. This means that it works along with enzymes, the catalysts for those reactions. Thiamin deficiency is called *beriberi* and affects primarily the heart and the nervous system. In the United States it occurs mainly in alcoholics, whereas in developing countries it occurs in people consuming mostly refined white flour or white rice. One study whose results have not been replicated showed lower blood levels of thiamin in glaucoma patients than in

In one study, glaucoma patients tended to have lower blood levels of thiamin.

people without glaucoma. Good sources of thiamin include whole or fortified grains, legumes (beans, peas, and lentils), nuts and seeds, and brewer's yeast.

Riboflavin (Vitamin B₂)

Riboflavin (vitamin B_2) helps catalyze a number of chemical reactions having to do with processes called *oxidation* and *reduction*. It also helps the body maintain adequate levels of the B vitamins niacin and pyridoxine. Therefore, to maintain a good antioxidant status, you have to consume a sufficient amount of riboflavin. Deficiency can produce skin changes, including soreness near the corners of the mouth (the most common cause of this, however, is the consumption of acidic drinks like orange juice), and cataract. Dairy and other animal products contain riboflavin, but mushrooms, asparagus, broccoli, collard greens, spinach, turnip greens, avocados, brewer's yeast, and grains (whole or fortified) are good sources as well.

Riboflavin deficiency can cause cataracts.

Niacin (Vitamin B₃)

Niacin (vitamin B_3) is part of a coenzyme that participates in the production and breakdown of carbohydrates, fatty acids, and amino acids. Niacin comes from the diet, but the body can also manufacture it from the amino acid tryptophan, with riboflavin helping out in the process.

Deficiency of niacin is called *pellagra* and is characterized by diarrhea and inflammation in the skin and mucous membranes. Meat contains niacin, but good plant sources include asparagus, avocados, broccoli, brussels sprouts, corn, kale, mushrooms, okra, peas, potatoes, pumpkin, rutabagas, squash, tomatoes, and brewer's yeast.

Niacin contributes to the antioxidant defense system against cataracts.

Pyridoxine (Vitamin B₆)

Pyridoxine (vitamin B_6) also participates in many chemical reactions, including those involved in the production of *neurotransmitters,* the chemical signaling agents of the nervous system. Pyroxidine aids in the formation of niacin (vitamin B_3) and is important for the functioning of red blood cells. It plays an especially important role in chemical reactions involving amino acids. The more protein you consume, the more pyridoxine you require. Therefore, someone who follows a healthy diet that avoids the excess protein characteristic of the typical Western

Vitamin B_6 may help prevent heart disease.

diet may need a little less pyridoxine than the average person needs. Deficiency in our society is uncommon but can cause seizures, skin changes, and anemia. It can also raise blood levels of the amino acid homocysteine, and such elevated levels represent an important risk factor for heart and other blood vessel diseases. There is some evidence that a diet rich in pyridoxine may even help prevent heart disease independent of its effect on homocysteine levels. Besides animal products, good sources of pyridoxine include whole grains and rice, soy products, peanuts, and walnuts.

Cobalamin (Vitamin B_{12})

Vitamin B_{12} is involved in manufacturing protein as well as DNA. Deficiency of this vitamin can cause irreversible damage to the brain and spinal cord. The earliest sign may be cognitive dysfunction—problems with memory and thinking. In the eye, damage may occur to the optic nerve, causing a decrease in vision. Anemia is often a late sign of the disease. The toxicity to the nervous system is attributed to a buildup of the amino acid homocysteine

Brain and nerve (including optic nerve) damage often occurs before the anemia.

and a reduction in the amino acid S-adenosyl methionine that occur when vitamin B_{12} levels become too low. Although a test can measure the vitamin B_{12} level in the blood, some people develop high homocysteine levels in the fluid bathing the brain and spinal cord before the level of vitamin B_{12} in the blood falls below the "normal" range (and sometimes even before the homocysteine level in the blood rises). Nevertheless, in people who have a borderline vitamin B_{12} level, the blood homocysteine level should be checked.

The dietary concern about vitamin B_{12} is that it is present almost exclusively in animal products, with beef and fish being the best sources. Dairy products and eggs contain some vitamin B_{12}, but the vitamin B_{12} from eggs does not appear to be as well absorbed as that from chicken. Small amounts may be present on some plants as a result of bacterial contamination, and organically grown vegetables may contain small amounts as well. Before the era of modern food processing, many people probably obtained adequate amounts of vitamin B_{12} from plant sources. For example, strict vegetarians in India may have no problem there but become vitamin B_{12} deficient when they move to England, where they consume a sanitized version of the same types of food.

Another potential source for vitamin B_{12} is the bacteria in our intestines. We have a large number of bacteria in our large intestines, and they do make some active vitamin B_{12}. Unfortunately, the large intestine cannot absorb this vitamin. Some people may have bacteria in their small intestines as well that can produce small amounts of vitamin B_{12}, but in this location it can be absorbed, aided by a protein called *intrinsic factor* that floats down from the stomach and facilitates vitamin B_{12} absorption. It would be foolish for most people to depend on these bacteria as their sole source of the vitamin, however.

Most people who develop vitamin B_{12} deficiency do so because of age-related changes in the stomach that reduce or eliminate acid production. Without acid, vitamin B_{12} cannot be cleaved from the protein in foods and is not absorbed. The lack of acid also allows bacteria to grow in the stomach, and these bacteria can consume any vitamin B_{12} that comes their way. Less commonly, the production of intrinsic factor may be reduced as well. With a normal stomach and small intestine, the amount of vitamin B_{12} required in the diet is extremely small. The recommended dietary allowance is 2.4 micrograms a day. Further, the body is extremely efficient at recycling vitamin B_{12}, so it can take years to use up the body's stores.

Nevertheless, since the consequences of vitamin B_{12} deficiency are serious, everyone should make sure to include a source of this vitamin in their diet. A nonanimal source

Some people may have to supplement with vitamin B_{12}.

that contains the active vitamin is the Red Star brand of nutritional yeast (vegetarian formula). Nutritional yeast has a nutty, cheesy taste and is good in soups and as a cheese substitute.

Cereals and soy milks may be fortified as well. The vitamin comes from bacterial cultures in these cases. Organically grown vegetables, as mentioned before, contain minute amounts of vitamin B_{12}. Dried sea vegetables and blue-green algae probably do not contain significant amounts of active vitamin B_{12} and should not be relied on as a source of this vitamin. They contain analogues of vitamin B_{12}, substances that are very similar to the actual vitamin but that do not function in the same way.

For people with no vitamin B_{12} sources in their diet, I recommend taking 1,000 micrograms of vitamin B_{12} once a week or 2,000 micrograms every two weeks. People who obtain a little from dairy and eggs but not from meat or fish should probably supplement with about half of the above amounts.

Folate

Folate (also *folic acid* or *folacin*) is another of the B vitamins that is active as a coenzyme in chemical reactions involving amino acids and DNA. Deficiency can cause anemia. Pregnant women who are deficient are at increased risk for certain birth defects (neural tube defects) in their off-spring. Leafy green vegetables, asparagus, beets, orange juice, and many beans are all rich sources of folate, although processing and heat can destroy some of it. Because of the problem with pregnant women, refined flour is now fortified with this vitamin. Predictably, studies show that vegetarians maintain significantly higher levels of folate than do nonvegetarians.

Folate deficiency can also cause optic nerve degeneration.

Biotin

Biotin is also a vitamin and is a coenzyme in chemical reactions involving sugars and fatty acids. Deficiency is rare, although it can be induced by eating a great deal of raw egg white, which contains a substance that binds to biotin. Some biotin is produced by the bacteria in our intestines, but it is also present in a number of foods. Animal products had been felt to be the best sources, but a study showed that strict vegetarians who ate no animal products, including dairy or eggs, had higher levels of biotin than vegetarians who ate dairy and eggs, who in turn had higher levels than people who ate mixed diets that included meat. Whether the extra biotin in the vegetarians came from their diets or from "healthier" bacteria in their intestines is unknown.

Pantothenic Acid

Pantothenic acid is a B vitamin that plays a role in the production of energy from carbohydrates and in fatty acid metabolism especially. Deficiency is virtually unknown. It is in a wide variety of foods, and intestinal bacteria may produce it as well. As with many other vitamins, food-processing techniques such as freezing and canning can destroy a significant amount of the pantothenic acid present in various foods.

Ascorbic Acid (Vitamin C)

Vitamin C has many functions in the body. It is necessary for the formation of *collagen*, a structural protein important for wound healing, and it plays a role in the formation of certain neurotransmitters. Vitamin C also influences white blood cell function and is important for a strong immune system. Its antioxidant properties are well known, and it restores vitamin E to its active state. Deficiency of vitamin C is called *scurvy*, which is marked by bleeding gums, fatigue, muscle ache, tiny hemorrhages in the skin, and joint pains.

Vitamin C is present in the lens and may help prevent cataract.

The best food sources of vitamin C are fruits and vegetables, including citrus fruits; red and green peppers; chili peppers; strawberries; kiwifruits; tropical fruits like papayas, mangoes, and guavas; cantaloupes; cruciferous vegetables; tomatoes; potatoes; sweet potatoes; and many more. Animal products contain minimal to no vitamin C. The current RDA is 75 milligrams a day for women and 90 milligrams a day for men, but the optimal level is probably much higher. I normally recommend at least 200 milligrams a day. People who consume a great deal of fruits and vegetables obviously obtain much more vitamin C than people who don't.

Eating plenty of fruits and vegetables will assure optimal amounts of vitamin C.

Two other warnings—vitamin C is easily destroyed by cooking, and smokers have significantly lower levels of vitamin C in their bloodstream than do nonsmokers.

Vitamin D

Vitamin D is really a steroid hormone rather than a vitamin. That is because the skin—the largest organ in the body—manufactures vitamin D from *7-dehydrocholesterol*, a form of cholesterol, after exposure to sunlight. Vitamin D aids in the absorption of calcium from the intestine, helps the kidney regulate calcium levels, and helps create and maintain strong bones. It helps support the immune system as well. One study showed that adequate sunlight exposure

Vitamin D is really a hormone, not a vitamin.

may reduce the risk of breast cancer, a finding that may be explained by the immune-enhancing effects of vitamin D. Deficiency of vitamin D can cause a bone problem called *rickets* in infants, and it may also contribute to osteoporosis in adults. Although vitamin D can be obtained from foods, sunlight exposure is a much more important factor for maintenance of adequate vitamin D levels. Hence, it is preferable to obtain vitamin D from sunlight rather than from dietary supplementation.

There are few dietary sources of vitamin D. Fatty fish, egg yolks, and mushrooms contain moderate amounts, but the main food source in the United States has been fortified food products. Dairy products naturally contain very little vitamin D, but they have usually been fortified by the time they reach the consumer, at least in the United States. Unfortunately, this fortification is not always done accurately, and consumers have occasionally been exposed to excessive amounts of vitamin D. Other foods and beverages, such as soy milk, are often fortified with vitamin D as well.

Vitamin E

Vitamin E is a major component of the body's antioxidant defense system. Deficiency can lead to sterility as well as muscle and nerve problems. Vitamin E is in the lens of the eye and may help prevent cataract. It is also present in the retina, where it may help prevent macular degeneration. Vitamin E in nature actually comprises eight different compounds: alpha-, beta-, gamma-, and delta-tocopherol; and alpha-, beta-, gamma-, and delta-tocotrienol. No one food source is rich in all of them, but wheat and soy oils together cover the spectrum fairly well. Most animal products provide small amounts of alpha-tocopherol and hardly any of the other forms.

Vitamin E is present in both the lens and the retina.

The average diet contains more gamma-tocopherol than alpha-tocopherol, but the bloodstream maintains higher levels of alpha-tocopherol. As a result, it has been assumed that alpha-tocopherol is the more important and the more biologically active. This may not always be the case, however. One study showed that gamma-tocopherol was more effective than alpha-tocopherol in detoxifying nitrogen dioxide, a powerful prooxidant in cigarette smoke. Gamma-tocopherol may also be more effective in preventing the development of cancer under some circumstances. A recent study found that higher blood levels of gamma-tocopherol may provide protection against heart disease. In addition, some of our body tissues may preferentially take up gamma-tocopherol as compared with alpha-tocopherol. The tocotrienols have important antioxidant properties as well and are being investigated for possible cholesterol-lowering effects.

We should try to ingest the full range of vitamin E compounds that we find in foods, as opposed to alpha-tocopherol alone, as is found in supplements (even most so-called mixed tocopherol vitamin E supplements contain over 95 percent alpha-tocopherol). Another problem with vitamin E supplements is that large dosages (over 400 IU a day) of alpha-tocopherol drastically lower the levels of gamma-tocopherol in the bloodstream, an action that may have harmful consequences. These findings may explain why a few studies have found beneficial effects from consuming vitamin E from foods as opposed to vitamin E from supplements.

Vitamin E is carried in the blood by the proteins that carry cholesterol. The ratio of vitamin E to cholesterol in the bloodstream may be important, especially with regard to the risk for developing hardening of the arteries. One study found that vegetarians have higher levels of vitamin E relative to cholesterol than do nonvegetarians. This can be explained by the fact that the foods richest in vitamin E are whole grains (containing the germ), sweet potatoes, green vegetables, soy products, peanuts and most nuts, mangoes, and, to some degree, apples, pears, and other fruits.

Vitamin K

Vitamin K is a group of substances involved in producing certain proteins, most notably those having to do with blood clotting. These substances, called *phylloquinone* and *menaquinones,* occur in plants, animals, and bacteria (including those in our intestines). Interestingly, there are vitamin K receptors on our bones, and maintaining an adequate vitamin K status may help prevent osteoporosis. Deficiency is marked by bleeding problems. Since vitamin K is a fat-soluble vitamin, deficiency may occur in people who have fat malabsorption problems. Chronic disease and long-term antibiotic therapy that wipes out many of the normal intestinal bacteria increase the risk of deficiency. Leafy green vegetables are considered the best sources of vitamin K.

Minerals

Minerals are crucial for all bodily functions. In addition to their obvious contribution to bone and cartilage development, minerals are required for the proper functioning of many enzymes and hormones. We require more of certain minerals than of others, but a deficiency of any of them can lead to serious problems. Therefore, maintaining adequate levels in the body is just as important for minerals as for vitamins. In some cases, it may be hard to determine whether a deficiency of a particular mineral is present, because the level of the mineral in the bloodstream may not reflect the level in the body tissues where it is most active. Let us now look at the major minerals and see what role they play in promoting good health, including the health of the eyes.

Iron

Iron is best known for being a part of the *hemoglobin* molecule, the oxygen carrier of red blood cells. However, it is also part of *myoglobin,* a similar type of protein in muscle cells, and it acts as a cofactor in conjunction with many enzymes. Fatigue and compromise of the immune system are early signs of mild iron deficiency. For example, an immune system slightly compromised from iron deficiency may increase the likelihood of recurrences of herpes infections in the eye. As the deficiency becomes more pronounced, a type of anemia occurs marked by small, pale red blood cells. Iron deficiency can *Too much iron in the body may promote oxidation, causing heart disease.* occur as the result of blood loss or because of inability to meet the increased need for iron caused by rapid growth or pregnancy. In the elderly, iron may not be absorbed as well as it is in younger people. And dietary factors can play a role. However, excessive iron intake and storage can cause serious problems. About 10 to 15 percent of the population has a tendency to store too much iron. This excess iron may promote oxidation reactions in the body, and some feel it is a major risk factor for heart disease. Thus, it is important to avoid both deficiencies and excesses of iron.

Absorption of iron from foods depends on many factors, including the amount and form of iron in food products, the amount of iron stores in an individual, and the presence of inhibitors or promoters of iron absorption in the foods consumed. Iron from animal products is in the form of *heme iron,* which is more readily absorbed than the nonheme iron derived from plant foods. Therefore, people who eat red meat often absorb more iron from their foods than people who do not eat red meat. There is evidence that people who switch to diets containing primarily nonheme iron adjust rapidly and begin to absorb a larger percentage of the nonheme iron than they were absorbing before. People at higher risk for iron deficiency who want to avoid meat consumption can improve their iron stores by paying attention to the factors that promote or inhibit iron absorption, which we will soon discuss. Even if not eating meat tends to lower the body's iron stores somewhat, it probably also decreases the risk of toxicity from too much iron.

Plant foods that contain good amounts of iron include whole and fortified grains, lentils, garbanzo beans, Swiss chard, spinach, potatoes, watermelon, strawberries, almonds, blackstrap molasses, kale, and broccoli. Seitan, a meat analogue (fake meat) made from the gluten (protein) portion of wheat, is often a very rich source.

Vitamin C, including that present naturally in foods, greatly enhances the absorption of nonheme iron. That is why foods like potatoes, watermelon, and strawberries are such good sources: They not only have a fair amount of iron but also contain vitamin C. Eating other vitamin C–rich foods at the same meal has the same effect.

Soy products contain moderate amounts of iron, but the iron is not well absorbed. Fermented soy products such as tempeh, which have less of an inhibitory substance called *phytate,* allow slightly better iron absorption than other soy products such as tofu, but it is still not very good. Some other inhibitory factor associated with the protein fraction of soy products seems to be responsible for the poor iron absorption. One study found that some young Buddhist adults in China who ate a diet very rich in soy products showed compromised iron status.

Tea contains inhibitors of iron absorption called *tannins,* so at-risk individuals should avoid drinking tea with meals. Excess fiber, as might be seen in bran-enriched breads or muffins, can also have an inhibitory effect.

Dairy products may promote iron deficiency in several ways. First, they contain almost no iron and are being substituted for foods that do contain iron. Second, their calcium content is high, and high concentrations of calcium in foods may inhibit iron absorption. Third, there has even been the suggestion that the types of proteins in dairy products may inhibit iron absorption somewhat. Therefore,

Dairy products contain minimal iron.

minimizing or eliminating dairy products should improve your iron status. Remember, there are many good sources of calcium besides dairy products.

Calcium

Calcium is the most abundant mineral in the body, and almost all of it is in the skeleton. However, it has other important functions as well, playing a role in blood clotting, nerve and muscle activity, and other areas. A calcium deficiency can lead to bone problems in both the young and the old. Adequate calcium intake is important in children because that is the period of life in which the bone mass, which must last a lifetime, is determined. A great deal of attention has been focused on calcium intake with regard to the development of osteoporosis in adults. However, there is a lack of evidence indicating that higher dietary calcium intakes in adults, especially in the form of dairy products, has any real impact on the incidence of bone fractures. Calcium intake is just one of many factors involved in osteoporosis.

Absorption of calcium from foods depends on the amount in the food and the type of food. About 30 percent of the calcium from milk is absorbed. By comparison, many of the dark, leafy green vegetables that are rich in calcium, such as kale, mustard greens, broccoli, and turnip greens, have a fractional absorption (percent absorbed) at least as high if not higher. Spinach is the exception: Although rich in calcium, only about 5 percent is absorbed. It contains some calcium absorption inhibitors. The majority of the

Most dark, leafy green vegetables represent the best source of calcium.

calcium from whole wheat bread is absorbed, indicating that the amount of fiber and other substances present does not interfere with absorption. Other good dietary sources include collard greens, bok choy (Chinese cabbage), almonds, figs, tofu processed with calcium sulfate, and blackstrap molasses. This form of molasses is rich in both iron and calcium, although bear in mind that the sugar in blackstrap molasses makes you lose much of the calcium in your urine. It is also worth mentioning the alternative grains amaranth, teff, and quinoa, which are being introduced into this country and are good sources of both calcium and iron.

Children should eat at least four or five servings of calcium-rich foods every day. At least one or two of these should be dark, leafy green vegetables. In older people, a good calcium intake is also important, but it may be even more important to avoid the things that make you lose calcium in the urine: excess protein, especially animal protein; excess salt and sugars; and, to a minor degree, caffeine.

Avoid the things that make you lose calcium.

When you lose more than you take in, we call this a *negative calcium balance*. The amount lost has to come from somewhere, so it comes from your bones. Supplementation with large amounts of calcium can often create a positive calcium balance, but large doses of calcium can interfere somewhat with absorption of iron, zinc, and other minerals.

Magnesium

Magnesium is the "forgotten" mineral. Although the dairy industry tries to remind us about calcium, and the meat industry about iron, who is there to stand up for magnesium? Magnesium interacts with over 300 enzymes and participates in many of the body's most important chemical reactions. High magnesium intake from food may help protect against high blood pressure, diabetes, certain heart problems, kidney stones, and osteoporosis, and deficiency may increase the risk of these diseases. In fact, magnesium is probably at least as important as, if not more

Magnesium may be at least as important as, if not more important than, calcium in preventing osteoporosis.

important than, calcium in preventing osteoporosis. In some situations, magnesium may either oppose or augment the effects of calcium, and its body levels must therefore maintain a balance with those of calcium.

Mild magnesium deficiency may be much more common than most people realize. That is because the richest sources are green vegetables (chlorophyll, the green coloring in plants, contains magnesium), whole grains (with emphasis on the "whole"), legumes, nuts, and seeds. Most animal products contain much less magnesium. Therefore, magnesium is one of those minerals in which vegetarians surpass meat eaters, and a meat-based diet without much vegetable and whole grain consumption may actually be considered a risk factor for magnesium deficiency. High sugar intake can

Magnesium deficiency may increase the risk of diabetic retinopathy.

increase loss of magnesium in the urine as well, as can high blood levels of sugar, as seen in diabetics. In fact, some people have speculated that magnesium deficiency may increase the risk of diabetic complications such as diabetic retinopathy.

Phosphorus

Phosphorus, usually in the form of phosphate, is involved in numerous chemical processes in the body, but most of it is located in the bones along with calcium. Deficiency in adults is very rare, although taking aluminum hydroxide antacids for long periods of time can tie up enough phosphate to actually produce a deficiency. In general, the amount of phosphate consumed should equal the amount of calcium consumed. Actually, most people in the United States consume significantly more phosphate than calcium. The reason is that animal products are quite high in phosphate, whereas green vegetables are low. Some phosphate also comes from the phosphoric acid often used in soft drinks. This excess phosphate may cause the parathyroid glands to secrete extra parathyroid hormone, producing a condition called *secondary hyperparathyroidism.* This extra parathyroid hormone may then cause loss of calcium from bone. Some studies have supported this scenario by showing that higher dietary phosphate intake is associated with lower bone mass. Thus, high phosphate intake may be a risk factor for osteoporosis.

Zinc

Zinc is another trace mineral that most people don't think about as often as they should. It acts as a cofactor for numerous enzymes and is important for a strong immune system and for growth. The eye and the prostate gland both contain high levels of zinc, and as discussed thoroughly in chapter 12, a high zinc intake may help prevent the progression of age-related macular degeneration, the number one cause of poor vision among the elderly. Zinc deficiency causes an impaired immune system, growth retardation in children, skin abnormalities, and other symptoms. The exact amount of zinc required is not certain, but the RDA is 11 milligrams for men and 8 milligrams for women. Zinc is one mineral that may be a little more difficult to obtain from a plant-based diet as compared with the average American diet.

Zinc keeps the immune system strong and may help prevent macular degeneration.

Meat contains zinc, but good plant sources include whole grains (especially rye), wheat germ, black-eyed peas, sesame and pumpkin seeds, most types of beans, lentils, peas, peanuts, pecans, almonds, cashews, chestnuts, pine nuts, asparagus, spinach, and mushrooms. Although *phytate,* a substance found in abundance in cereal grains and some vegetables, may inhibit zinc absorption in a plant-based diet, it is probably not a major problem in the United States as compared with countries where flat breads predominate. The reason is that the yeast in leavened breads produces a phytase enzyme that eliminates much of the phytate. Nevertheless, because of the potential for mild zinc deficiency, it is important to pay attention to its dietary sources.

Toxicity from too much zinc can occur as the result of high-dose supplementation. Potential problems include deficiencies of copper, iron, manganese, and other minerals; lowering of HDL cholesterol, the "good" form; immune system impairment; and perhaps accelerated development of Alzheimer's disease.

Copper

Copper is important for many bodily functions, including blood cell production and maintenance of healthy nervous and cardiovascular systems. Copper deficiency can cause anemia, low white blood cell counts, and possibly even heart disease. Mild deficiency, which cannot be detected by a simple measurement of the copper level in the blood, can depress the activity of important antioxidant and other enzymes, such as superoxide dismutase and glutathione peroxidase (important in the eye). The RDA for adults is 0.9 milligrams per day.

Although some organ meats and some types of seafood are good sources of copper, plant sources provide abundant amounts as well. Soy foods, other beans, lentils, nuts, and seeds are especially rich sources. Consequently, people who follow a plant-based diet have a higher copper intake than do people following the typical diet.

Manganese

Manganese is most heavily concentrated in the mitochondria of our cells. *Mitochondria* are specialized cell parts that act as their powerhouses, creating energy to meet cell demands. One mitochondrial enzyme that contains manganese is superoxide dismutase. This enzyme, which inactivates potentially harmful oxygen free radicals, is different from the other superoxide dismutase (found outside mitochondria), which depends on copper (primarily) and zinc for its activity. Severe manganese deficiency is extremely rare, although it is difficult to determine the incidence of mild deficiency. The blood levels of manganese are fairly low and do not necessarily reflect its concentration in the organs. The liver, kidney, and pancreas are quite rich in manganese, but it is obviously a lot more difficult to biopsy an organ to determine its manganese level than it is to obtain a blood sample!

The richest sources of manganese are whole grains, legumes, nuts, and tea. Fruits and leafy vegetables contain moderate amounts. As expected, then, vegetarians and others who consume a lot of these foods maintain much better levels of manganese in their bodies than do people whose consumption of plant foods is lower. Whether the poorer manganese status in people eating a meat-based diet has any adverse effect on the activity of enzymes like mitochondrial superoxide dismutase remains to be determined.

Selenium

Selenium plays an important role in the body's antioxidant defense system. It replaces a sulfur atom in the essential amino acid cysteine to form selenocysteine. Selenocysteine becomes part of the glutathione peroxidase enzyme in the eye, which can detoxify hydrogen peroxide. Some people have theorized that maintaining adequate amounts of selenium in the body can help prevent certain types of cancer, and several studies support this theory.

Selenium is part of an important antioxidant enzyme in the eye.

Selenium deficiency has also been implicated as a risk factor for an unusual type of heart problem that strikes young people in China.

THE EYE CARE SOURCEBOOK

Animal products, especially organ meats and seafood, tend to contain more selenium than other foods. Whole grains can be a good source, but the selenium content generally depends on the amount of selenium in the soil, which can vary greatly from one area to another. Nevertheless, the selenium status of vegetarians appears to be about the same as that of nonvegetarians.

Iodine

The thyroid hormones contain *iodine*. An iodine deficiency results in a hypothyroid (underactive thyroid) state marked by a *goiter* (enlargement of the thyroid gland). At present, most cases of hypothyroidism are due to a disorder of the thyroid gland itself rather than to an iodine deficiency. Seafood and sea vegetables are rich sources of iodine. Plants contain some iodine, but the amount varies greatly depending on the concentration of iodine in the soil. The use of iodized salt has greatly reduced the incidence of iodine deficiency. It still remains a problem, though, especially in the developing countries. People who consume no sea vegetables or other seafood and who do not use iodized salt are at some risk for deficiency. Therefore, a plant-based diet should include either sea vegetables or iodized salt. Eating large amounts of raw cruciferous vegetables (broccoli, cauliflower, and so on) can also suppress thyroid function because of the presence of chemicals called *goitrogens*.

Phytochemicals

It is obvious that eating a wide variety of fruits and vegetables in quantity reduces the risk of many diseases, such as cataract, cancer, and cardiovascular disease, but that's not good enough for some people. They need to know *why*. This is where *phytochemicals* (plant chemicals) come into the picture. Fruits and vegetables contain much more than just vitamin C, vitamin E, and beta-carotene. They contain a wide range of substances with diverse

Phytochemicals help prevent heart disease, cancer, and inflammation.

effects, helping to prevent cancer by interfering with virtually every step in the chain of events that leads to the formation of a cancer cell. Many have antioxidant properties that may also protect against heart disease and stroke, keeping the harmful LDL cholesterol from being oxidized to a more *atherogenic* (promoting hardening of the arteries) form. Some have anti-inflammatory properties as well.

Flavonoids and other polyphenols represent a large group of phytochemicals found throughout the plant kingdom. Red wine and grape juice have been found to contain this type of chemical, and some people feel that it may be what is behind the "French paradox," the low incidence of coronary artery disease among the French. Tea, especially the green variety, contains catechins and other polyphenols that may prevent cancer. Tea consumption was also correlated with a lower incidence of cataracts in one study. Another polyphenol, ellagic acid, is found in high concentration in walnuts, strawberries, and some other berries and is strongly suspected of protecting against cancer by a variety of mechanisms.

Most people are aware that cruciferous vegetables, such as broccoli and cauliflower, may be cancer protective because they contain compounds like *indoles* and *isothiocyanates*. But have you heard about the *umbelliferous* vegetables? This is the group to which carrots, parsley, celery, and parsnips belong. Those of you who are chemists will be glad to know that they contain phthalides, polyacetylenes, polyphenols, monoterpenes, and many other compounds. They are probably at least as important as the cruciferous vegetables. An old-fashioned celery tonic may make you nostalgic, but try a drink combining apple, carrot, and celery juices for a nice refresher.

Soy products such as tofu and tempeh have become more in vogue as a result of the publicity about their cholesterol-lowering and possible cancer-protective effects. They contain substances such as isoflavones (also known as phytoestrogens), saponins, phytates, and lignans, all of which are being actively studied. Many spices also contain powerful phytochemicals. For example, rosemary contains antioxidants that appear to be more potent than vitamin E. And turmeric (an ingredient in mustard) is yellow because of curcumin, another potential cancer preventer.

The list goes on and on, and we have just begun to scratch the surface in discovering the array of phytochemicals present in plants. But we don't really need more studies to tell us what to eat. Studies of phytochemicals are done to satisfy scientific curiosity, as a way to screen for new drugs, and with the goal of some researchers to supplement unhealthy foods with phytochemicals to make them less unhealthy. For example, people who don't want to eat their vegetables might one day be able to eat hamburgers fortified with a number of phytochemicals.

There are a number of drawbacks to this approach, however. First, virtually all the studies done on phytochemicals have been test tube or animal studies. The weakness of animal studies is that they cannot be extrapolated directly to the human situation, since different species of animals metabolize substances in different ways. And test tube experiments cannot simulate the human condition very well either.

Phytochemicals represent the greatest deficiency in the average American diet.

Another drawback to studying individual phytochemicals is that a given phytochemical may not have much of an effect when used alone but may have a synergistic effect when certain other phytochemicals are present. Plants are endowed with certain combinations of phytochemicals, and the human body is adapted to the phytochemical mixtures as they exist in nature.

What all this means is that most of the money being spent on phytochemical research would probably be better spent on educating people to eat their dark leafy greens along with all the other fruits and vegetables, thereby preventing macular degeneration, cataract, and the whole slew of chronic diseases that plague our society. The health benefits derived from eating whole foods greatly exceed that associated with chemical supplementation of unhealthy food products.

Perhaps the most important reason, though, for discussing the subject of phytochemicals is that they represent the most prevalent deficiency in the average American diet. A plant-based diet with minimal or no animal products can easily meet your nutritional needs while avoiding the phytochemical deficiency that characterizes the standard meat-based diet.

Notes

Chapter Five

1. J. J. Perez-Santonja, M. J. Ayala, H. F. Sakla, J. M. Ruiz-Moreno, and J. L. Alio. "Retreatment After Laser in Situ Keratomileusis." *Ophthalmology* 106 (1999): 21–28.

2. G. O. Waring III, J. D. Carr, R. D. Stulting, W. M.Wiley, D. Huang, and K. P. Thompson. "LASIK for Myopia and Astigmatism in 2,100 Consecutive Eyes Using a Nidek EC-5000 Excimer Laser." *Investigative Ophthalmology and Visual Science* 40 (1999): S588.

3. R. D. Stulting, J. D. Carr, K. P. Thompson, G. O. Waring III, W.M. Wiley, and J. G. Walker. "Complications of Laser in Situ Keratomileusis for the Correction of Myopia." *Ophthalmology* 106 (1999): 13–20.

4. J. Ben-nun. "Photorefractive Keratectomy and Laser in Situ Keratomileusis: A Word from the Devil's Advocate." *Archives of Ophthalmology* 118 (2000): 1706–7.

5. P. S. Hersh, S. F. Brint, R. K. Maloney, D. S. Durrie, M. Gordon, M. A. Michelson, V. M. Thompson, R. D. Berkeley, O. D. Schein, and R. F. Steinert. "Photorefractive Keratectomy Versus Laser in Situ Keratomileusis for Moderate to High Myopia." *Ophthalmology* 105 (1998): 1512–23.

6. D. J. Schanzlin, P. A. Asbell, T. E. Burris, and D. S. Durrie. "The Intrastromal Corneal Ring Segments." *Ophthalmology* 104 (1997): 1067–78.

Chapter Nine

1. A. Taylor, P. F. Jacques, T. Nowell, G. Perrone, J. Blumberg, G. Handelman, B. Jozwiak, and D. Nadler. "Vitamin C in Human and Guinea Pig Aqueous, Lens and Plasma in Relation to Intake."*Current Eye Research* 16 (1997): 857–64.

2. K.- J. Yeum, F. Shang, W. Schalch, R. M. Russell, and A. Taylor. "Fat-Soluble Nutrient Concentrations in Different Layers of Human Cataractous Lens." *Current Eye Research* 19 (1999): 502–5.

3. C. J. Bates, S. Chen, A. MacDonald, and R. Holden. "Quantitation of Vitamin E and a Carotenoid Pigment in Cataractous Human Lenses, and the Effect of a Dietary Supplement." *International Journal for Vitamin and Nutrition Research* 66 (1996): 316–21.

4. L. Chasan-Taber, W. C. Willett, J. M. Seddon, M. J. Stampfer, B. Rosner, G. A. Colditz, F. E. Speizer, and S. E. Hankinson. "A Prospective Study of Carotenoid and Vitamin A Intakes and Risk of Cataract Extraction in U. S. Women. *The American Journal of Clinical Nutrition* 70 (1999): 509–16.

5. L. Brown, E. B. Rimm, J. M. Seddon, E. L. Giovannucci, L. Chasan-Taber, D. Spiegelman, W. C. Willett, and S. E. Hankinson. "A Prospective Study of Carotenoid Intake and Risk of Cataract Extraction in U. S. Men." *The American Journal of Clinical Nutrition* 70 (1999): 517–24.

6. H. W. Skalka and J. T. Prchal. "Cataracts and Riboflavin Deficiency." *The American Journal of Clinical Nutrition* 34 (1981): 861–3.

7. S. E. Hankinson, M. J. Stampfer, J. M. Seddon, G. A. Colditz, B. Rosner, F. E. Speizer, and W. C. Willett. "Nutrient Intake and Cataract Extraction In Women: A Prospective Study." BMJ (*British Medical Journal*) 305 (1992): 335–39.

8. J. M. Robertson, A. P. Donner, and J. R. Trevithick. "A Possible Role for Vitamins C and E in Cataract Prevention." *American Journal of Clinical Nutrition* 53 (1991): 346S–51S.

9. P. F. Jacques and L. T. Chylack, Jr. "Epidemiologic Evidence of a Role for the Antioxidant Vitamins and Carotenoids in Cataract Prevention." *The American Journal of Clinical Nutrition* 53 (1991): 352S–5S.

10. H. W. Skalka and J. T. Prchal. "Presenile Cataract Formation and Decreased Activity of Galactosemic Enzymes." *Archives of Ophthalmology* 98 (1980): 269–73.

11. [1]M. J. Elman, M. T. Miller, and R. Matalon. "Galactokinase Activity in Patients with Idiopathic Cataracts." *Ophthalmology* 93(1986): 210–15.

12. P. F. Jacques, J. Phillips, S. C. Hartz, and L. T. Chylack, Jr. "Lactose Intake, Galactose Metabolism and Senile Cataract." *Nutrition Research* 10 (1990): 255–65.

Chapter Ten

1. M. S. Passo, L. Goldberg, D. L. Elliot, and E. M. Van Buskirk. "Exercise Training Reduces Intraocular Pressure Among Subjects Suspected of Having Glaucoma." *Archives of Ophthalmology* 109 (1991): 1096–98.
2. E. J. Higginbotham, H. A. Kilimanjaro, J. T. Wilensky, R. L. Batenhorst, and D. Hermann. "The Effect of Caffeine on Intraocular Pressure in Glaucoma Patients." *Ophthalmology* 96 (1989): 624–26.
3. K. Lotfi and J. E. Grunwald. "The Effect of Caffeine on the Human Macular Circulation." *Investigative Ophthalmology and Visual Science* 32 (1991): 3028–32.
4. C. Pissarello. "La curva giornaliera della tensione nell'occhio normale e nell'occhio glaucomatoso e influenza di fattori diversi (miotici, iridectomia, irido-sclerectomia, derivativi, pasti) determinata con il Tonometro di Schiotz." *Annali di Ottalmologia* 44 (1915): 544–636.
5. F. W. Stocker, L. B. Holt, and J. W. Clower. "Clinical Experiments with New Ways of Influencing Intraocular Tension. I. Effect of Rice Diet." *Archives of Ophthalmology* 40 (1948): 46–55.
6. N. Naveh-Floman and M. Belkin. "Prostaglandin Metabolism and Intraocular Pressure. *British Journal of Ophthalmology* 71 (1987): 254–56.
7. J. H. J. Klaver, E. L. Greve, H. Goslinga, H. C. Geijssen, and J. H. A. Heuvelmans. "Blood and Plasma Viscosity Measurements in Patients with Glaucoma." *British Journal of Ophthalmology* 69 (1985): 765–70.
8. P. Garcia-Salinas, G. E. Trope, and M. Glynn. "Blood Viscosity in Ocular Hypertension." *Canadian Journal of Ophthalmology* 23 (1988): 305–7.
9. H. S. Chung, A. Harris, J. K. Kristinsson, T. A. Ciulla, C. Kagemann, and R. Ritch. "Ginkgo Biloba Extract Increases Ocular Blood Flow Velocity." *Journal of Ocular Pharmacology and Therapeutics* 15 (1999): 233–40.

Chapter Eleven

1. J. Karjalainen, J. M. Martin, M. Knip, J. Ilonen, B. H. Robinson, E. Savilahti, H. K. Åkerblom, and H.-M. Dosch. "A Bovine Albumin

Peptide as a Possible Trigger of Insulin-Dependent Diabetes Mellitus." *The New England Journal of Medicine* 327 (1992): 302–7.

2. M. G. Cavallo, D. Fava, L. Monetini, F. Barone, and P. Pozzilli. "Cell-Mediated Immune Response to Beta-Casein in Recent-Onset Insulin-Dependent Diabetes: Implications for Disease Pathogenesis." *The Lancet* 348 (1996): 926–28.

3. J. W. Anderson, J. A. Zeigler, D. A. Deakins, T. L. Floore, D. W. Dillon, C. L. Wood, P. R. Oeltgen, and R. J. Whitley. "Metabolic Effects of High-Carbohydrate, High-Fiber Diets for Insulin-Dependent Diabetic Individuals." *The American Journal of Clinical Nutrition* 54 (1991): 936–43.

4. Early Treatment Diabetic Retinopathy Study Research Group. "Photocoagulation for Diabetic Macular Edema." *Archives of Ophthalmology* 103 (1985): 1796–1806.

5. M. S. Roy, G. Stables, B. Collier, A. Roy, and E. Bou. "Nutritional Factors in Diabetics with and Without Retinopathy." *The American Journal of Clinical Nutrition* 50 (1989): 728–30.

6. American Diabetes Association. "Nutritional Recommendations and Principles for Individuals with Diabetes Mellitus: 1986." *Diabetes Care* 10 (1987): 126–32.

7. E. Y. Chew, M. L. Klein, F. L. Ferris III, N. A. Remaley, R. P. Murphy, K. Chantry, B. J. Hoogwerf, and D. Miller; for the ETDRS Research Group. "Association of Elevated Serum Lipid Levels with Retinal Hard Exudate in Diabetic Retinopathy." *Archives of Ophthalmology* 114 (1996): 1079–84.

8. W. F. Van Eck. "The Effect of a Low Fat Diet on the Serum Lipids in Diabetes and Its Significance in Diabetic Retinopathy." *American Journal of Medicine* 27 (1959): 196–211.

9. I. Ernest, E. Linner, and A. Svanborg. "Carbohydrate-Rich, Fat-Poor Diet in Diabetes." *American Journal of Medicine* 39 (1965): 594–600.

10. B. Gordon, S. Chang, M. Kavanagh, M. Berrocal, L. Yannuzzi, C. Robertson, and A. Drexler. "The Effects of Lipid Lowering on Diabetic Retinopathy." *American Journal of Ophthalmology* 112 (1991): 385–91.

11. P. McNair, C. Christiansen, S. Madsbad, E. Lauritzen, O. Faber, C. Binder, and I. Transbøl. "Hypomagnesemia, a Risk Factor in Diabetic Retinopathy." *Diabetes* 27 (1978): 1075–77.

12. A. Ceriello, D. Giugliano, P. Dello Russo, and N. Passariello. "Hypomagnesemia in Relation to Diabetic Retinopathy." *Diabetes Care* 5 (1982): 558–59.

13. American Diabetes Association. "Magnesium Supplementation in the Treatment of Diabetes." *Diabetes Care* 15 (1992): 1065–67.
14. J. Kleijnen and P. Knipschild. "Ginkgo Biloba." *The Lancet* 340 (1992): 1136–39.
15. F. V. DeFeudis. *Ginkgo Biloba Extract (EGb 761): Pharmacological Activities and Clinical Applications.* Paris: Elsevier, 1991.

Chapter Twelve

1. D. A. Newsome, M. Swartz, N. C. Leone, R. C. Elston, and E. Miller. "Oral Zinc in Macular Degeneration." *Archives of Ophthalmology* 106 (1988): 192–98.
2. M. Stur, M. Tittl, A. Reitner, and V. Meisinger. "Oral Zinc and the Second Eye in Age-Related Macular Degeneration." *Investigative Ophthalmology and Visual Science* 37 (1996): 1225–35.
3. C. Kies. "Bioavailability of Manganese." In D. J. Klimis-Tavantzis, ed., *Manganese in Health and Disease.* Boca Raton, Fla.: CRC Press, 1994, 45–47.
4. Eye Disease Case-Control Study Group. "Antioxidant Status and Neovascular Age-Related Macular Degeneration." *Archives of Ophthalmology* 111 (1993): 104–9.
5. J. M. Seddon, U. A. Ajani, R. D. Sperduto, R. Hiller, N. Blair, T. C. Burton, M. D. Farber, E. S. Gragoudas, J. Haller, D. T. Miller, L. A. Yannuzzi, and W. Willett; for the Eye Disease Case-Control Study Group. "Dietary Carotenoids, Vitamins A, C, and E, and Advanced Age-Related Macular Degeneration." *JAMA (Journal of the American Medical Assocation)* 272 (1994): 1413–20.
6. N. I. Krinsky, M. D. Russett, G. J. Handelman, and D. M. Snodderly. "Structural and Geometrical Isomers of Carotenoids in Human Plasma." *The Journal of Nutrition* 120 (1990): 1654–62.
7. J. A. Mares-Perlman, W. E. Brady, R. Klein, G. M. VandenLangenberg, B. E. K. Klein, and M. Palta. "Dietary Fat and Age-Related Maculopathy." *Archives of Ophthalmology* 113 (1995): 743–48.
8. C. Eunyoung, S. E. Hankinson, W. C. Willett, M. J. Stampfer, D. Spiegelman, F. E. Speizer, E. B. Rimm, and J. M. Seddon. "Prospective Study of Alcohol Consumption and the Risk of Age-Related Macular Degeneration." *Archives of Ophthalmology* 118 (2000): 681–88.

Chapter Thirteen

1. P.-J. Lamey and P. A. Biagioni. "Relationship Between Iron Status and Recrudescent Herpes Labialis." *European Journal of Clinical Microbiology and Infectious Diseases* 14 (1995): 604–5.
2. American Academy of Pediatrics Committee on Nutrition. "The Use of Whole Cow's Milk in Infancy." *Pediatrics* 89 (1992): 1105–9.
3. D. R. Hoffman, E. E. Birch, D. G. Birch, and R. D. Uauy. Effects of Supplementation with Omega-3 Long-Chain Polyunsaturated Fatty Acids on Retinal and Cortical Development in Premature Infants." *The American Journal of Clinical Nutrition* 57 (suppl.) (1993): 807S–12S.
4. M. Makrides, K. Simmer, M. Goggin, and R. A. Gibson. "Erythrocyte Docosahexaenoic Acid Correlates with the Visual Response of Healthy, Term Infants." *Pediatric Research* 33 (1993): 425–27.
5. A. Lucas, R. Morley, T. J. Cole, G. Lister, and C. Leeson-Payne. "Breast Milk and Subsequent Intelligence Quotient in Children Born Preterm." *The Lancet* 339 (1992): 261–64.
6. S. E. Carlson, S. H. Werkman, J. M. Peeples, and W. M. Wilson. "Long-Chain Fatty Acids and Early Visual and Cognitive Development of Preterm Infants." *European Journal of Clinical Nutrition* 48 (suppl. 2) (1994): S27–S30.
7. A. J. M. Burton, A. Reynolds, and D. O'Neill. "Sildenafil (Viagra) a Cause of Proliferative Diabetic Retinopathy?" *Eye* 14 (2000): 785–86.

Chapter Fourteen

1. D. Ornish, S. E. Brown, L. W. Scherwitz, J. H. Billings, W. T. Armstrong, T. A. Ports, S. M. McLanahan, R. L. Kirkeeide, R. J. Brand, and K. L. Gould. "Can Lifestyle Changes Reverse Coronary Heart Disease?" *The Lancet* 336 (1990): 129–33.
2. *Diet, Nutrition, and the Prevention of Chronic Diseases.* Geneva: World Health Organization, 1990.
3. A. Birkett, J. Muir, J. Phillips, G. Jones, and K. O'Dea. "Resistant Starch Lowers Fecal Concentrations of Ammonia and Phenols in Humans." *The American Journal of Clinical Nutrition* 63 (1996): 766–72.

Glossary

Accommodation The process by which the eye changes the shape of the lens to change its focus from distance to near. The alteration in the shape of the lens is brought about by contraction of the ciliary muscle.

Amblyopia (am-blee-oh´-pee-a) Reduced vision in any eye not caused by any disease of the eye itself. Amblyopia may occur in young children (1) as a result of a misalignment of the two eyes, (2) when the difference between the refractive errors of the two eyes is large, or (3) when an eye has been prevented from seeing because it has been kept covered for an extended period or because of opacities in certain parts of the eye.

Angle The junction of the cornea with the iris, where the trabecular mesh-work is located. A narrow angle may predispose a person to angle-closure glaucoma.

Aqueous humor The watery fluid secreted by the ciliary body. It fills the posterior and anterior chambers of the eye.

Astigmatism A refractive error generally caused by a cornea that is not curved to the same degree in all directions.

Autoimmune disease A disease in which the immune system, which normally defends the body against infection, turns against some of the body's own tissues.

Background diabetic retinopathy (ret-i-nop´-a-thee) Damage to the retina caused by weakening of the walls of blood vessels in diabetics. The damage results from leakage of fluid from the vessels and from the shutdown of small blood vessels.

Bacterium (plural: bacteria) A primitive, microscopic, single-celled organism that can cause infection.

Bifocal A type of eyeglass lens correction in which a special segment on the lower part of the lens allows focusing at near.

Bleb A blisterlike elevation of the conjunctiva containing aqueous humor that has percolated out of the eye. May be intentional, as in glaucoma filtering surgery, or unintentional, as may occur after cataract surgery.

Blepharitis (blef-a-ry´-tis) An inflammation of the eyelid, as may occur at the margins of the eyelids when the oil glands become irritated.

Canaliculus (can-a-lick´-you-lus) The narrow canal in the lower and upper lids that transports the tears from the eye to the lacrimal sac.

Cataract A condition in which the lens of the eye has become cloudy.

Cataract extraction Removal of the eye's lens by surgery.

Cellophane maculopathy (mak-you-lah´-pa-thee) Wrinkling of a membrane on the surface of the macula. Causes distortion of vision. Also known as *macular pucker*.

Central retinal artery The main artery that supplies the inner layers of the retina with blood.

Central retinal vein The main vein that drains blood from the inner layers of the retina out of the eye.

Chalazion (plural: chalazia) (ka-lay´-zee-un, not cha-lay´-zee-un) An inflamed, distended oil gland in the eyelid, also known as an *internal hordeolum*.

Chlamydia (kla-mid´-ee-a) A microscopic organism that can cause infection. One species causes trachoma, a cause of blindness in developing countries. A more benign strain is transmitted as a venereal infection in Western countries.

Choroid (kaw´-roid) The blood vessel–rich layer of the eye between the sclera and the retina. Supplies blood to the outer layers of the retina.

Ciliary body Part of the uveal tract of the eye, located between the iris and the choroid. It secretes aqueous humor into the eye and contains the *ciliary muscle*, which is involved in accommodation.

Conjunctiva (con-junk-ty´-va) The transparent mucous membrane that covers the sclera toward the front of the eye and that also lines the inside of the eyelids.

Conjunctivitis (con-junk″-ti-vy′-tis) Inflammation of the conjunctiva. May be of any cause, but the term is commonly applied to infections.

Contact lens A rigid or soft lens that fits over the cornea and is used as a substitute for eyeglasses.

Cornea The transparent, curved structure on the front of the eye that focuses incoming light rays.

Corneal abrasion An eye injury marked by the loss of some or all of the cornea's epithelial cells, its outermost layer.

Corneal transplant An operation in which the central portion of the cornea from an eye donor is used to replace the central cornea of someone with a clouded cornea. Also known as *keratoplasty*.

Corneal ulcer Area of loss of the epithelium and at least part of the stroma (middle layer) of the cornea. Often associated with infection.

Cortical cataract A cloudiness in the cortex, the outer layers of the lens.

Corticosteroid (cawr-ti-coh-stee′-roid) A class of medication used to treat inflammation. Cortisone is the body's natural form; prednisone, prednisolone, and dexamethasone are commonly used synthetic forms.

Cortisone A hormone produced by the adrenal gland. Has anti-inflammatory properties.

Cycloplegic (cy-cloh-plee′-jik) A medication, usually in eyedrop form, that temporarily paralyzes the ciliary muscle and dilates the pupil.

Dendrite An area of loss of corneal epithelium that has the shape of a branching figure. Characteristic of herpes infections.

Diabetes mellitus A disease of the pancreas marked by elevated blood sugar levels.

Diopter A unit of measurement of refractive error or lens power. Over six diopters is considered a high refractive error.

Diplopia (di-ploh′-pee-a) Double vision.

Dry eye syndrome A drying out of the surface of the eyes caused by a lack of tears or by a chemical imbalance in the tears.

Ectropion (ek-troh′-pee-un) A turning out of the eyelid.

Edema (a-dee′-ma) Fluid buildup.

Endothelium The cell layer forming the inside lining of certain structures, such as the cornea or the blood vessels. In the cornea, this cell layer helps prevent fluid from getting into the cornea and causing edema.

Entropion (en-troh′-pee-un) A turning in of the eyelids. May cause the eyelashes to abrade the cornea.

Enucleation Surgical removal of the eyeball.

Epiphora (a-pif´-a-ra) Overflow of tears from the eye.

Episcleritis (ep-ee´-skla-ry´-tis) Inflammation between the sclera and the conjunctiva, often due to a derangement of the immune system.

Epithelium The outermost layer of cells on the cornea. The *retinal pigment epithelium* is the deepest layer of the retina.

Esophoria (ee-so-for´-ee-a) A tendency for the eyes to turn in. May cause eyestrain.

Esotropia (ee-so-troh´-pee-a) A condition in which an eye turns in. May be intermittent or constant.

Exophoria A tendency for the eyes to turn out. May cause eyestrain.

Exophthalmos Forward protrusion of one or both eyes.

Exotropia A condition in which an eye turns out. May be intermittent or constant.

Filtering procedure A glaucoma operation to allow the aqueous humor to bypass the trabecular meshwork. Creates a drainage channel through the sclera, allowing aqueous humor to form under a conjunctival bleb.

Floaters Spots, lines, or "cobwebs" that people may see in their vision. Occur at one time or another in half the population. Caused by clumps of cells or other material in the vitreous. Occur as part of posterior vitreous face detachment, a normal part of aging, but may also occur with retinal tears or detachment, vitritis, or other problems in the vitreous.

Fluorescein (floo´-ra-seen) A yellow dye used to detect loss of corneal epithelial cells. Can also be injected into a vein as part of fluorescein angiography, a photographic test to evaluate the circulation of the retina.

Fundus The structures on the inside surface of the back wall of the eye. Includes the optic disk, the retina, and the retinal blood vessels.

Glaucoma A chronic degeneration of the optic nerve often associated with an elevated intraocular pressure.

Hordeolum An inflamed and sometimes infected oil gland of the eyelids. External hordeola are also known as *styes*, while internal hordeola are also known as *chalazia*.

Hyperopia (hy-per-oh´-pee-a) A refractive error in which light rays focus behind the retina. Commonly known as *farsightedness*.

Hypertension High blood pressure.

Hyphema (hy-fee´-ma) Bleeding into the anterior chamber of the eye.

Intraocular pressure The fluid pressure inside the eye, regulated by the secretion of aqueous humor into the eye and drainage of aqueous humor through the trabecular meshwork out of the eye. Elevated intraocular pressure is the main risk factor for glaucoma.

Iridocyclitis (ir″-i-doh-cy-cly′-tis) A form of uveitis characterized by inflammation of the iris and ciliary body. Inflammatory cells and protein can be seen in the aqueous humor and in the front part of the vitreous.

Iridotomy (ir″-i-dah′-ta-mee) An opening created in the iris by either laser or conventional surgery.

Iris Part of the uveal tract of the eye. It is the brown or blue ring of tissue surrounding the pupil.

Iritis (eye-ry′-tis) A form of uveitis in which the iris is inflamed. Characterized by inflammatory cells and protein in the aqueous humor.

Keratitis (ker-a-ty′-tis) Inflammation of the cornea.

Keratoconus (ker-a-ta-coh′-nus) An eye disease marked by bulging and thinning of the cornea.

Keratopathy (ker-a-tah′-pa-thee) A disease or problem of the cornea.

Keratoplasty (ker′-a-to-plas″-tee) A corneal transplant.

Lacrimal (lak′-ri-mul) **gland** The tear gland. Produces tears to lubricate the eye.

Lacrimal sac The tear sac. Located in a depression on the side of the nose near the bridge. Collects the tears from the eye, which then travel down through the nasolacrimal duct, where they empty into the nose.

Laser A powerful light beam that can perform surgery by burning or by creating miniature explosions in the tissues of the eyes.

Lens The clear, disklike structure behind the pupil that focuses light onto the retina. When it becomes cloudy, the condition is called *cataract*. The term also refers to the glass or plastic material in eyeglasses.

Lens implant An artificial lens placed inside the eye during cataract surgery to take the place of the eye's natural lens.

Macula (mak′-yu-la) The central portion of the retina.

Macular degeneration A degeneration of the macula that distorts or causes blind spots in the center of the field of vision. The most common form is known as *age-related macular degeneration*.

Macular edema Fluid buildup in the macula. May occur in many conditions, including diabetic retinopathy, retinal vein occlusions, inflammations in the eye, and as a side effect of certain medications.

Macular pucker A distortion of the center of the macula caused by the contraction of a membrane on its surface. Also known as *cellophane maculopathy*.

Meibomian gland (my-boh´-mee-an) An oil gland near the margins of the eyelids.

Myopia (my-oh´-pee-a) A refractive error in which the light rays come to a focus in front of the retina. Commonly known as *nearsightedness*.

Nasolacrimal (nay˝-zoh-lak´-ri-mul) **duct** The passageway through the bone of the nose that carries the tears from the lacrimal sac to the interior of the nose. Commonly known as the *tear duct*.

Neovascularization A condition in which abnormal blood vessels develop, sometimes in response to a lack of oxygen from poor circulation. When it occurs in the retina, as in diabetics, it is also known as *proliferative retinopathy*. When it occurs on the iris, it is also known as *rubeosis iridis*.

Nuclear sclerosis A form of cataract in which there is a diffuse clouding of the nucleus, the central portion of the lens.

Nystagmus (na-stag´-mus) A movement disorder of the eyes characterized by rapid back-and-forth jiggly movements.

Ophthalmologist A physician (M.D.) who specializes in the care of the eyes. Ophthalmologists perform refractions, fit patients with contact lenses, diagnose eye problems and systemic problems that have eye or visual manifestations, and treat by medical and surgical means.

Ophthalmoscope A special instrument used to examine the interior of the eye.

Optic cup The central depressed area in the optic disk of most eyes. It enlarges in size when the optic disk is damaged by glaucoma.

Optic disk The optic nerve at its termination in the back wall of the eye. So-called because it is shaped like an oval disk.

Optician A specially trained professional who fills prescriptions for eyeglass lenses.

Optic nerve The cranial nerve (extension of the brain) that carries visual signals from the eye to the brain.

Optic neuritis Inflammation of the optic nerve.

Optic neuropathy A disease or problem of the optic nerve.

Optometrist A non-M.D. specialist who performs refractions and determines contact lens prescriptions, examines eyes to detect disease, and may, where permitted by law, treat certain eye problems.

Orbit The bony socket in which the eyeball rests.

Perimetry Determination of the visual field using special instruments known as *perimeters*.

Phacoemulsification A technique of cataract surgery in which the nucleus of the lens is pulverized by ultrasonic (high-frequency sound wave) energy.

Pinguecula (pin-gwek´-yu-la) A yellowish-white degeneration of the conjunctiva, usually located near the cornea.

Posterior chamber The small space in the eye between the lens and the iris, containing aqueous humor.

Posterior subcapsular cataract A type of cataract marked by a cloudy spot located just within the back surface of the lens.

Prednisone A synthetic corticosteroid drug used to treat inflammation. When used as eyedrops, an activated form called *prednisolone* is needed.

Presbyopia (prez´-bee-oh´-pee-a) Decline in accommodation, the near focusing mechanism of the eye, that is expected with aging.

Prism A special lens that bends light rays. Occasionally used to treat eye straightness problems.

Proliferative diabetic retinopathy Growth of abnormal blood vessels on the retina and optic nerve of diabetics. These vessels may bleed into the vitreous and cause serious problems.

Pterygium (ta-rij´-ee-um) (plural: pterygia) A benign, degenerative growth beginning in the conjunctiva and extending onto the cornea.

Ptosis (toh´-sis) A drooping of an eyelid.

Punctum (plural: puncta) The tiny porelike opening in the margin of the upper and lower eyelids toward the nose. Tears drain from the eye through these puncta into the canaliculi as they travel to the lacrimal sac.

Pupil The dark opening in the center of the iris through which light rays travel on their way to the retina.

Refraction The procedure for determining refractive error and eyeglass prescription.

Refractive error A problem in which the light rays entering the eye fail to come to a focus on the retina, thereby causing blurred vision. Hyperopia, myopia, and astigmatism are forms of refractive errors.

Retina The delicate lining of the back wall of the eye. Images are focused on the retina and transmitted to the brain via the optic nerve.

Retinal detachment A disorder in which the retina balloons forward, separating itself from its deepest layer, the pigment epithelium. Retinal detachments are most commonly caused by fluid that travels through retinal tears and then dissects between the pigment epithelium and the other layers.

Tractional retinal detachments occur when scar tissue in the vitreous pulls the retina forward.

Retinitis Inflammation of the retina, most commonly the result of infection.

Retinopathy A disease or disorder of the retina.

Rubeosis iridis (roo-bee-oh´-sis ir´-i-dis) Neovascularization (abnormal blood vessel growth) on the iris, often seen with diabetes and with retinal vein occlusions. May cause neovascular glaucoma.

Sclera (sklehr´-a) The white outer coat of the eyeball.

Scleral buckle A surgical procedure used to repair retinal detachments in which a band or sponge is sewn onto the sclera to indent it.

Scleritis An inflammation of the sclera associated with autoimmune disease (a turning of the immune system against one's own tissues).

Scotoma (ska-toh´-ma) A blind spot.

Seborrhea (seb´-a-ree´-a) An oil gland disorder marked by an increased amount and thickness of oil gland secretions. It is associated with one form of blepharitis.

Sjögren's (shoh´-grinz or zha-grinz´) **syndrome** Dry eye syndrome associated with rheumatic diseases.

Staphylococcus (staf´´-a-lo-cok´-us) A bacterium commonly associated with eye infections. Often called "staph" for short. Some forms live in the skin.

Strabismus (stra-biz´-mus) A misalignment of the eyes. Examples include esotropia (turning in) and exotropia (turning out).

Stye An inflamed, often infected, oil gland that points toward the margin of the eyelid. Also called an *external hordeolum*.

Tear duct The passageway through the bone of the nose that carries the tears from the lacrimal sac to the interior of the nose. Also called *nasolacrimal duct*.

Tear film The layer of tears that coats the cornea. Consists of an outer oily layer, a middle watery layer, and an inner mucin (mucous) layer.

Tear gland A gland that produces tears. Consists of the main tear gland and the small, accessory tear glands located in the upper eyelids. Also called *lacrimal gland*.

Temporal arteritis An autoimmune disease of elderly people marked by inflammation and closure of arteries, especially those of the head. May cause optic neuropathy as well as central retinal artery occlusions.

Thyroid ophthalmopathy (of-thal-mah´-pa-thee) Disorders of the eyes seen in people with hyperthyroidism.

Trabecular (tra-bek´-yoo-ler) **meshwork** The channels located in the angle where aqueous humor drains out of the anterior chamber.

Trabeculectomy A surgical procedure for glaucoma in which a channel is created in the sclera to allow the aqueous humor to bypass the trabecular meshwork. The aqueous humor collects under a conjunctival bleb. Also called *filtering procedure*.

Trabeculoplasty A glaucoma procedure performed with the argon laser in which tiny burn spots are applied over the trabecular meshwork to facilitate the outflow of aqueous humor and thereby lower the intraocular pressure.

Ultrasound High-frequency, inaudible sound waves that sometimes can be used in a manner similar to X rays for diagnosis. Also used in phacoemulsification to pulverize the lens nucleus.

Ultraviolet A form of invisible light that comes from the sun and from some artificial light sources.

Uveal tract The iris, ciliary body, and choroid. These heavily pigmented structures of the eye are also known as the *uvea*.

Uveitis (yoo-vee-eye´-tis) Inflammation of part or all of the uveal tract. Forms of uveitis include iritis, iridocyclitis, cyclitis, vitritis, and choroiditis.

Virus A primitive, infectious particle consisting of DNA or RNA with a protein coat.

Visual acuity The ability to see tiny details in the center of one's field of vision.

Visual field The full extent of one's vision, including both central vision and peripheral version.

Vitrectomy An operation to remove some of the vitreous from the eye. Sometimes performed in diabetics to remove blood and scar tissue but also used for other indications.

Vitreous humor The gel-like material that fills the cavity of the eye between the retina and the lens. Partially liquefies with age. Usually called "vitreous" for short.

Vitritis Inflammation in the vitreous caused by uveitis.

Selected Resources

American Foundation for the Blind
11 Penn Plaza, Suite 300
New York, NY 10001
(212) 502-7600 www.afb.org

Advocate and provider of resources for the blind and visually impaired.

Lighthouse International
111 East 59th Street
New York, NY 10022-1202
(212) 821-9200 or (800) 829-0500 www.lighthouse.org

Rehabilitation services, education, research, and advocacy for the partially sighted and blind.

National Library Service for the Blind and Physically Handicapped (NLS)
The Library of Congress
1291 Taylor Street NW
Washington, DC 20542
(202) 707-5100 www.loc.gov/nls

Provides a wealth of information and resources for the vision impaired.

Recording for the Blind & Dyslexic
20 Roszel Road
Princeton, NJ 08540
(609) 452-0606 www.rfbd.org

Educational library for those people with "print disabilities."

Talking Tapes/Textbooks on Tape
16 Sunnen Drive, Suite 162
St. Louis, MO 63143-3800
(314) 646-0500 or (877) 926-0500 www.talkingtapes.org

Records and provides tapes for people with visual and other disabilities.

Bibliography

American Academy of Pediatrics Committee on Nutrition. "The Use of Whole Cow's Milk in Infancy." *Pediatrics* 89 (1992): 11059.

American Diabetes Association. "Nutritional Recommendations and Principles for Individuals with Diabetes Mellitus: 1986." *Diabetes Care* 10 (1987): 126–32.

———. "Magnesium Supplementation in the Treatment of Diabetes." *Diabetes Care* 15 (1992): 1065–67.

Anderson, James W., Jeri A. Zeigler, Dee A. Deakins, Tammy L. Floore, Debra W. Dillon, Constance L. Wood, Peter R. Oeltgen, and Ronald J. Whitley. "Metabolic Effects of High-Carbohydrate, High-Fiber Diets for Insulin-Dependent Diabetic Individuals." *The American Journal of Clinical Nutrition* 54 (1991): 936–43.

Bates, C. J., Su-jing Chen, A. MacDonald, and R. Holden. "Quantitation of Vitamin E and a Carotenoid Pigment in Cataractous Human Lenses, and the Effect of a Dietary Supplement." *International Journal for Vitamin and Nutrition Research* 66 (1996): 316–21.

Ben-nun, Joshua. "Photorefractive Keratectomy and Laser in Situ Keratomileusis: A Word from the Devil's Advocate." *Archives of Ophthalmology* 118 (2000): 1706–7.

Birkett, Anne, Jane Muir, Jodi Phillips, Gwyn Jones, and Kerin O'Dea. "Resistant Starch Lowers Fecal Concentrations of Ammonia and Phenols in Humans." *The American Journal of Clinical Nutrition* 63 (1996): 766–72.

Brown, Lisa, Eric B. Rimm, Johanna M. Seddon, Edward L. Giovannucci, Lisa Chasan-Taber, Donna Spiegelman, Walter C. Willett, and Susan E. Hankinson. "A Prospective Study of Carotenoid Intake and Risk of Cataract Extraction in U.S. Men." *The American Journal of Clinical Nutrition* 70 (1999): 517–24.

Burton, Anthony J. M., Anita Reynolds, and Damian O'Neill. "Sildenafil (Viagra) a Cause of Proliferative Diabetic Retinopathy?" *Eye* 14 (2000): 785–86.

Carlson, Susan E., S. H. Werkman, J. M. Peeples, and W. M. Wilson. "Long-Chain Fatty Acids and Early Visual and Cognitive Development of Preterm Infants." *European Journal of Clinical Nutrition* 48(suppl. 2) (1994): S27–S30.

Cavallo, Maria Gisella, Danila Fava, Laura Monetini, Fortunata Barone, and Paolo Pozzilli. "Cell-Mediated Immune Response to Beta-Casein in Recent-Onset Insulin-Dependent Diabetes: Implications for Disease Pathogenesis." *The Lancet* 348 (1996): 926–28.

Ceriello, A., D. Giugliano, P. Dello Russo, and N. Passariello. "Hypomagnesemia in Relation to Diabetic Retinopathy." *Diabetes Care* 5 (1982): 558–59.

Chasan-Taber, Lisa, Walter C. Willett, Johanna M. Seddon, Meir J. Stampfer, Bernard Rosner, Graham A. Colditz, Frank E. Speizer, and Susan E. Hankinson. "A Prospective Study of Carotenoid and Vitamin A Intakes and Risk of Cataract Extraction in U.S. Women." *The American Journal of Clinical Nutrition* 70 (1999): 509–16.

Chew, Emily Y., Michael L. Klein, Frederick L. Ferris III, Nancy A. Remaley, Robert P. Murphy, Kathryn Chantry, Byron J. Hoogwerf, and Dayton Miller; for the ETDRS Research Group. "Association of Elevated Serum Lipid Levels with Retinal Hard Exudate in Diabetic Retinopathy." *Archives of Ophthalmology* 114 (1996): 1079–84.

Chung, Hak Sung, Alon Harris, Johannes Kari Kristinsson, Thomas A. Ciulla, Carol Kagemann, and Robert Ritch. "Ginkgo Biloba Extract Increases Ocular Blood Flow Velocity." *Journal of Ocular Pharmacology and Therapeutics* 15 (1999): 233–40.

DeFeudis, Francis V. *Ginkgo Biloba Extract (EGb 761): Pharmacological Activities and Clinical Applications*. Paris: Elsevier, 1991.

Diet, Nutrition, and the Prevention of Chronic Diseases. Geneva: World Health Organization, 1990.

Early Treatment Diabetic Retinopathy Study Research Group. "Photocoagulation for Diabetic Macular Edema." *Archives of Ophthalmology* 103 (1985): 1796–1806.

Elman, Michael J., Marilyn T. Miller, and Reuben Matalon. "Galactokinase Activity in Patients with Idiopathic Cataracts." *Ophthalmology* 93 (1986): 210–15.

Ernest, Ingrid, Erik Linner, and Alvar Svanborg. "Carbohydrate-Rich, Fat-Poor Diet in Diabetes." *American Journal of Medicine* 39 (1965): 594–600.

Eunyoung, Cho, Susan E. Hankinson, Walter C. Willett, Meir J. Stampfeer, Donna Spiegelman, Frank E. Speizer, Eric B. Rimm, and Johanna M. Seddon. "Prospective Study of Alcohol Consumption and the Risk of Age-Related Macular Degeneration." *Archives of Ophthalmology* 118 (2000): 681–88.

Eye Disease Case-Control Study Group. "Antioxidant Status and Neovascular Age-Related Macular Degeneration." *Archives of Ophthalmology* 111 (1993): 104–9.

Garcia-Salinas, Paul, Graham E. Trope, and Max Glynn. "Blood Viscosity in Ocular Hypertension." *Canadian Journal of Ophthalmology* 23 (1988): 305–7.

Gordon, Bruce, Stanley Chang, Mary Kavanagh, Maria Berrocal, Lawrence Yannuzzi, Carolyn Robertson, and Andrew Drexler. "The Effects of Lipid Lowering on Diabetic Retinopathy." *American Journal of Ophthalmology* 112 (1991): 385–91.

Hankinson, Susan E., Meir J. Stampfer, Johanna M. Seddon, Graham A. Colditz, Bernard Rosner, Frank E. Speizer, and Walter C. Willett. "Nutrient Intake and Cataract Extraction in Women: A Prospective Study." *BMJ (British Medical Journal)* 305 (1992): 335–39.

Hersh, Peter S., Stephen F. Brint, Robert K. Maloney, Daniel S. Durrie, Michael Gordon, Marc A. Michelson, Vance M. Thompson, Ralph B. Berkeley, Oliver D. Schein, and Roger F. Steinert. "Photorefractive Keratectomy Versus Laser in Situ Keratomileusis for Moderate to High Myopia." *Ophthalmology* 105 (1998): 1512–23.

Higginbotham, Eve J., Heidi A. Kilimanjaro, Jacob T. Wilensky, Randal L. Batenhorst, and David Hermann. "The Effect of Caffeine on Intraocular Pressure in Glaucoma Patients." *Ophthalmology* 96 (1989): 624–26.

Hoffman, Dennis R., Eileen E. Birch, David G. Birch, and Ricardo D. Uauy. "Effects of Supplementation with Omega-3 Long-Chain Polyunsaturated Fatty Acids on Retinal and Cortical Development in Premature Infants." *The American Journal of Clinical Nutrition* 57 (suppl.) (1993): 807S–12S.

Jacques, Paul F., and Leo T. Chylack, Jr. "Epidemiologic Evidence of a Role for the Antioxidant Vitamins and Carotenoids in Cataract Prevention." *The American Journal of Clinical Nutrition* 53 (1991): 352S–55S.

Jacques, Paul F., Judy Phillips, Stuart C. Hartz, and Leo T. Chylack, Jr. "Lactose Intake, Galactose Metabolism, and Senile Cataract." *Nutrition Research* 10 (1990): 255–65.

Karjalainen, Jukka, Julio M. Martin, Mikael Knip, Jorma Ilonen, Brian H. Robinson, Erkki Savilahti, Hans K. Åkerblom, and Hans-Michael Dosch. "A Bovine Albumin Peptide as a Possible Trigger of Insulin-Dependent Diabetes Mellitus." *The New England Journal of Medicine* 327 (1992): 302–7.

Kies, Constance. "Bioavailability of Manganese." In Dorothy J. Klimis-Tavantzis, ed., *Manganese in Health and Disease.* Boca Raton, Fla.: CRC Press, 1994: 45–47.

Klaver, J. H. J., E. L. Greve, H. Goslinga, H. C. Geijssen, and J. H. A. Heuvelmans. "Blood and Plasma Viscosity Measurements in Patients with Glaucoma." *British Journal of Ophthalmology* 69 (1985): 765–70.

Kleijnen, Jos, and Paul Knipschild. "Ginkgo Biloba." *The Lancet* 340 (1992): 1136–39.

Krinsky, Norman I., Mark D. Russett, Garry J. Handelman, and D. Max Snodderly. "Structural and Geometrical Isomers of Carotenoids in Human Plasma." *The Journal of Nutrition* 120 (1990): 1654–62.

Lamey, P.-J., and P. A. Biagioni. "Relationship Between Iron Status and Recrudescent Herpes Labialis." *European Journal of Clinical Microbiology and Infectious Diseases* 14 (1995): 604–5.

Lotfi, Karan, and Juan E. Grunwald. "The Effect of Caffeine on the Human Macular Circulation." *Investigative Ophthalmology and Visual Science* 32 (1991): 3028–32.

Lucas, A., R. Morley, T. J. Cole, G. Lister, and C. Leeson-Payne. "Breast Milk and Subsequent Intelligence Quotient in Children Born Preterm." *The Lancet* 339 (1992): 261–64.

Makrides, M., K. Simmer, M. Goggin, and R. A. Gibson. "Erythrocyte Docosahexaenoic Acid Correlates with the Visual Response of Healthy, Term Infants." *Pediatric Research* 33 (1993): 425–27.

Mares-Perlman, Julie A., William E. Brady, Ronald Klein, Gina M. VandenLangenberg, Barbara E. K. Klein, and Mari Palta. "Dietary Fat and Age-Related Maculopathy." *Archives of Ophthalmology* 113 (1995): 743–48.

McNair, P., C. Christiansen, S. Madsbad, E. Lauritzen, O. Faber, C.. Binder, and I. Transbøl. "Hypomagnesemia, a Risk Factor in Diabetic Retinopathy." *Diabetes* 27 (1978): 1075–77.

Naveh-Floman, Nava, and Michael Belkin. "Prostaglandin Metabolism and Intraocular Pressure." *British Journal of Ophthalmology 71* (1987): 254–56.

Newsome, David A., Mano Swartz, Nicholas C. Leone, Robert C. Elston, and Earl Miller. "Oral Zinc in Macular Degeneration." *Archives of Ophthalmology* 106 (1988): 192–98.

Ornish, Dean, Shirley E. Brown, Larry W. Scherwitz, James H. Billings, William T. Armstrong, Thomas A. Ports, Sandra M. McLanahan, Richard L. Kirkeeide, Richard J. Brand, and K. Lance Gould. "Can Lifestyle Changes Reverse Coronary Heart Disease?" *The Lancet* 336 (1990): 129–30.

Passo, Michael S., Linn Goldberg, Diane L. Elliot, and E. Michael Van Buskirk. "Exercise Training Reduces Intraocular Pressure Among Subjects Suspected of Having Glaucoma." *Archives of Ophthalmology* 109 (1991): 1096–98.

Perez-Santonja, Juan J., Maria J. Ayala, Hani F. Sakla, Jose M. Ruiz-Moreno, and Jorge L. Alio. "Retreatment After Laser in Situ Keratomileusis." *Ophthalmology* 106 (1999): 21–28.

Pissarello, Carlo. "La Curva Giornaliera della Tensione Nell'occhio Normale e Nell'occhio Glaucomatoso e Influenza di Fattori Diversi (Miotici, Iridectomia, Irido-sclerectomia, Derivativi, Pasti) Determinata con il Tonometro di Schiotz." *Annali di Ottalmologia* 44 (1915): 544–636.

Robertson, James M., Allan P. Donner, and John R. Trevithick. "A Possible Role for Vitamins C and E in Cataract Prevention." *The American Journal of Clinical Nutrition* 53 (1991): 346S–51S.

Roy, Monique S., Gloria Stables, Bronwyn Collier, Alec Roy, and Ernestina Bou. "Nutritional Factors in Diabetics with and Without Retinopathy." *The American Journal of Clinical Nutrition* 50 (1989): 728–30.

Schanzlin, David J., Penny A. Asbell, Terry E. Burris, and Daniel S. Durrie. "The Intrastromal Corneal Ring Segments." *Ophthalmology* 104 (1997): 1067–78.

Seddon, Johanna M., Umed A. Ajani, Robert D. Sperduto, Rita Hiller, Norman Blair, Thomas C. Burton, Marilyn D. Farber, Evangelos S. Gragoudas, Julia Haller, Dayton T. Miller, Lawrence A. Yannuzzi, and Walter Willett; for the Eye Disease Case-Control Study Group. "Dietary Carotenoids, Vitamins A, C, and E, and Advanced Age-Related Macular Degeneration." *JAMA (Journal of the American Medical Association)* 272 (1994): 1413–20.

Skalka, Harold W., and Josef T. Prchal. "Presenile Cataract Formation and Decreased Activity of Galactosemic Enzymes." *Archives of Ophthalmology* 98 (1980): 269–73.

———— "Cataracts and Riboflavin Deficiency." *The American Journal of Clinical Nutrition* 34 (1981): 861–63.

Stocker, Frederick W., Lawrence B. Holt, and James W. Clower. "Clinical Experiments with New Ways of Influencing Intraocular Tension. I. Effect of Rice Diet." *Archives of Ophthalmology* 40 (1948): 46–55.

Stulting, R. Doyle, Jonathan D. Carr, Keith P. Thompson, George O. Waring III, Wendy M. Wiley, and Judy G. Walker. "Complications of Laser in Situ Keratomileusis for the Correction of Myopia." *Ophthalmology* 106 (1999): 13–20.

Stur, Michael, Michael Tittl, Andreas Reitner, and Vanee Meisinger. "Oral Zinc and the Second Eye in Age-Related Macular Degeneration." *Investigative Ophthalmology and Visual Science* 37 (1996): 1225–35.

Taylor, Allen, Paul F. Jacques, T. Nowell, G. Perrone, J. Blumberg, G. Handelman, B. Jozwiak, and D. Nadler. "Vitamin C in Human and Guinea Pig Aqueous, Lens and Plasma in Relation to Intake." *Current Eye Research* 16 (1997): 857–64.

Van Eck, William F. "The Effect of a Low-Fat Diet on the Serum Lipids in Diabetes and Its Significance in Diabetic Retinopathy." *American Journal of Medicine* 27 (1959): 196–211.

Waring, George O., III, Jonathan D. Carr, R. Doyle Stulting, Wendy M. Wiley, David Huang, and Keith P. Thompson. "LASIK for Myopia and Astigmatism in 2,100 Consecutive Eyes Using a Nidek EC-5000 Excimer Laser." *Investigative Ophthalmology and Visual Science* 40 (1999): S588.

Yeum, Kyung-Jin, Fu Shang, Wolfgang Schalch, Robert M. Russell, and Allen Taylor. "Fat-Soluble Nutrient Concentrations in Different Layers of Human Cataractous Lens." *Current Eye Research* 19 (1999): 502–5.

Index

incision size in, 140–41
indications for, 137–38
procedure for, 139–40
types of
  cortical, 16, 123, 124
  nuclear sclerotic, 16, 123, 124, 135
  posterior subcapsular, 123, 134, 135, 138, 271
  secondary, 142, 211
in uveitis, 238
Cellophane maculopathy, 215
Chalazia
  defined, 64
  and oil gland tumors, 74–75
  susceptibility to, 64–65
  treatment of, 65–66
Chemicals in eyes, 5
Children
  amblyopia in, 111–12
  esotropia in, 2, 108–11
  exotropia in, 113–14
  getting eyedrops into eyes, 98
  glaucoma in, 150
  hyperopia in, 109, 110, 111
  nutrition in eye health, 268–71
  ptosis in, 79–80
  tear duct problems in, 70–71
Chlamydial conjunctivitis, 96–97
Cholesterol
  drugs to lower, 182, 275
  and macular degeneration, 203–5
  and retinopathy, 180–82
  and zinc, 194–95
Choroid, 9, 10, 16–17, 188, 235
Choroiditis, 17
Chronic angle-closure glaucoma, 149, 274
Chronic open angle glaucoma
  blood circulation in, 151
  defined, 14, 149, 150
  effect of medications on, 273–74
  and omega-3 fatty acids in, 165
  surgery for, 168–70
Ciliary body
  description of, 9, 10, 14, 235
  partial destruction of, 170
Clindamycin, 225, 226
CMV. See Cytomegalovirus
Cobalamin (vitamin B_{12}), 233, 289–90
Colitis
  pseudomembranous, 226
  ulcerative, 242
Color vision, 36
Cones, 17, 188, 269
Congenital disorders
  dacryostenosis, 70–71

esotropia, 108, 109–11
glaucoma, 150
Conjunctiva. See also Conjunctivitis
  anatomy of, 10, 12–13
  disorders of
    allergies, 98–101
    episcleritis, 101–3
    pinguecula, 105
    pterygium, 103–4
    subconjunctival hemorrhage, 105–6
  examination of, 33
  foreign bodies in, 6, 85–86
Conjunctivitis
  bacterial, 94, 97–98
  caused by herpes simplex, 96, 257
  causes of, 93
  in children, 98
  chlamydial, 96–97
  defined, 13
  giant papillary, 50–51
  phlyctenular, 61–62
  viral, 93–96
Contact lenses, 45–51
  advantages/disadvantages of, 45–46
  after cataract surgery, 140
  bandage lens, 85, 88–89
  choosing, 48–49
  costs of, 49
  examination for, 49
  and eyes changing, 2
  fittings, 49–50
  follow-up care, 50
  in presbyopia, 47–48
  problems with, 7, 11, 50–51, 91
  types of, 46–47
Convergence amplitudes, 36–37, 115
Convergence insufficiency, 113–15, 244
Copper, 191–93, 300–301
Cornea
  abrasions of, 11, 83–85, 91
  anatomy of, 9, 10–12, 10
  clouding of, 87–90, 141
  edema of, 11–12, 46, 51, 87–89
  effect of diabetes on, 176
  endothelial cell loss in, 87–88
  examination of, 32–33
  foreign bodies in, 6, 85–87
  infections of, 90–93, 257–59
  lacerations to, 11, 85
  scarring of, 11
  transplantation of, 89
  ulcers of, 11, 50, 90–93
Cortex of lens, 15–16, 123
Cortical cataracts, 16, 123, 124